Controlled Release Delivery Systems

Controlled Release Delivery Systems

EDITED BY

Theodore J. Roseman
The Upjohn Company
Kalamazoo, Michigan

S. Z. Mansdorf
S. Z. Mansdorf and Associates
Akron, Ohio

MARCEL DEKKER, INC. New York and Basel

Library of Congress Cataloging in Publication Data

Main entry under title:

Controlled release delivery systems.

"Outgrowth of the 8th International Symposium on Controlled Release of Bioactive Materials held July 26-29, 1981 in Fort Lauderdale, Florida"--Pref.

Includes index.

1. Drugs--Controlled release--Congresses. I. Roseman, Theodore J., [date]. II. Mansdorf, S. Z. (S. Zack), [date]. III. International Symposium on Controlled Release of Bioactive Materials (8th : 1981 : Fort Lauderdale, Fla.)

RS201.C64C658 1983 615'.191 82-25513

ISBN 0-8247-1728-7

MARCEL DEKKER, INC.
270 Madison Avenue, New York, New York 10016

Current printing (last digit):
10 9 8 7 6 5 4 3 2 1

PRINTED IN THE UNITED STATES OF AMERICA

Preface

The rapid growth of the controlled release field is evidenced by the publication of at least eight books on the subject in the last seven years. This proliferation of interest is a reflection of the recognition that controlled release delivery systems offer significant advantages over conventional modes of delivery or administration of bioactive agents. Mass transport theories are utilized to design matrix systems which release the bioactive species at preselected release rates. An intriguing aspect of this continuously expanding field is its diversification across a variety of disciplines since there is a common application of basic physicochemical principles. These systems are being explored for therapeutic agents in medicine as well as agricultural and veterinary products. Specific emphasis has been placed on drugs, pesticides, herbicides, pheromones, molluscicides, and antifouling agents. The commitment to this area of research has resulted in several successful products in both the medical and nonmedical fields.

The Controlled Release Society, Inc. was formed in 1978 to promote the rapid dissemination of information and exchange of ideas on an international level through an annual symposium. This book is an outgrowth of the 8th International Symposium on Controlled Release of Bioactive Materials held July 26-29, 1981 in Fort Lauderdale, Florida. The chapters in this book are selected full manuscripts from among the 65 papers which were presented at the meeting. Each manuscript was independently reviewed by a leading expert in the field. This book provides the reader with the latest research developments in liposomes, microencapsulation, reservoir and monolithic devices, biodegradable and swellable matrices, the characterization of the delivery systems, the use of molecular modification (prodrugs) to optimize drug delivery, and magnetically controlled systems. In addition, it provides a review of the current status and future prospects of the field.

Extensive bibliographies are provided throughout the book. It is our belief that this book will provide the reader with a technically current perspective of the controlled release field as well as a solidly referenced text of previous research.

Theodore J. Roseman
S. Z. Mansdorf

Contributors

Mounir M. Abd El-Malek, Ph.D., M.Sc., B.Sc. Assistant Research Professor, Laboratory of Polymers and Pigments, National Research Centre, Dokki, Cairo, Egypt

Magdy H. Ayoub, M.Sc., B.Sc. Research Assistant, Laboratory of Polymers and Pigments, National Research Centre, Dokki, Cairo, Egypt

Joseph A. Bakan, B.S. Director of Research and Development, Eurand America, Inc., Dayton, Ohio

David C. Baker, Ph.D. Associate Professor, Department of Chemistry, The University of Alabama, University, Alabama

Richard W. Baker, Ph.D.* Director of Research, Bend Research, Inc., Bend, Oregon

William R. Brade, Ph.D. Research Engineer, Department of Polymer Chemistry, Armak Company, McCook, Illinois

Frederick G. Burton, Ph.D., M.A., B.A. Senior Research Scientist, Biology and Chemistry Department, Pacific Northwest Laboratory, Richland, Washington

Dominic A. Cataldo, Ph.D., M.Ph., M.S. Staff Scientist, Department of Environmental Sciences, Pacific Northwest Laboratory, Richland, Washington

---

**Present affiliation*: President, Membrane Technology and Research, Inc., Palo Alto, California

S. Kumar Chandrasekaran, Ph.D., B.S.* Principal Scientist and Director of Physical Sciences, ALZA Corporation, Palo Alto, California

John F. Cline, B.S. Senior Research Specialist, Department of Environmental Sciences, Pacific Northwest Laboratory, Richland, Washington

O. I. Corrigan, Ph.D., M.A., B.Sc. (Pharm.), M.P.S.I. Senior Lecturer, Department of Pharmaceutics, Trinity College School of Pharmacy, Dublin, Ireland

Clarence C. Dannelly, M.S.† Research Associate, Health and Nutrition Research Division, Eastman Chemicals Division, Eastman Kodak Company, Kingsport, Tennessee

Timothy D. Davis, Ph.D. Section Head, Department of Polymer Chemistry, Armak Company, McCook, Illinois

Stephen A. de Keczer, A.A., B.A., M.S.‡ Research Scientist, Department of Organic Chemistry, Dynapol, Palo Alto, California

Albert Dorsky, M.S., B.S.§ Senior Research Scientist, Radiochemistry Department, Dynapol, Palo Alto, California

R. O. Drummond, Ph.D., A.B. Laboratory Director, United States Livestock Insects Laboratory, United States Department of Agriculture, Kerrville, Texas

Adrian Dunne, Ph.D., B.Sc. Lecturer, Department of Pharmacology, University College, Dublin, Ireland

Nnochiri Ekwuribe Department of Macromolecular Science, Case Western Reserve University, Cleveland, Ohio

---

Present affiliations
*Director of Research and Development, Abcor, Inc., Wilmington, Massachusetts
†Retired
‡Senior Chemist, Institute of Organic Chemistry, Syntex (U.S.A.), Inc., Palo Alto, California
§Research Chemist, Cooper-Lipotech, Inc., South San Francisco, California

A. Kirk Field, Ph.D. Senior Investigator, Department of Virology and Cell Biology, Merck Sharp & Dohme Research Laboratories, West Point, Pennsylvania

Jeffrey L. Fox, Ph.D., B.S. Assistant Professor, The University of Michigan College of Pharmacy, Ann Arbor, Michigan

Bruce K. Fritzinger, B.A. Polymer Chemist, Department of Polymer Sciences, SRI International, Menlo Park, California

Hiroshi Fuyama Master of Technology, Institute for Biological Science, Sumitomo Chemical Company, Ltd., Takarazuka, Hyogo, Japan

Edward O. Gangstad, Ph.D., M.S., B.S. Botanist, Department of the Army, Office Chief of Engineers, Washington, D.C.

Norman L. Gauthier, Ph.D., B.S. Entomologist, Chittenango, New York

Edward J. Geoghegan, B.Sc. Technical Director, Elan Corporation, Ltd., Monksland, Athlone, Ireland

Nadim A. Ghanem, D.Sc., Ph.D., M.Sc., B.Sc. Department of Chemical Engineering, College of Engineering, King Saud University, Riyad, Saudi Arabia

Neal A. Gordon, Ph.D., B.S.* Research Assistant, Department of Pharmaceutical Chemistry, The University of Michigan College of Pharmacy, Ann Arbor, Michigan

Ron L. Hale, Ph.D., M.S., B.S. Associate Director, Radiochemistry Department, Dynapol, Palo Alto, California

Richard J. Harwood, Ph.D., M.Sc., B.Sc.† Research Fellow, Pharmaceutical Research, Merck Sharp & Dohme Research Laboratories, West Point, Pennsylvania

Jorge Heller, Ph.D., B.S. Director, Polymer Sciences Department, SRI International, Menlo Park, California

---

Present affiliations

*Senior Scientist, Pharmacy Research and Development, Revlon Health Care Group, Tuckahoe, New York

†Section Manager, Pharmaceutical Sciences, New Product Development, William H. Rorer, Inc., Fort Washington, Pennsylvania

Robert F. Helwing, B.S.* Polymer Chemist, Department of Polymer Sciences, SRI International, Menlo Park, California

William I. Higuchi, Ph.D.† Professor of Pharmaceutical Chemistry, The University of Michigan College of Pharmacy, Ann Arbor, Michigan

Norman F. H. Ho, Ph.D. Professor, The University of Michigan College of Pharmacy, Ann Arbor, Michigan

Dean S. T. Hsieh, Ph.D.‡ Instructor, Surgery, Harvard Medical School and Children's Hospital Medical Center, Boston, Massachusetts

Chung-Chiang Hsu, Ph.D. Research Scientist, Pharmaceutical Products Division, Abbott Laboratories, North Chicago, Illinois

H. Huikeshoven, Ph.D. Scientific Officer, Department of Tropical Hygiene, Royal Tropical Institute, Amsterdam, The Netherlands

Chrissie A. Killian, B.Sc., H.D.E. Manager, Biochemistry Division, Elan Corporation, Ltd., Monksland, Athlone, Ireland

A. J. P. Klein-Szanto, M.D. Medical Staff Scientist, Biology Division, Oak Ridge National Laboratory, Oak Ridge, Tennessee

Richard W. Korsmeyer, M.S., B.A. School of Chemical Engineering, Purdue University, West Lafayette, Indiana

Akira Kusai§ Visiting Associate Research Scientist, The University of Michigan College of Pharmacy, Ann Arbor, Michigan

Agis Kydonieus, Ph.D. Executive Vice President, Hercon Division, Health-Chem Corporation, New York, New York

Robert Langer, Sc.D. Associate Professor, Nutrition and Food Science, Massachusetts Institute of Technology, Cambridge, Massachusetts

D. L. Leiker, M.D. Scientific Officer, Department of Tropical Hygiene, Royal Tropical Institute, Amsterdam, The Netherlands

---

Present affiliations

*Chemist, Department of Development Engineering, Memorex Corporation, Santa Clara, California

† Professor of Pharmaceutics, College of Pharmacy, University of Utah, Salt Lake City, Utah

‡ Assistant Professor of Pharmaceutics, Department of Pharmaceutics, College of Pharmacy of Rutgers, The State University of New Jersey, Piscataway, New Jersey

§ Product Development Laboratory, Sankyo Corporation, Tokyo, Japan

Harold K. Lonsdale, Ph.D., B.S. President, Bend Research, Inc., Bend, Oregon

Hugh McLaughlin, M.D., M.Sc. Lecturer, Department of Pathology, University College, Dublin, Ireland

F. W. H. M. Merkus, Ph.D. Professor and Chairman, Department of Biopharmaceutics, Schools of Pharmacy and Medicine, University of Amsterdam, Amsterdam, The Netherlands

J. Allen Miller, Ph.D., M.S., B.S. Research Agricultural Engineer, United States Livestock Insects Laboratory, United States Department of Agriculture, Kerrville, Texas

E. S. M. Modderman, Pharm. D. Senior Scientist, Department of Biopharmaceutics, Schools of Pharmacy and Medicine, University of Amsterdam, Amsterdam, The Netherlands

Yasuo Ninomiya, Ph.D. Assistant Chief Researcher, Technical Research Laboratory, Nitto Electric Industrial Co., Ltd., Ibaraki, Osaka, Japan

D. D. Oehler, B.A., M.S. Chemist, United States Livestock Insects Laboratory, United States Department of Agriculture, Kerrville, Texas

Bimal C. Pal, Ph.D. Senior Scientist, Biology Division, Oak Ridge National Laboratory, Oak Ridge, Tennessee

Donald E. Panoz Chairman, Elan Corporation, Ltd., Monksland, Athlone, Ireland

Jung Y. Park, Ph.D. Research Scientist, Pharmaceutical Research, Boehringer Ingelheim, Ridgefield, Connecticut

Bruce L. Parker, Ph.D., M.S., B.S. Associate Professor, Associate Research Entomologist, Plant and Soil Science Department, University of Vermont, Burlington, Vermont

D. W. H. Penhale Assistant, Chemical Engineering, Polymer Sciences Department, SRI International, Menlo Park, California

Nikolaos A. Peppas, Sc.D., Dipl. Eng. Professor, School of Chemical Engineering, Purdue University, West Lafayette, Indiana

Helen Carol B. Perry, B.S. M.T. (A.S.C.P.) Research Virologist, Department of Virus and Cell Biology, Merck Sharp & Dohme Research Laboratories, West Point, Pennsylvania

Thomas C. Powell, B.ChE. Senior Scientist, Research and Development, Eurand America, Inc., Dayton, Ohio

Theodore J. Roseman, Ph.D., M.S., B.S. Senior Research Scientist, Pharmaceutical Research and Development, The Upjohn Company, Kalamazoo, Michigan

Roger M. Rowell, Ph.D., M.S., B.S. Research Chemist, United States Department of Agriculture, Forest Products Laboratory, Madison, Wisconsin

Brenda E. Ryman, M.A., Ph.D., F.R.S.C., F.R.C.Path. Professor, Department of Biochemistry, Charing Cross Hospital Medical School (University of London), London, England

Pongpen Sa-Nguankul, Department of Biology, Faculty of Science, Mahidol University, Bangkok, Thailand

William M. Shannon, Ph.D. Senior Virologist, Chemotherapy Research Department, Southern Research Institute, Birmingham, Alabama

Goro Shinjo, Research Scientist, Master, Household and Public Health Pesticides Development Section, Sumitomo Chemical Company, Ltd., Takarazuka, Hyogo, Japan

W. Eugene Skiens, PH.D., B.S. Senior Research Scientist, Materials Department, Pacific Northwest Laboratory, Richland, Washington

Kelly L. Smith, M.S., B.S. Director, Controlled Release Division, Bend Research, Inc., Bend, Oregon

Randall V. Sparer, Ph.D.* Research Fellow, Department of Macromolecular Science, Case Western Reserve University, Cleveland, Ohio

Charles H. Spilman, Ph.D. Senior Research Scientist, Fertility Research, The Upjohn Company, Kalamazoo, Michigan

Nouwarath Sukhapanth, Department of Biology, Faculty of Science, Mahidol University, Bangkok, Thailand

---

**Present affiliation*: Senior Research Chemist, INTERx Research Corporation, Lawrence, Kansas

Kozo Tsuji, Doctor of Engineering, Research Department, Pesticides Division, Sumitomo Chemical Company, Ltd., Takarazuka, Hyogo, Japan

Mark Edward Tuttle, M.S., B.S. Research Chemist, Polymer Synthesis, Bend Research, Inc., Bend, Oregon

E. S. Upatham, Department of Biology, Faculty of Science, Mahidol University, Bangkok, Thailand

Alan G. Walton,* Professor, Department of Macromolecular Science, Case Western Reserve University, Cleveland, Ohio

Rose M. Wright, B.S. Research Scientist, Technical Information and Publications, ALZA Corporation, Palo Alto, California

Stephen Hong-wei Wu, Ph.D. Senior Research Chemist, Health and Nutrition Research Division, Research Laboratories, Eastman Chemicals Division, Eastman Kodak Company, Kingsport, Tennessee

M. James Yuen, A.B. Technical Editor, Technical Information and Publications, ALZA Corporation, Palo Alto, California

J. Zuidema, Ph.D. Senior Scientist, Department of Biopharmaceutics, Schools of Pharmacy and Medicine, University of Amsterdam, Amsterdam, The Netherlands

---

* *Present affiliation* : President, University Genetics Company, Norwalk, Connecticut

Contents

Controlled Release Delivery Systems

Chapter 1

Controlled Release: Status and Future Prospects

S. KUMAR CHANDRASEKARAN,* ROSE M. WRIGHT, and M. JAMES YUEN
ALZA Corporation, Palo Alto, California

Controlled release technology is a relatively new field, and as a consequence, research in the field has been extremely fertile and has produced many discoveries. New and more sophisticated controlled release delivery systems are constantly being developed and tested. This chapter has three main objectives: (1) to set the stage and develop a rationale for the field of controlled delivery, (2) to highlight recent work in the field, and (3) to project future needs and developments in the field.

SELECTIVITY OF ACTION

Particular delivery rates of a drug elicit specific pharmacologic actions. Table 1 illustrates the relationship between delivery rate and pharmacologic action normally elicited by pilocarpine and scopolamine. Pilocarpine delivered at very low rates produces ocular hypotension; at higher rates it causes miosis, myopia, and browache; and at very high levels it induces systemic effects. Scopolamine, on the other hand, causes slight bradycardia at very low rates; inhibits motion sickness at slightly higher rates; and induces dry mouth, tachycardia, and drowsiness at progressively higher rates. Thus, if a particular pharmacologic effect is desired, the rate of delivery must be controlled within a specific range. Higher rates produce not only the desired

---

**Present affiliation*: Abcor, Inc., Wilmington, Massachusetts

Table 1 Two Examples of Rate-Controlled Pharmacology

Drug delivery rate	Rank order of actions elicited as delivery rate rises	
	Pilocarpine[a]	Scopolamine
Lowest	Ocular hypotension	Slight bradycardia
↓	Miosis	Inhibition of motion sickness
	Myopia	Dry mouth
	Browache, ciliary spasm	Slight tachycardia Drowsiness Cycloplegia
Highest	Systemic effects, (e.g., salivation, intestinal cramping)	Amnesia Hallucinations

[a]Topical, to the eye.
Source: Ref. 1.

therapeutic action of the drug but also unwanted pharmacologic effects. These two cases exemplify the preliminary list of agents (Table 2) whose selectivity of action relates to the rate of administration rather than the dose administered.

In the agricultural area, Allan and coworkers [3] monitored the growth of trees following the application of varying amounts of controlled release herbicide. They found that the factors controlling tree growth are complicated (Fig. 1) and that the cumulative growth rate does reach a peak. Since the various factors do not increase linearly with the amount or rate of application, herbicide application for trees must be controlled in order to elicit a particular beneficial effect.

BIOLOGICAL INTERFACE AND THE PHARMACOKINETIC PROCESS

The interface between the delivery system and the biological or agricultural environment, and the pharmacokinetic processes taking place therein, must be considered jointly. The pharmacokinetic process in the biological environment depends greatly on the volume of distribution and clearance of a particular drug [4]. In the case of agricultural chemicals, the pharmacokinetic process may involve environmental parameters, such as surface runoff, rainfall, and temperature. Certain enzymatic actions, which may occur in the soil, can be considered in a more generic sense to be pharmacokinetic in themselves.

Table 2 Examples of Agents Whose Selectivity of Therapeutic or Physiological Action Is Related to the Rate of Administration

Acetazolamide	Hydrochlorothiazide
Adrenocorticotropic hormone (ACTH)	Insulin
Angiotensin II	Methoxyflurane
Bleomycin	Minocycline
Chlordiazepoxide	Morphine
Cytosine arabinoside	Nitrofurantoin
Diethylcarbamazine	Nitroglycerin
Diphenhydramine	Nitroprusside
Dopamine	Norepinephrine
Estradiol	Parathormone
Ether	Phenacetin
Furosemide	Pilocarpine
Glucagon	Scopolamine
Gonadotropin-releasing hormone (GnRH)	Vasopressin
Heparin	

Source: Ref. 2.

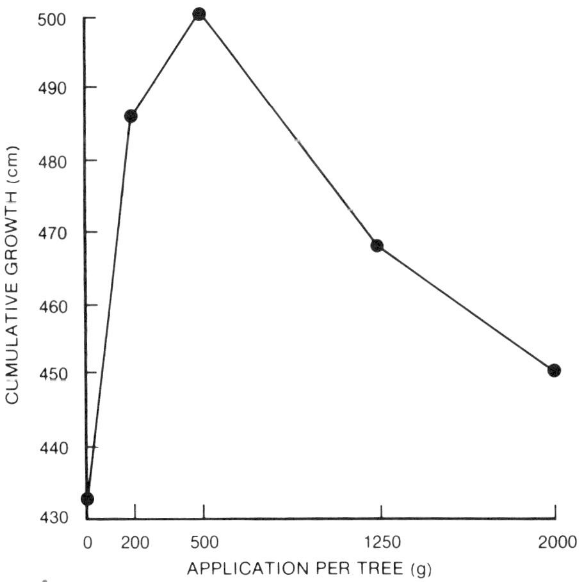

Figure 1 Cumulative growth of trees receiving different amounts of a controlled release herbicide. (From Ref. 3.)

Simplistically, the rate of change of plasma concentration of a particular drug entity relates to two factors: infiltration—the rate at which matter and drug are delivered to the biological environment—and outfiltration or excretion—the rate at which drug gets excreted from the environment or from the body. Excretion depends on K_D, the excretion rate constant. The relationship between the infiltration and excretion rates and the pharmacokinetic parameters dictates the plasma concentration.

DELIVERY RATE PROFILE

Consider a delivery system whose delivery profile could be depicted by any of the profiles shown in Fig. 2. In the curve in which 20% of the drug is delivered at zero order, the initial rate is very high, followed by a declining rate [5]. In the second profile (i.e., 40%), a declining rate follows a steady-state period. The third profile (i.e., 60%) shows a slightly longer steady-state period, and the fourth profile (i.e., 80%) represents an essentially flat steady state over an extended time period.

The fate of the drug when delivered to a biological environment using these four profiles is greatly dependent on the drug's biological half-life. In the case where the biological half-life of the drug is extremely short, the distinction between these curves is very predominant with respect to drug in the body (Fig. 3). If a significant portion of the drug is delivered at a constant steady-state rate, the subsequent profile within the systemic circulation assumes steady state during this period. Furthermore, if the drug delivery curve is even flatter, the profile within the systemic circulation becomes relatively flat. Bear in mind, however, that this simulation is done for a very short biological half-life. If the biological half-life is much longer (e.g., either 4 or 8 hr), the distinction between these curves becomes much smaller and the significance of the delivery profile to obtain a particular steady state of the biological environment becomes less critical (Figs. 4, 5). If a drug entity has a relatively small therapeutic index (i.e., the range between toxic and therapeutic levels is relatively small), the significance of the drug delivery rate is of utmost importance, especially for agents with short biological half-lives.

PATENT PROTECTION

Figure 6 shows the number of parent patents issued per year in the area of controlled delivery research. The number of pharmaceutical patents issued per year has been ascending steadily since 1970. The number of agricultural patents peaked in the early 1970s and has remained constant since then. Parent patents issued in both the

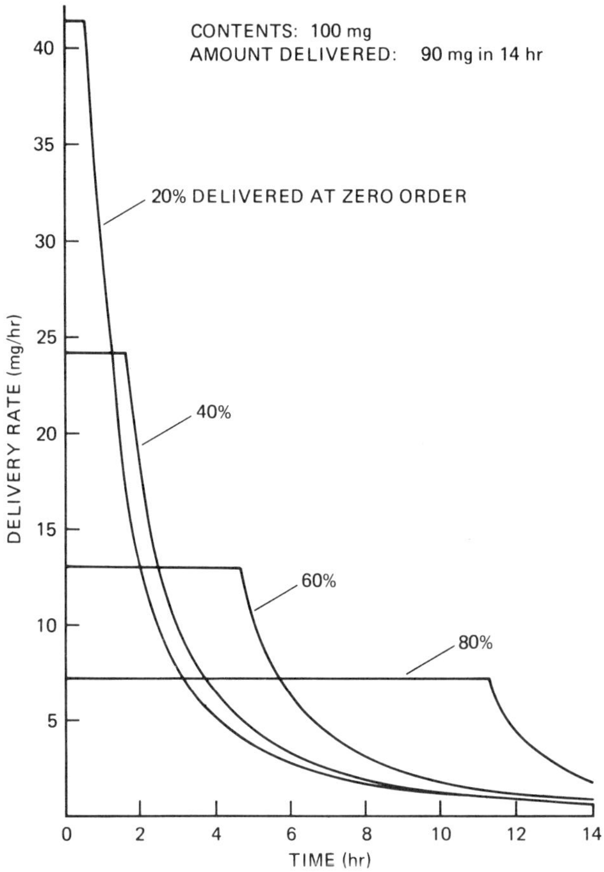

Figure 2 Delivery rate profile of elementary osmotic pumps characterized by the percentage of drug delivered at zero order. (From Ref. 5.)

agricultural and pharmaceutical areas number about 1200-1400 over the last 20 years.

The use of polymers in the area of controlled delivery really began in the 1960s when Long and Folkman [6] were granted a patent for their work dealing with use of a polysiloxane carrier for the controlled release of drugs and other agents (Fig. 7). The carrier comprised a Silastic tubing core that could be filled with pharmaceutical agent and plugged on both ends; the drug diffused from the core, through the membrane tubing, and into the biological environment. This work initiated rapid developments in the area of controlled delivery.

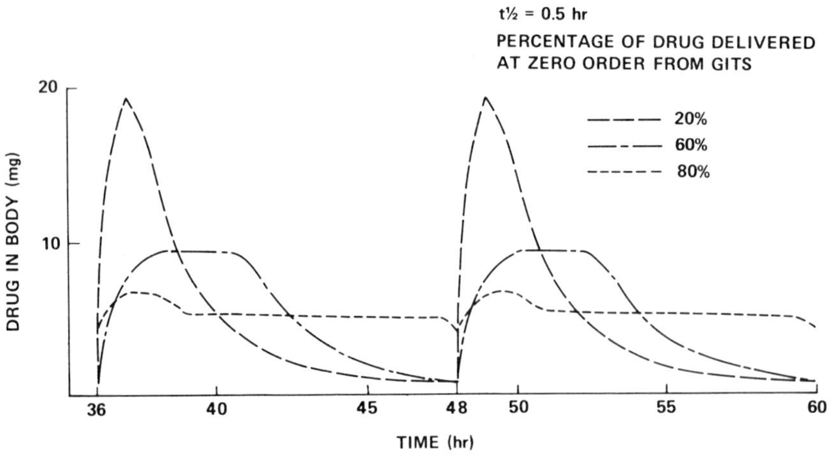

Figure 3 Simulated amounts of drug ($t_{1/2}$ = 0.5 hr) in the body at steady state following repetitive administration of elementary osmotic pumps delivering different percentages of the drug content at zero order. (From Ref. 5.)

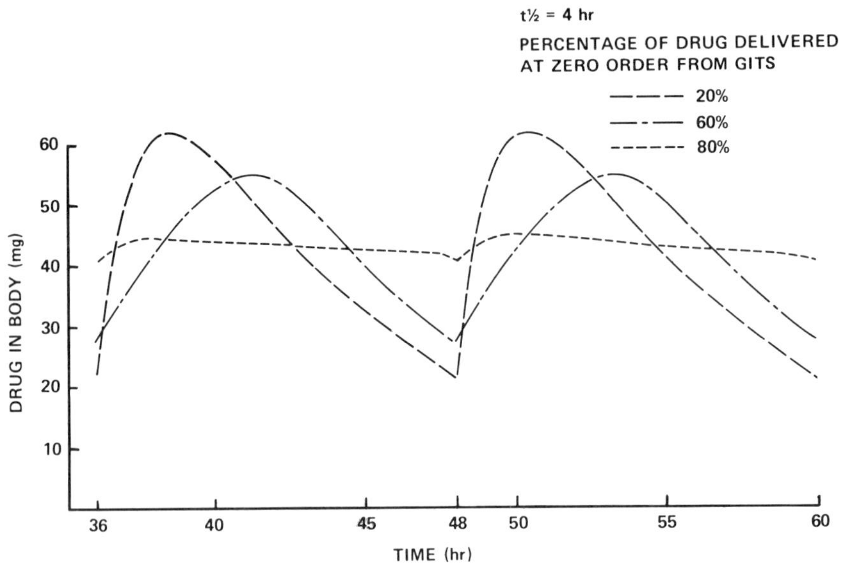

Figure 4 Simulated amounts of drug ($t_{1/2}$ = 4 hr) in the body at steady state following repetitive administration of elementary osmotic pumps delivering different percentages of the drug content at zero order. (From Ref. 5.)

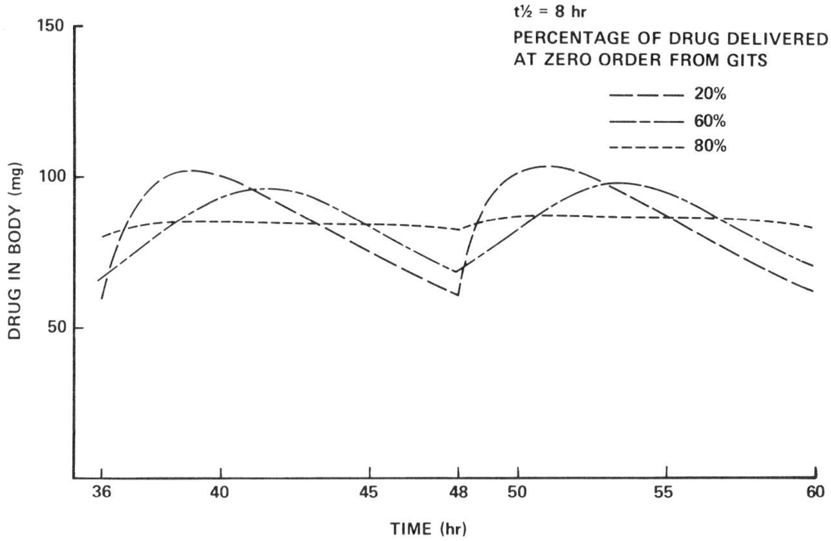

Figure 5 Simulated amounts of drug ($t_{1/2}$ = 8 hr) in the body at steady state following repetitive administration of elementary osmotic pumps delivering different percentages of the drug content at zero order. (From Ref. 5.)

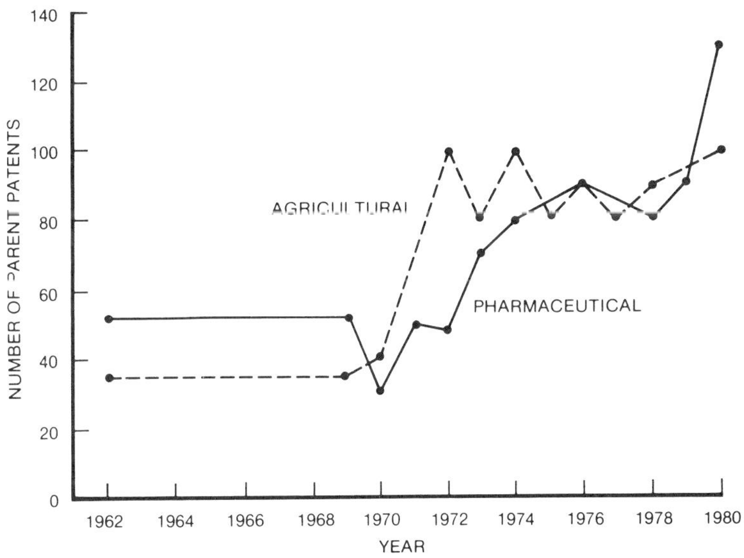

Figure 6 Number of parent patents issued per year for the controlled release of pharmaceutical and agricultural agents from 1970 to 1980 (averaged from 1962 to 1969).

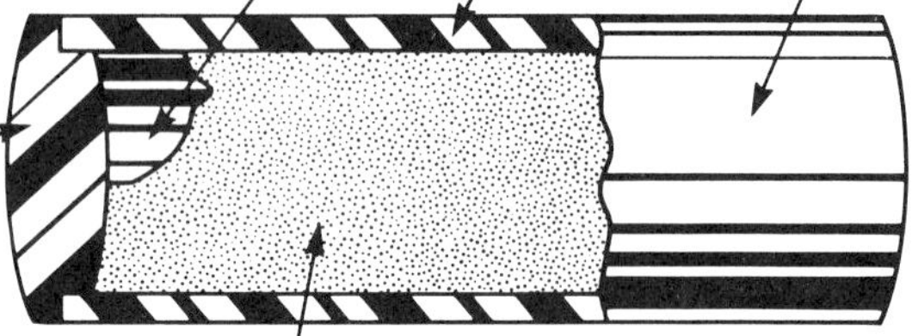

Figure 7 Schematic representation of a polysiloxane carrier for the controlled release of drugs and other agents. (From Ref. 6.)

OPEN-LOOP SYSTEMS

To date, most research on controlled release has involved open-loop drug delivery systems [7]. These systems (Fig. 8) comprise a drug platform; a reservoir, where the drug is stored; an energy source; and in more sophisticated systems, a therapeutic program, which meters the amount of agent passing through the rate-controlling mechanism. Once the agent gets into the biological environment, a pharmacokinetic process occurs before distinguishable therapeutic and side actions manifest themselves.

Many innovative systems for controlled delivery of pharmaceutical agents have been developed over the last few years, a few of which will be discussed here.

Drug in Polymer Matrices

Much discussion revolves around the innovative work of Higuchi [8], which uses polymeric matrices to deliver drug agents. One drawback of dispersing drugs within a matrix is the inability to deliver drug to a particular site and to achieve a steady state. The release rate declines continuously in a manner that essentially follows the square root of time.

Researchers at the University of Utah dispersed progesterone in a base of acrylate polymers [9]. Figure 9 shows typical release rate profiles with this type of drug delivery. The devices were soaked in varying concentrations of ethylene glycol dimethacrylate and the surfaces of these matrices were then irradiated with ultraviolet light in order to achieve an element of crosslinking and to form a rate-controlling membrane within the matrix surface. Depending on the extent of crosslinking, the resistance to drug passage offered by this crosslinked layer may actually increase. With increased crosslinking,

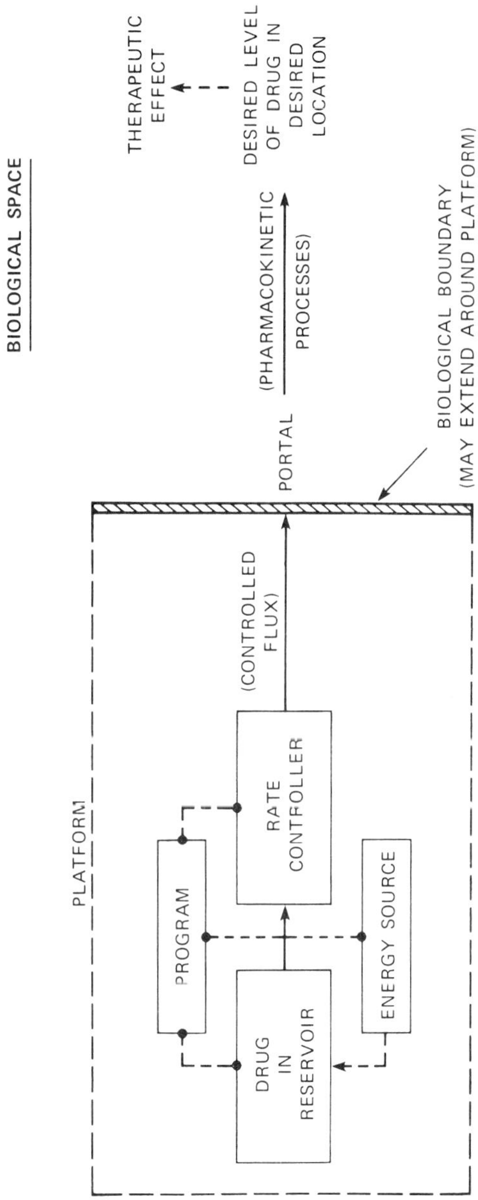

Figure 8 Schematic representation of an open-loop controlled delivery system. (From Ref. 7.)

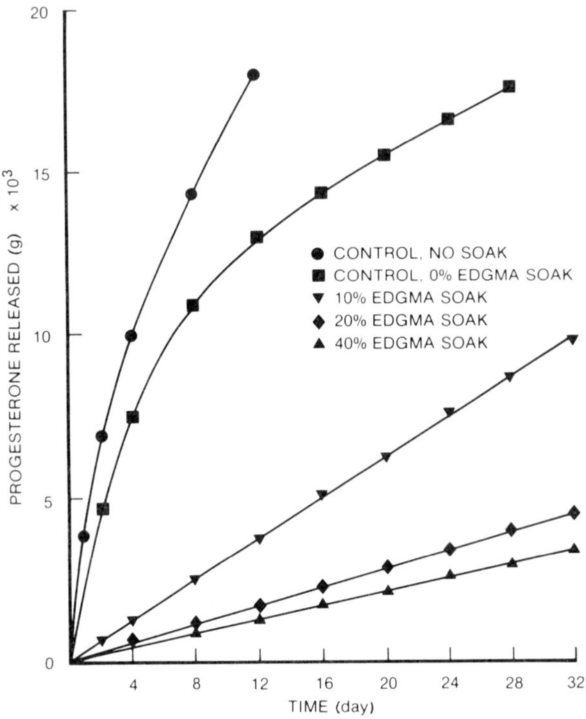

Figure 9 Progesterone release from a polymeric delivery system comprising progesterone dispersed in a polyhydroxyethyl methacrylate (HEMA) matrix. The 9.1%-progesterone HEMA devices were soaked in varying concentrations of ethylene glycol dimethacrylate (EGDMA) for 4 hr and exposed to ultraviolet light for 3 hr. (From Ref. 9.)

the release rate curve (Fig. 9) becomes much flatter, and drug delivery approaches zero order. Thus control of drug release from drug-dispersed matrices can be achieved by adjusting the extent of cross-linking of the in situ membrane.

Coated Ion Exchange Membrane

Raghunathan and colleagues [10] used ion exchange in polymers and membranes to control the delivery of the drug dextromethorphan. They coated ion exchange membranes with different concentrations of ethylcellulose in order to get a selectively permeable rate-controlling membrane at the surface. The curves in Fig. 10 represent the drug delivery rates of several ethylcellulose-coated dextromethorphan-resin complexes.

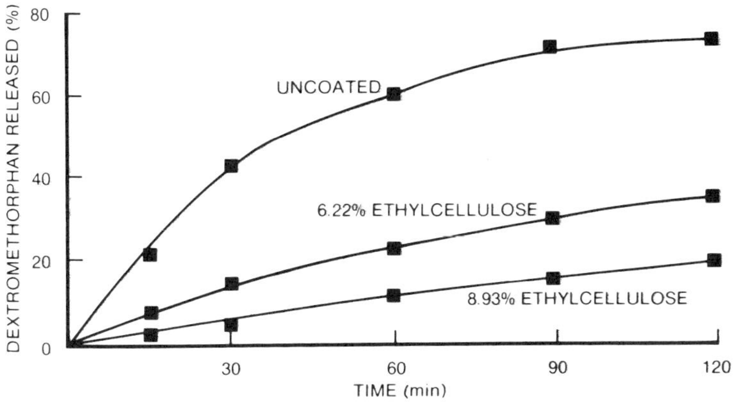

Figure 10 Mean release profile of dextromethorphan in 0.1 N hydrochloric acid at 60 rpm from a fine-particle dextromethorphan-resin complex at various coating levels of ethylcellulose. (From Ref. 10.)

Matrix with Magnetic Particles

Langer and associates [11] dispersed magnetic particles within the matrix system, which they energized externally, and obtained an increased delivery rate. Figure 11 shows the delivery rates they obtained with and without magnetic particles dispersed within the matrix; their results are indeed interesting and suggestive of numerous applications.

Bioerodible Polymers

Considerable work has been done with bioerodible polymers. Benagiano and colleagues discussed several bioerodible systems that were used to administer fertility regulating agents [12]. Units containing the drug norethindrone dispersed in bioerodible polymers were implanted in baboons [13]. Figure 12 shows serum levels of norethindrone in baboons implanted with either one or three systems, each containing 25 mg of drug. The curves are relatively flat for a long duration—6 months—and the mass balance between one and three systems is very good (differing by a factor of 3).

Osmotic Pumps

A miniaturized osmotic pump has been developed for use in pharmacokinetic experiments in animals [14]. The mini-osmotic pump, which can be filled with agent and implanted in animals as small as mice, delivers drug continuously at a constant rate to the body. Figure 13 shows the release rate profile of insulin delivered to diabetic rats with

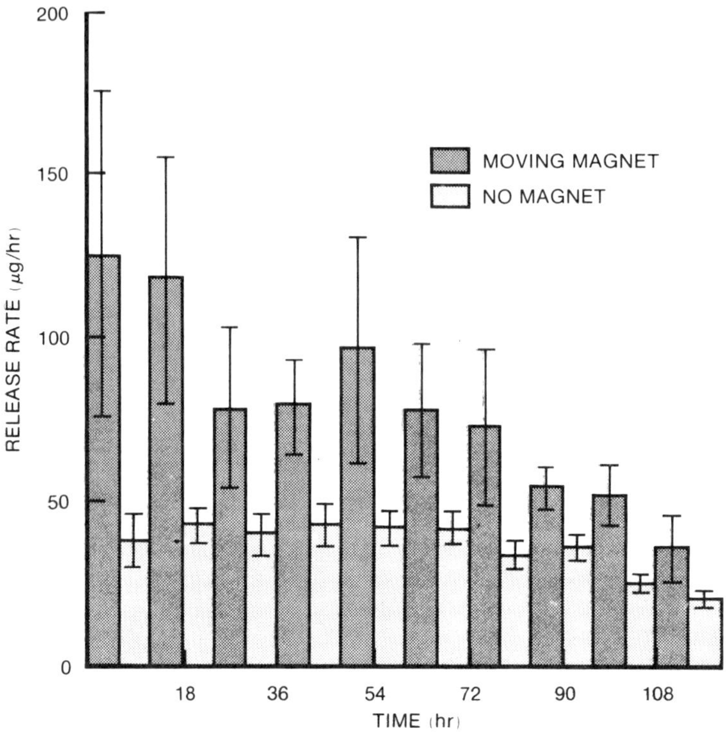

Figure 11 Magnetically induced, modulated sustained release of bovine serum albumin from polymeric vehicles. Each bar represents the average release rate of eight polymer squares. The graph shows cyclic shifting between triggering and nontriggering for alternating 6-hr periods. (From Ref. 11.)

an osmotic pump. Before administration of insulin by the mini-osmotic pump, the rat was extremely hypoglycemic; however, following administration of various concentrations of insulin at a constant rate using the pump, the serum glucose level declined sharply and remained steady during the time of administration. Thus the degree of hypoglycemia can be controlled by varying the concentration of insulin.

Radio-Controlled Pills

Zimmer and colleagues [16] performed some innovative work using radio-controlled pills in their attempt to find preferential pathways for absorption in the gastrointestinal tract. They wired a capsule with suitable heating elements and then localized the capsule within the gastrointestinal tract by using x-ray measurements. They then

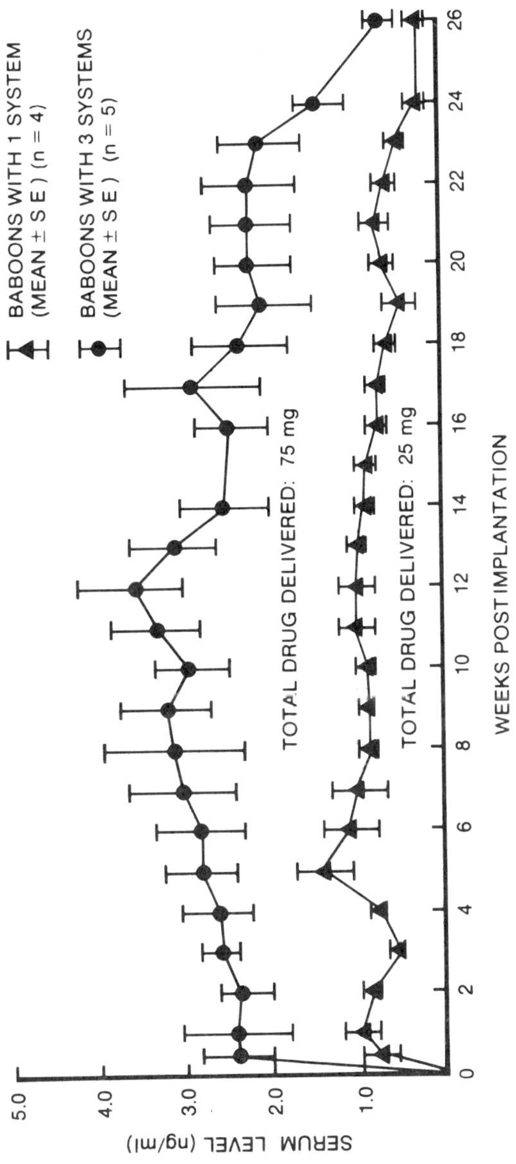

Figure 12 Serum levels of norethindrone after implantation in baboons of one or three norethindrone-containing bioerodible delivery systems. (From Ref. 13.)

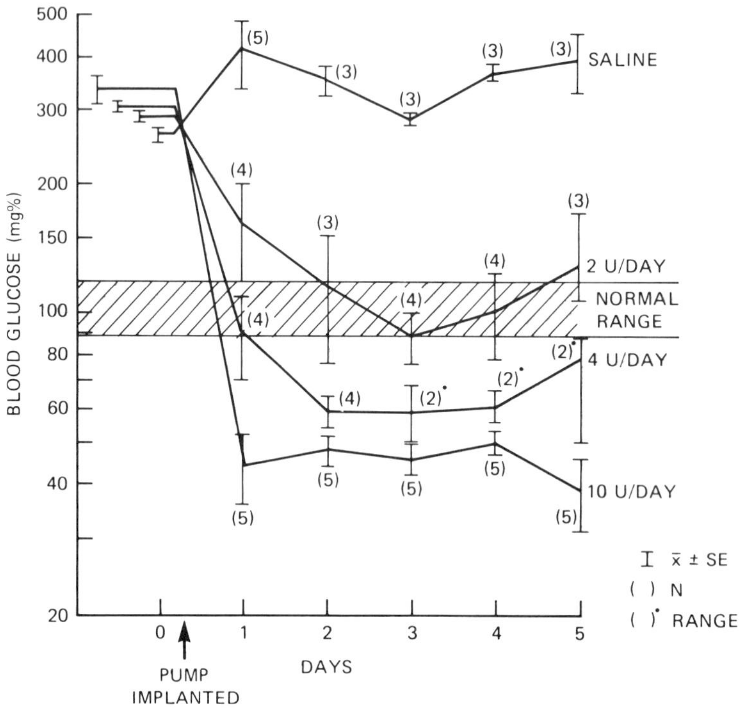

Figure 13 Delivery-rate-response curves of insulin in the streptozotocin-diabetic rat. Osmotic pumps were filled with different concentrations of unmodified crystalline bovine insulin in isotonic saline and implanted subcutaneously to infuse either 2, 4, or 10 U/day per 200-g rat. A 2-U/day dose was sufficient to return the streptozotocin-diabetic rat in normoglycemic levels of 90-120 mg %. (From Ref. 15.)

energized the capsule externally and caused it to self-destruct and release its contents to the specified area of the gastrointestinal tract.

Multiple Pellets

Beckett and coworkers [17] studied a controlled release oral dosage form containing multiple pellets. Rogers and colleagues [18] recently published an article on an osmotically controlled delivery system for indomethacin that achieves steady-state profiles within the systemic circulation.

These examples only scratch the surface on drug candidates and techniques that researchers have used to design delivery systems that provide specific delivery profiles within the in vitro and in vivo setup. But how well do in vitro tests predict delivery profile?

IN VIVO/IN VITRO CORRELATION

Hess and colleagues [19] showed that a correlation does exist between the in vitro rate and the in vivo absorption rate of the drug (Fig. 14). There is a 2-hr time delay between the curves, which are essentially identical. This finding suggests a time delay between the time when the drug is delivered to the biological environment and the time when steady state is achieved.

CORRELATION BETWEEN RATES OF ADMINISTRATION

Skin also can act as a portal for drug entry. The transdermal therapeutic system, a round patch, delivers drug through intact skin into the systemic circulation [20]. Figure 15 compares the rate of drug delivery within the systemic circulation when drug is applied either to the skin surface or intravenously. The amount of drug excreted corresponds to the amount absorbed by the body. The curves in Fig. 15 show an agreement between drug excretion after administration via the intravenous and transdermal routes. Since there is agreement between the two routes of administration and because the in vitro and

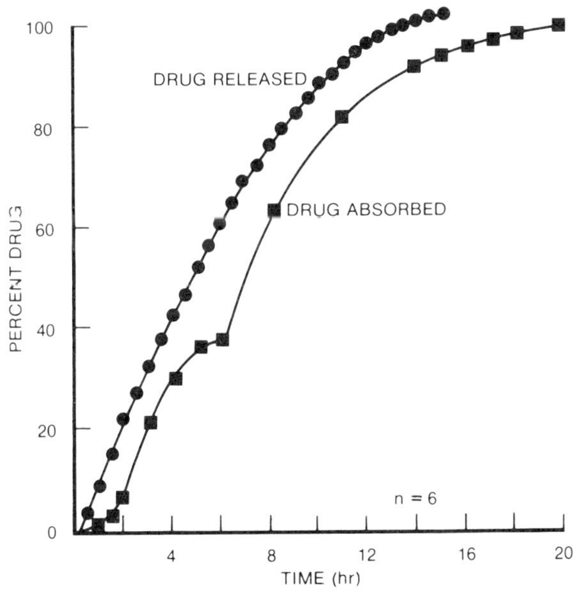

Figure 14 Correlation between in vitro dissolution and in vivo absorption of metoprolol fumarate delivered from an elementary osmotic pump. (From Ref. 19.)

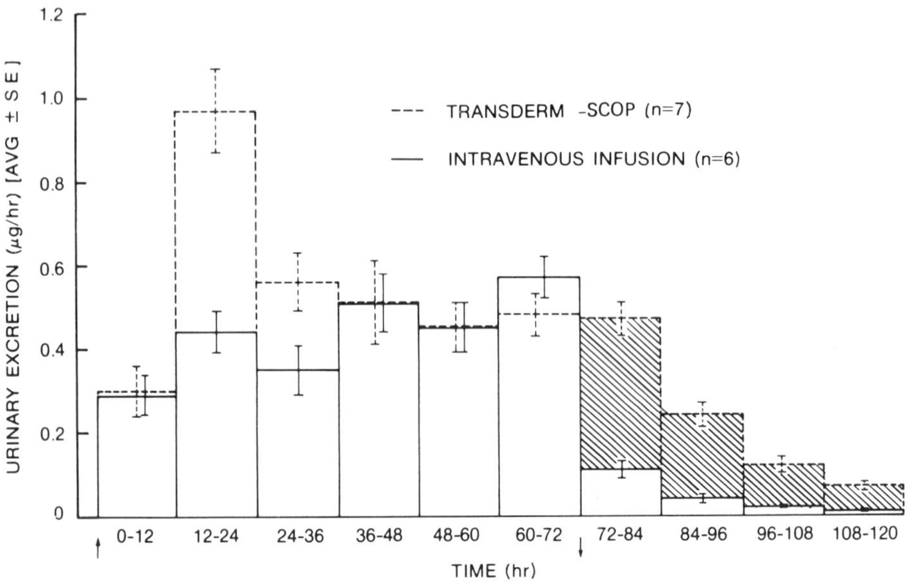

Figure 15 Urinary excretion of scopolamine during and following application of a transdermal system releasing scopolamine or during controlled continuous intravenous infusion of the drug. (From Ref. 21.)

in vivo release rates agree, the specifications of controlled delivery systems must be determined—that is, how tight should the release rate profile be?

RELEASE RATE SPECIFICATIONS

If one wants to achieve a certain constancy within the biological environment, one needs to determine the types of fluctuations one could tolerate in the release rate [5]. Equation (1) shows the in vitro release rate that applies for a linear system:

$$R = V_d \frac{dC_p}{dt} + \dot{V}_c C_p \tag{1}$$

where R is the release rate, V_d the volume of distribution, C_p the plasma concentration, and $\dot{V}_c$ the total body clearance.

Figure 16 graphically represents the ratio of the rate of change of plasma concentration to the rate of change in release rate (gain), as a function of noise frequency (i.e., fluctuations) for a set of varied drug

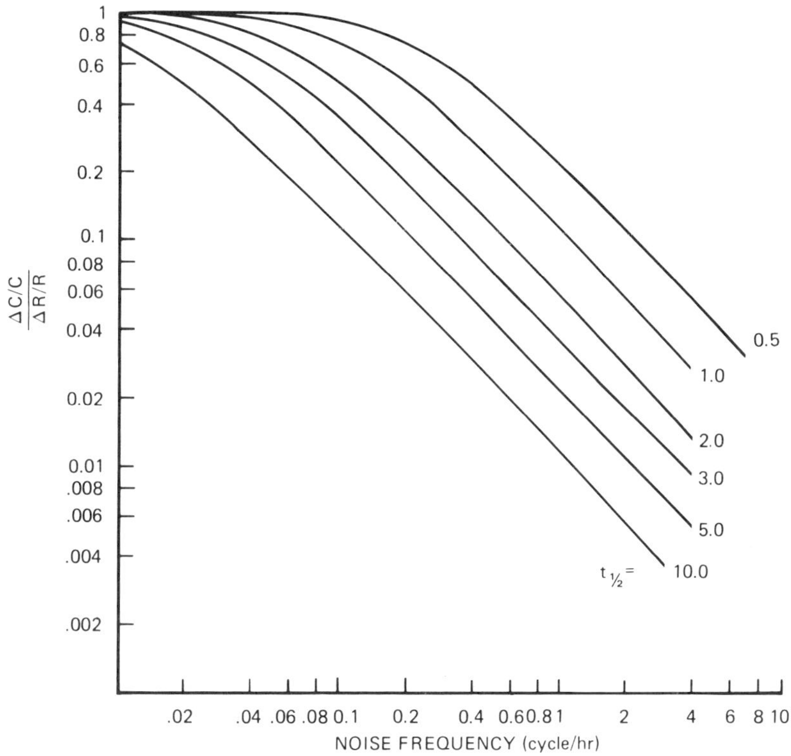

Figure 16 Magnitude of plasma concentration fluctuations $\Delta C/C$ as a function of the magnitude of release rate fluctuations $\Delta R/R$ of indicated frequency. (From Ref. 5.)

half-lives. This graph, called a Bode plot, can guide specification setting in vitro for controlled release dosage forms, because it permits one to calculate the allowable fluctuations on the rate $\Delta R/R$ from an allowable plasma concentration $\Delta C/C$. For example, assume that the drug half-life is 0.5 hr and the noise frequency is 0.5 cycle/hr or greater, and thus the gain is 0.5 at most. Assuming a narrow therapeutic index for the drug, and allowing a maximum plasma fluctuation $\Delta C/C$ of 10%, we have

$$\frac{\Delta R}{R} = \frac{0.1}{0.5} = 0.2 \qquad (2)$$

Thus release rate fluctuations should be limited to a maximum of 20%.

CLOSED-LOOP SYSTEMS

So far simple open-loop systems have been discussed, that is, systems where drug is delivered to a biological environment with little or no control on the subsequent effects. In the more complex closed-loop systems [7], the pharmacokinetic process taking place systemically is fed back to the drug delivery system (negative feedback system; Fig. 17). This mechanism instructs the delivery system to alter its therapeutic program appropriately. These systems are more complicated than open-loop systems because they require a very sensitive sensor in the biological environment that is capable of sending a negative feedback signal to the delivery system.

Glucose Monitor

The Biostator (Miles Labs), a glucose monitor, provides an example of a negative feedback system [22]. The monitor continuously removes blood from the patient, passes it through a glucose analyzer, a microcomputer, and an infusion pump, and then, depending on the glucose level within the systemic circulation, infuses either insulin or dextrose. Figure 18 shows schematically the glucose analyzer. This glucose monitor is expensive, selling for around $35,000, and only 8 to 10 units have been sold to date. In addition, the unit presently is sold under rather rigid constraints because its efficacy has only been tested for periods up to 24 hr.

Schade and colleagues [23] have done work on a totally implantable insulin delivery system (Fig. 19). This system has a reservoir, which is filled from an external portal. The drug goes through a pump, a monitor, and a remote electronic controlling facility that controls the subsequent rate of drug administration.

NEW PORTALS FOR DRUG DELIVERY

Many new portals for drug delivery are being explored, including the rectum, brain, buccal mucosa, and nasal passages. Discussion of the former two portals follows.

Rectal Delivery of Drug

Figure 20 shows data using the rectal portal for delivery of theophylline to the systemic circulation. The drug was monitored in the plasma and in the saliva. For theophylline, concentrations monitored in the saliva and the plasma agree reasonably well. In addition, a relatively flat profile is achieved using the rectal platform. Control of drug delivery from the rectal route is not that simple, however, because the location of the vital circulation between the rectum and the systemic circulation remains in question.

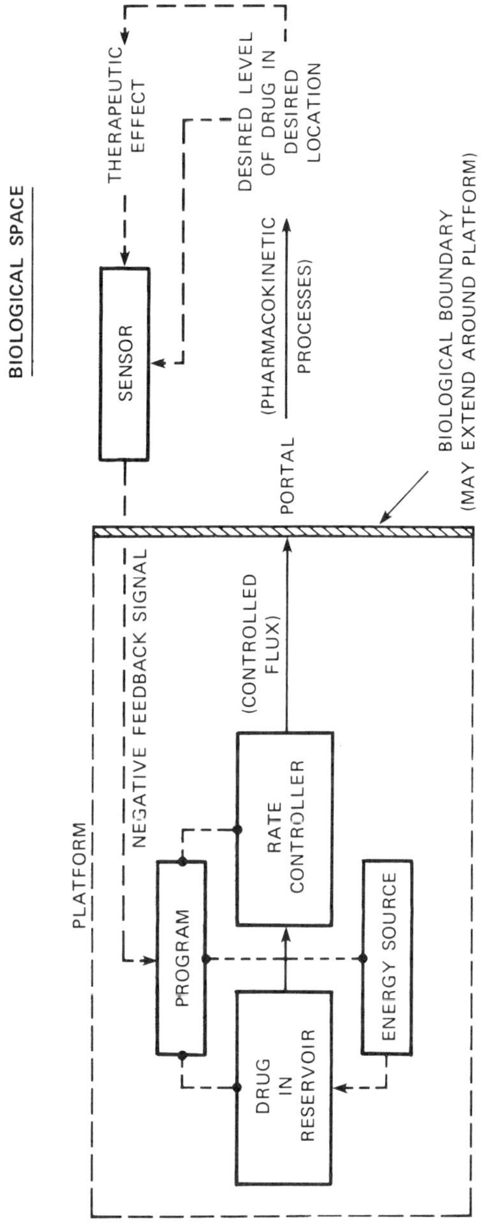

Figure 17 Schematic representation of a closed-loop controlled delivery system. (From Ref. 7.)

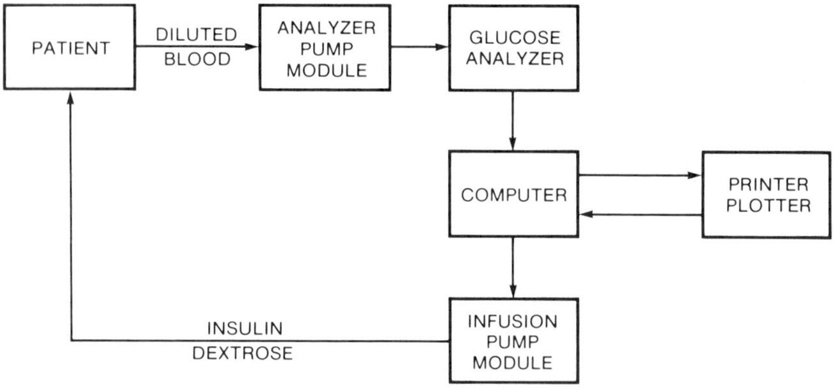

Figure 18 Diagram of the control of the Biostator and the computer control. (From Ref. 22.)

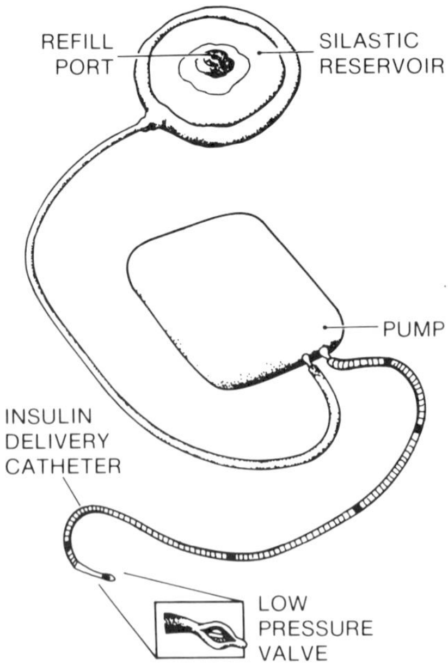

Figure 19 Schematic diagram of the implantable insulin delivery system. (From Ref. 23.)

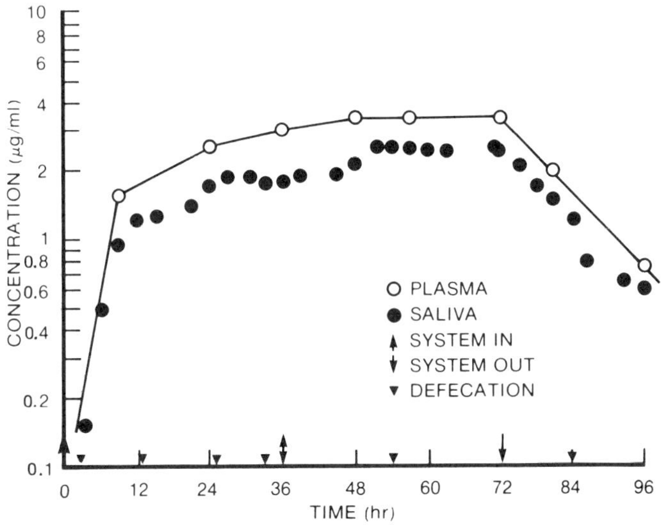

Figure 20 Plasma and saliva concentrations of theophylline after administration of theophylline (11 mg/hr) from rectal osmotic systems in humans. Large arrows indicate administration or removal of systems, and small arrows indicate defecation. (From Ref. 24.)

De Boer and colleagues [25] studied blood concentrations of the drug lidocaine delivered at a controlled rate within the rectal cavity of rats. They monitored the distance from the anus of the exit portal within the rectum. Drug was delivered first 2 cm from the anus and then at 4 cm. Figure 21 shows that for a set delivery rate, the concentration can vary considerably depending on the pump's distance from the anus. They hypothesized that either a certain amount of vital circulation occurs within the rectal cavity when drug moves between the portal and systemic circulations, or drug bypasses the portal circulation altogether. By circumventing the portal circulation, the drug avoids the enzymatic action of the liver the first time through; as a consequence, a greater amount of drug reaches the body.

Brain

The brain, too, has been studied as a possible portal for drug entry. In one study angiotensin II was delivered to the third ventricle of rat brains to evaluate the drug's dipsogenic effect [26]. The water uptake showed a constant increase (Fig. 22) during administration of angiotensin II. When the pumps were changed to deliver saline, the dipsogenic effect fell to nearly control baseline values. Thus it is now

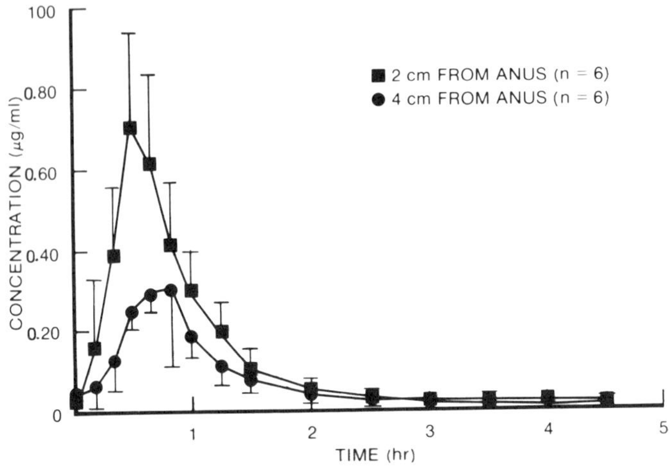

Figure 21 Mean blood concentration of lidocaine following rectal infusion of lidocine at either 2 or 4 cm from the anus of rats. (From Ref. 25.)

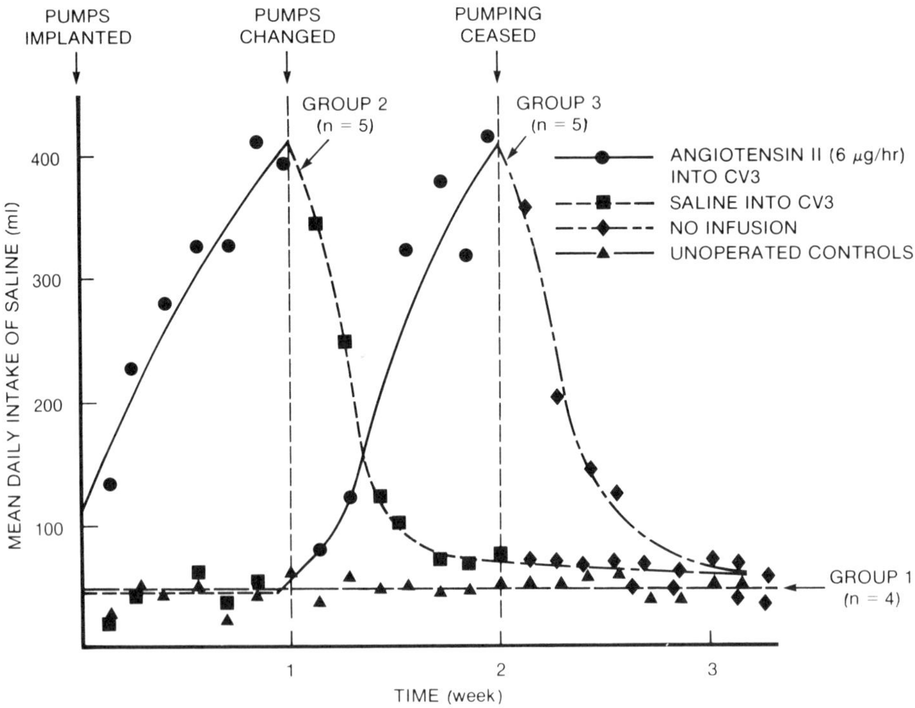

Figure 22 Chronic dipsogenic effect of angiotension II infused continuously into the third cerebral ventricle of rats by mini-osmotic pumps. (From Ref. 26.)

possible to control systemic drug concentrations and achieve a pharmacologic effect by delivering drug directly to the third ventricle.

Figure 23 shows the effect of the chronic infusion of angiotensin II on systolic blood pressure when delivered via the osmotic pump to the third ventricle of rats. Hypertension increased constantly. The systoles of rats infused with saline were similar to those of the controls. Once again, drug delivery directly to the brain elicits a controllable pharmacologic response.

CONTROLLED DELIVERY IN THE FUTURE

Technology in the field of controlled delivery has gone forward at a rapidly accelerating pace, and the future promises many new and exciting developments.

Research on oral dosage forms will focus on increasing gastric retention or gastrointestinal absorption for people taking drugs orally. Currently, retention time is quite variable and depends on the individual. Gastric platforms may be developed that will adhere to the

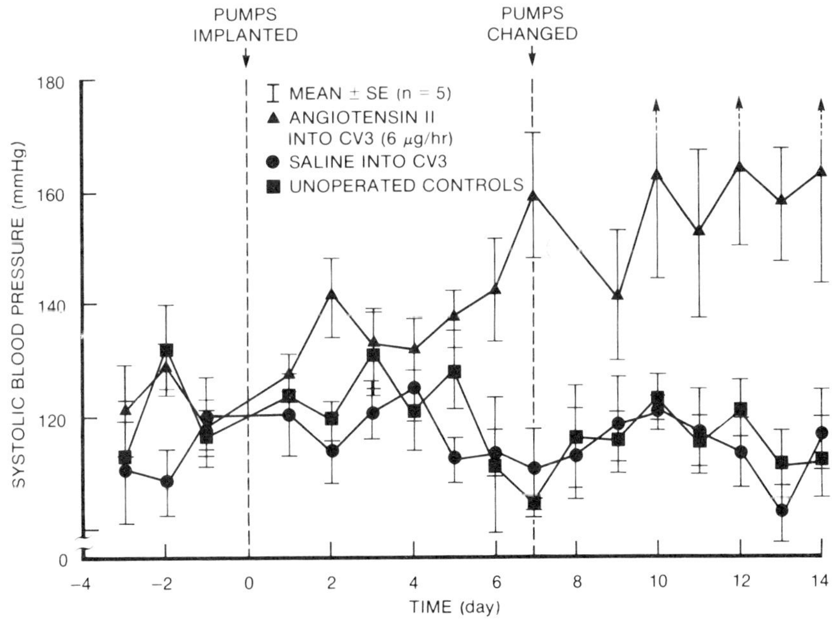

Figure 23 Hypertension induced in rats by chronic infusion of angiotensin II into the third cerebral ventricle (CV3) by mini-osmotic pumps. (From Ref. 27.)

stomach wall, thereby increasing gastric residence time and allowing for prolonged duration of therapy. Nishihata and colleagues [28] recently studied the use of salicylates as permeation enhancers to increase rectal absorption of theophylline.

Research on topical routes of administration will be diverse, depending on the site of administration (e.g., ocular or vaginal). Topical routes could utilize vaginal, buccal, or transdermal platforms.

Research on delivery systems using macromolecules and liposomes will investigate drugs with very short biological half-lives, will study and localize drug action, and will attempt to infuse drugs in a manner to achieve prolonged duration of delivery.

ACKNOWLEDGMENT

The authors appreciate the assistance and support given by Dr. Harriet Benson in the preparation of this manuscript.

REFERENCES

1. J. Urquhart, *Proc. Nat. Acad. Sci., Inst. Med., Conf. Pharmaceuticals for Developing Countries*, January 29-31, 1979.
2. J. Urquhart, in *Controlled-Release Pharmaceuticals* (J. Urquhart, ed.), American Pharmaceutical Association, Academy of Pharmaceutical Science, Washington, D.C., 1981.
3. G. G. Allan, J. W. Beer, and M. J. Cousin, *Proc. 4th Annu. Controlled Release Pestic. Symp.*, Corvallis, Oreg., August 22-24, 1977.
4. S. K. Chandrasekaran, *Proc. 4th Annu. Controlled Release Pestic. Symp.*, Corvallis, Oreg., August 22-24, 1977.
5. F. Theeuwes and W. Bayne, in *Controlled-Release Pharmaceuticals* (J. Urquhart, ed.), American Pharmaceutical Association, Academy of Pharmaceutical Sciences, Washington, D.C., 1981.
6. D. M. Long, Jr., and M. J. Folkman, U.S. Patent No. 3,279,996 (October 18, 1966).
7. F. E. Yates, H. Benson, R. Buckles, J. Urquhart, and A. Zaffaroni, in *Advances in Biomedical Engineering*, Vol. 5 (J. H. Brown and J. F. Dickson III, eds.), Academic Press, New York, 1975.
8. T. Higuchi, *J. Pharm. Sci.*, *50*:874 (1961).
9. E. S. Lee, S. W. Kim, S. H. Kim, J. R. Cardinal, and H. Jacobs, *J. Membr. Sci.*, *7*:293 (1980).
10. Y. Raghunathan, L. Amsel, O. Hinsvark, and W. Bryant, *J. Pharm. Sci.*, *70*:379 (1981).
11. R. Langer, *Chem. Eng. Commun.*, *6*:1 (1980).

12. G. Benagiano, E. Schmitt, D. Wise, and M. Goodman, in *Medical Polymers: Chemical Problems* (B. Sedláček, C. G. Overberger, and H. F. Mark, eds.), Journal of Polymer Science, Polymer Symposia No. 66, Interscience, New York, 1979.
13. B. Pharriss and E. Schmitt, *Int. Symp. Medicated IUDs and Polymeric Delivery Syst.*, Amsterdam, June 27-30, 1979.
14. F. Theeuwes and S. I. Yum, *Ann. Biomed. Eng.*, *4*:343 (1976).
15. S. K. Chandrasekaran, R. Capozza, and P. S. L. Wong, *J. Membr. Sci.*, *3*:271 (1978).
16. A. Zimmer, W. Roth, B. Hugemann, W. Spieth, and F. W. Koss, in *Biopharmaceutics*, Vol. 2 (J. M. Aiache and J. Hirtz, eds.), Technique et Documentation, Paris, 1981.
17. A. H. Beckett, in *Biopharmaceutics*, Vol. 1 (J. M. Aiache and J. Hirtz, eds.), Technique et Documentation, Paris, 1981.
18. J. D. Rogers, R. B. Lee, P. R. Webster, R. K. Ferguson, R. O. Davies, F. Theeuwes, and K. C. Kwan, in *Biopharmaceutics*, Vol. 1 (J. M. Aiache and J. Hirtz, eds.), Technique et Documentation, Paris, 1981.
19. H. Hess, J. Fara, J. Godbillon, and V. A. John, in *Biopharmaceutics*, Vol. 1 (J. M. Aiache and J. Hirtz, eds.), Technique et Documentation, Paris, 1981.
20. J. Shaw and J. Urquhart, *Trends Pharmacol. Sci.*, *1*:208 (1980).
21. J. E. Shaw and S. K. Chandrasekaran, in *Drug Absorption* (L. F. Prescott and W. S. Nimmo, eds.), ADIS Press, Balgowlah, Australia, 1981.
22. A. H. Clemens, *Med. Prog. Technol.*, *6*:91 (1979).
23. D. S. Schade, R. P. Eaton, G. A. Carlson, R. E. Bair, J. I. Gaona, Jr., J. T. Love, R. S. Urenda, and W. J. Spencer, *Diabetes Care*, *4*:319 (1981).
24. L. G. J. De Leede, A. G. De Boer, S. L. Van Velsen, and D. D. Breimer, in *Biopharmaceutics*, Vol. 1 (J. M. Aiache and J. Hirtz, eds.), Technique et Documentation, Paris, 1981.
25. A. G. De Boer, L. G. J. De Leede, P. J. Roos, C. P. J. M. Roozen, and D. D. Breimer, in *Biopharmaceutics*, Vol. 1 (J. M. Aiache and J. Hirtz, eds.), Technique et Documentation, Paris, 1981.
26. F. E. Yates, ed., Driving rats to drink: dipsogenic effect of angiotensin II during continuous infusion into the third cerebral ventricle (CV3 infusion) for seven days, *Special Delivery*, *1*(3):1 (1977).
27. F. E. Yates, ed., Hypertension induced by chronic intracerebral infusion of angiotensin II, *Special Delivery*, *2*(2):1 (1978).
28. T. Nishihata, J. H. Rytting, and T. Higuchi, *J. Pharm. Sci.*, *70*: 71 (1981).

Chapter 2

Liposomes: Possible Potential in Drug Delivery

BRENDA E. RYMAN Charing Cross Hospital Medical School (University of London), London, England

Liposomes are small (25 nm–4 μm diameter) phospholipid vesicles which are formed when dried, naturally occurring phospholipids swell, hydrate, and form bilayers in the presence of an aqueous phase. Such structures have for some 12 years been used mainly for studying membrane behavior, since the phospholipid bilayers formed are oriented in a similar way in biological membranes, as well as membrane-mediated processes such as those that occur in immunological phenomena. More recently, liposomes have been studied extensively as a possible carrier of therapeutic agents since both aqueous and lipid-soluble material may be entrapped (either in the aqueous space between the phospholipid bilayers or within the phospholipid itself).

The delivery of enzymes into defective cells in genetically inherited diseases in which a specific enzyme is absent was the earliest approach in which the carrier was used, and during the intervening years the potential of liposomes in drug delivery has extended to many areas, including anticancer chemotherapy, in the treatment of tropical diseases, and in iron and heavy metal accumulation. Their use in immunological research continues, and the potential of these small biodegradable vesicles, the properties of which may be readily manipulated, in vaccine preparation and adjuvant production is attracting considerable interest.

In the field of molecular biology the encapsulation of informational molecules such as DNA, RNA, plasmids, chromosomes, and viruses into liposomes with a view to delivery of the entrapped material to cells is another area of active research. Liposome potential in drug administration has also extended to hormones and the possibility of utilizing insulin via the oral route or cortisol esters by the intra-articular route have both been explored, as have the possibilities of using liposomes (or the dried phospholipid) in the treatment and/or diagnosis of myocardial infarction, in respiratory distress of the newborn, or in the early detection of metastatic spread in lymph nodes.

The literature concerning liposomal potential in drug delivery is now extensive, and rather than reiterate a survey the reader is referred to three review articles which cover the periods 1969-1976 [1], 1976-1979 [2], and 1979-1980 [3], and other useful reviews [4-6] give full reference to the areas mentioned briefly above. Only recent work will be discussed and will concern the following topics:

1. Reappraisal of the use of liposome-entrapped antitumor drugs in cancer chemotherapy
2. Entrapment of antibodies in liposomes for treatment of drug overdose, or in the early detection of tumors
3. The use of liposomes in the introduction of drugs into the lymphatic circulation and their use in detecting lymph nodes involved in metastatic spread
4. Possible placental transfer of drugs entrapped in liposomes

REAPPRAISAL OF THE USE OF LIPOSOME-ENTRAPPED ANTITUMOR DRUGS IN CANCER CHEMOTHERAPY

The literature abounds with reports of entrapment of antitumor drugs in liposomes [4,5] and the change in pharmokinetics of the drug which are observed following entrapment in liposomes compared with the free drug. Not unsurprisingly, the drug in the entrapped form persists much longer in the circulation than the free (relatively smaller molecular weight) form, which is frequently quickly filtered by the kidney and excreted in the urine. However, despite the earlier evidence that many tumor cell lines are penetrated by liposomes in vitro, there is less clear-cut evidence in vivo. Although several workers, including our own laboratory, have shown that small negatively charged liposomes appear to gain access to certain tumors in animals, we have been unable to detect any such uptake into a wide variety of tumors in humans [7-9].

It will be appreciated that if liposomally entrapped drugs in anticancer chemotherapy are to be regarded as superior to treatment employing *free* drug, then a change in the therapeutic index (TI) of that drug must be observable. The TI is a measure of the ratio of the LD_{50} to the minimal effective dose (MED), and clearly if both parameters change simultaneously there is no change in TI and hence no advantage in the formulation. If only one aspect of TI is measured, no conclusion can be reached regarding the superiority or otherwise of the entrapped drug. Although there are many claims in the literature (see Ref. 3) that entrapment of antitumor drugs in liposomes results in a lowering of toxicity of the drug and increased survival time of tumor-bearing animals, it must be noted that in most studies only *one* of these parameters of TI has been studied.

In an attempt to clarify the effect of entrapment in liposomes of a commonly used antitumor drug on TI over a wide dose range, Kaye et al. [10] have used in AKR mice the highly actinomycin D-sensitive mouse Ridgway osteosarcoma, which exhibits an orderly dose-response curve for the drug [11]. Tissue distribution of the free and entrapped drug was also followed and confirmed other work in which, using a variety of antitumor drugs, it has been shown that entrapment results in reduced peak concentrations in many organs. Of particular interest in this respect are the small intestine and bone marrow, which are normally unwanted targets for the drug. Liver and spleen, as was to be expected (since liposomes are taken up avidly by reticuloendothelial elements in these organs), exhibited high levels of the drug when it was administered in the entrapped form. As was predictable, the liposome-associated drug persisted much longer in the circulation.

The data on survival time of animals and drug effectiveness against the tumor are shown in Fig. 1a. The mean tumor weight at 10 days of nine control untreated mice is shown, together with tumor weight at 10 days, over a dose range of actinomycin D (0.125-8.0 µg/g). All control animals were given empty liposomes and liposomes for control and experimental animals were composed of phosphatidylcholine: cholesterol:stearylamine in 18:4:5 molar ratio.

Figure 1a shows that whereas liposomally entrapped drug (x----x) is far less toxic than free drug (x——x), nevertheless the efficacy of the drug is greatly diminished. Thus the antitumor activity, expressed as the minimum effective dose (inhibition to 10% of control tumor weight) of free drug (●——●) is 0.3 µg/g, whereas the entrapped actinomycin D in doses up to 8 µg/g fails to inhibit tumor growth to less than 68% of the untreated tumors (●——●). While the LD_{50} for free actinomycin D is 0.8 µg/g even at the highest dose of entrapped drug (8 µg/g), survival of the animals is 83%.

The treatment with empty liposomes alone showed some fall in tumor weight, which can probably be explained by the inhibitory effect on the tumor of the cationic (stearylamine-containing) liposomes.

Similar experiments were performed again using AKR mice bearing the Ridgway osteosarcoma [10] but using methotrexate as the drug. The results are shown in Fig. 1b and are somewhat different in that entrapped methotrexate (x----x) was more toxic than free drug (x——x), and was more effective against the tumor as assessed by the drop in tumor weight in the entrapped form (●----●), compared with the free drug (●——●), but in neither of the experiments described (i.e., using actinomycin D or methotrexate) is there any change in TI and thus no evidence of advantageous properties of administering the drugs in liposomes.

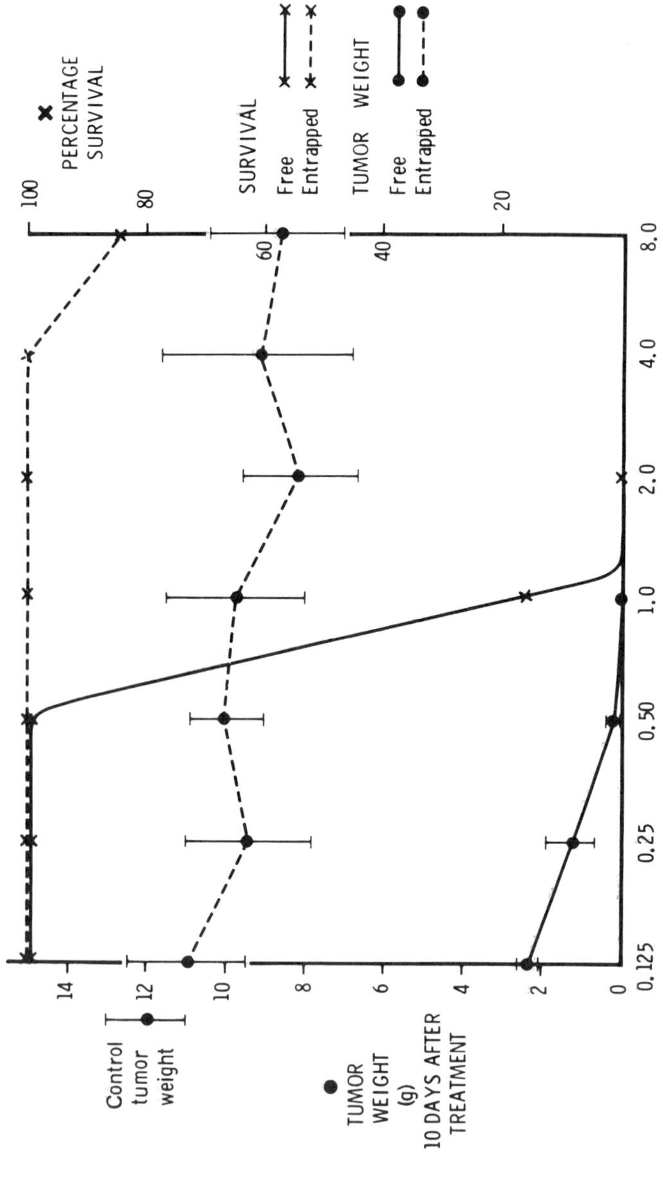

PERCENTAGE SURVIVAL
SURVIVAL
Free
Entrapped
TUMOR WEIGHT
Free
Entrapped
100
80
60
40
20
Control tumor weight
TUMOR WEIGHT (g) 10 DAYS AFTER TREATMENT
14
12
10
8
6
4
2
0
0.125
0.25
0.50
1.0
2.0
4.0
8.0
ACTINOMYCIN-D (μg/g)

(a)

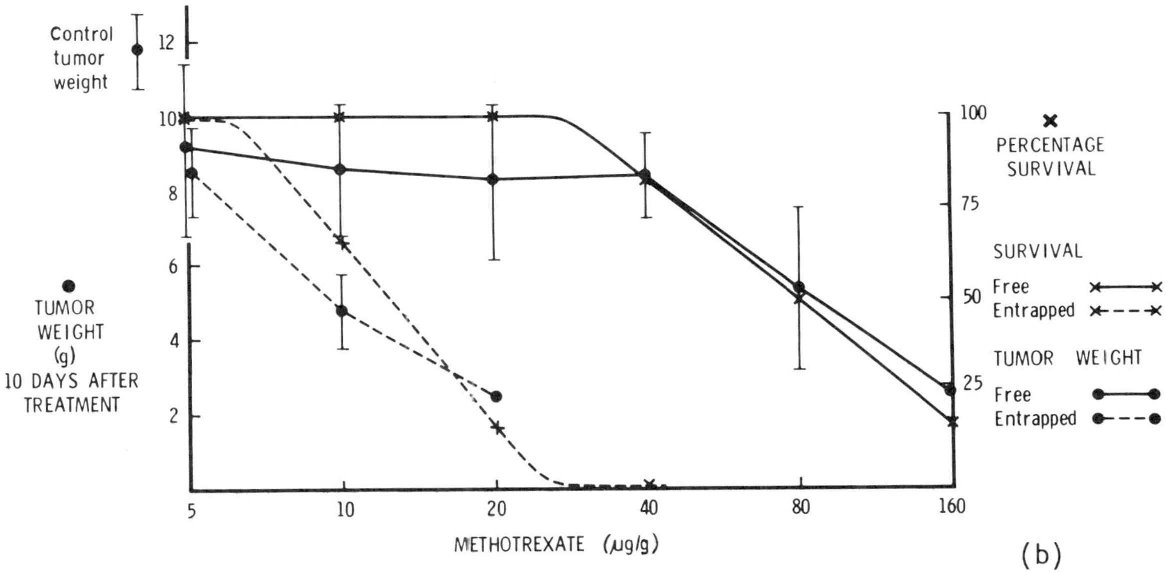

Figure 1 Therapeutic-toxicity data on the treatment of Ridgway osteogenic sarcoma-bearing AKR mice with actinomycin D (a) and methotrexate (b) in the free and (cationic) liposome-entrapped form. Liposome composition was phosphatidylcholine: cholesterol: stearylamine in the molar ratio 18:4:5. Each point refers to the mean for six mice with the standard error shown. Untreated control tumor weight at 10 days (11.8 ± 1.0 g) is also shown. For actinomycin D in the free form, the LD_{50} is 0.8 μg/g and the MED_{10} (dose inhibiting tumor growth to 10% of control) is 0.3 μg/g. Neither LD_{50} nor MED_{10} is reached using liposome-entrapped actinomycin D in doses up to 8 μg/g. In contrast, for methotrexate in the free form the LD_{50} is 80 μg/g and the MED_{20} (20% control tumor growth inhibition) is 160 μg/g, whereas for methotrexate in the liposome-entrapped form, the LD_{50} is 12 μg/g and the MED_{20} is 20 μg/g; that is, there is no significant improvement in the therapeutic index. (From Ref. 3.)

Does Entrapment Overcome Drug Resistance?

An actinomycin D-resistant Ridgway osteosarcoma was derived by successive passages of tumor fragments in the phase of regrowth after repeated treatment of the animals with actinomycin D commencing at a dose of 0.25 μg/g (given four times at 14-day intervals and progressively increasing the dose in successive generations). After passaging tumors through seven generations of treated mice, the tumors grew despite treatment with 0.8 μg/g of intravenous actinomycin D (the LD_{50} for the free drug). When animals bearing the resistant tumor were treated with liposomally entrapped actinomycin D it was clear that the drug was ineffective (Table 1).

The distribution of free and entrapped drug remained similar to that observed with the actinomycin D-sensitive tumor, implying a similar method of drug handling. However, a major difference is seen in tumor drug concentration following injection of free actinomycin D in the sensitive and resistant tumor (Fig. 2). Whereas the initial levels are similar, there is a difference between the sensitive and resistant sublines of the tumors in that the resistant one shows a rapid and consistent fall in actinomycin D, whereas in the sensitive line the drug is retained efficiently.

Table 1 Therapeutic-Toxicity Study Using Liposome-Entrapped Actinomycin D in the Treatment of Resistant Ridgway Osteosarcoma Subline

Dose (μg/g body wt)	Mean tumor weight (g) on day of treatment (SEM)	Mean tumor weight (g) 10 days after treatment (SEM)	Number of survivors at 10 days / Number of treated animals
a	1.31 (0.09)	9.77 (0.64)	6/6
0.125	1.21 (0.20)	10.19 (1.35)	6/6
0.25	1.10 (0.19)	10.75 (2.54)	6/6
0.5	1.22 (0.18)	10.77 (2.54)	6/6
1.0	1.38 (0.18)	9.33 (1.85)	6/6
2.0	1.17 (0.24)	10.10 (2.81)	6/6
4.0	1.21 (0.28)	9.53 (2.59)	5/5
8.0	1.39 (0.37)	9.39 (3.43)	5/5

[a]Empty liposomes equivalent to 12.5 mg of lipid.
Source: Ref. 10.

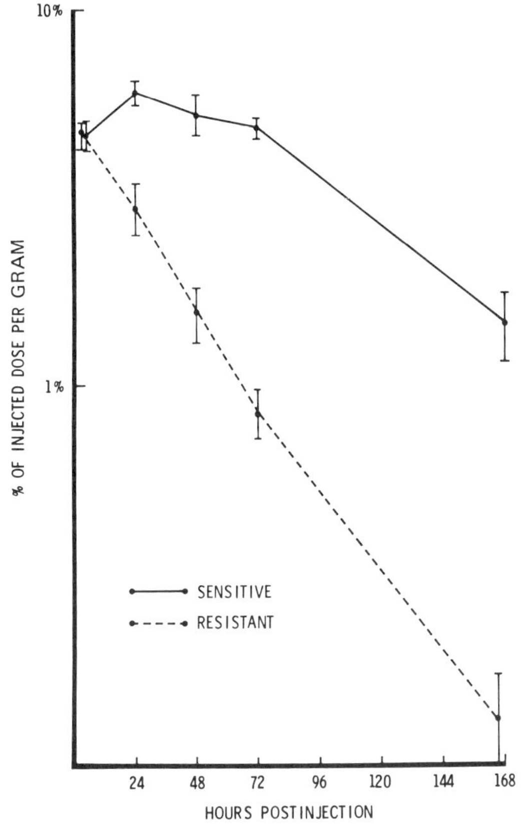

Figure 2 Concentration of [^{3}H]actinomycin D (AD) in the sensitive and resistant Ridgway osteosarcoma from 3 hr to 7 days following injection of free AD (500 μg/kg). (From Ref. 10.)

The claims that drug resistance can be overcome by entrapment of the drug in liposomes [12,13] perhaps emphasize the difficulties in translating the in vitro to the in vivo situation, and furthermore the method of inducing the resistance may be very important if one is attempting to mimic the situation that exists in drug resistance in humans [10]. While liposomes may fulfill a role in transporting a drug into resistant cells where there is a defect in the entry process of the drug, in our model this appears not to be the case.

In summary, therefore, from our work we must conclude that in the case of actinomycin D, a non-phase-specific drug, we can find no evidence that entrapment in liposomes changes the TI of the drug. In a resistant subline no evidence could be found that liposomally entrapped actinomycin D overcomes the resistance.

No change in TI could be observed when methotrexate was examined in the free and entrapped form in the Ridgway osteogenic sarcoma in mice. The reported work by Rustum et al. [14] on cytosine arabinoside (another phase-specific drug) has also suggested that the apparent increased efficacy of this drug in the entrapped form may reflect the slow release due to its leakage from the liposome in the body, and it will be necessary to compare the performance of such drugs given in this way with the currently used form of administration, i.e., slow infusion in cancer chemotherapy.

It is perhaps of some interest that Rustum et al. [14] and Mayhew [15] concluded from their studies of entrapped cytosine arabinoside (ara-C) that in the mouse L1210 leukemia long-term survivors were observed when the drug was given in liposomes compared with a 3 × daily treatment with nonentrapped drug, where no long-term survivors were found. Layton and Trouet [16], comparing free and liposomally encapsulated vincristine in leukemic mice, concluded that encapsulation did not provide any advantage either in terms of reduced toxicity or increased therapeutic index over the free drug for the treatment of lymphocytic leukemia. The liposome as a carrier of antitumor drugs therefore does not as yet appear to have achieved the first-promised potential. It may prove to be a useful method of administering some anticancer drugs in a slow release form, but insufficient evidence exists at the moment to make such a suggestion a reality.

ENTRAPMENT OF ANTIBODIES IN LIPOSOMES

For the Treatment of Drug Overdose

Antidigoxin Antibodies: Digoxin Overload Treatment Digoxin overload can be treated by giving the patient intravenous antibodies to digoxin. However, the long-circulating immune complexes which are formed pose problems. We have incorporated sheep digoxin antibodies into liposomes made of a 10:2:1 weight ratio, phosphatidylcholine (PC): cholesterol (C): phosphatidic acid (PA) with a view to overcoming this problem. Liposomes are removed rapidly from the circulation and are taken up by liver lysosomes and spleen [17,18]; it thus seemed logical to us to try to dispose of the excess digoxin by liposomally entrapped digoxin antibodies rather than antibody alone. This appears to be a successful approach [19].

This principle may have value in the treatment of overdoses of drugs other than digoxin: for example, clinically toxic compounds such as cytotoxic drugs, paraquat, and compounds active on the central nervous system.

Antibodies to Tumor Products: Improvement in Localization to Tumors?

The intravenous administration of radiolabeled antibodies to tumor products has been used to localize human tumor by scanning techniques [20,21]. Although this technique is very promising, problems of high background (due to circulating antibody) exist and in its present form the method requires the injection of [^{99m}Tc]serum albumin as well as [^{99m}Tc]O_4 so that suitable subtraction can be made from the imaging obtained with ^{131}I-labeled antibody (primary antibody, 1°). This subtraction is not entirely satisfactory. We have been investigating the possibility of entrapping an antibody to the primary antibody (secondary antibody, 2°) to "clear" the background, and hopefully allow retention of attachment of 1° antibody to tumor-bound products by incorporation of the 2° antibody into liposomes which would quickly be cleared from the circulation to liver and spleen. Experimental evidence suggests that so far this method of approach is worthy of further investigation [22].

The 1° antibody preparation was an anti-CEA (carcinoembryonic antigen) which was raised in goats. An immunoglobulin G fraction isolated from horse antiserum to the goat IgG was entrapped in sonicated, negatively charged liposomes. Although a considerable amount of 2° antibody was associated with the liposomes, only 4% of this would bind radiolabeled 1° antibody when incubated in vitro. Thus one must assume that most of the binding sites are "hidden" within the liposomes.

In experiments using AKR mice in which intravenous injections of ^{125}I-labeled anti-CEA (1°) were given, followed 24 hr later by liposomes containing the 2° antibody, there was good evidence of a considerable lowering of blood and kidney levels of the isotope, while liver and spleen showed enhanced radioactivity. Such a result would be anticipated if the liposome containing the 2° antibody were interacting with the anti-CEA (1°) and the complex was being removed by liver and spleen (the natural fate of intravenous liposomes). Some of the results are summarized in Fig. 3. Similar results were obtained using an extra marker by labeling the liposomes with ^{99m}Tc (Fig. 4). Rapid clearance of labels resulted in only 9% of liposome labels being detectable in the blood after 30 min following intravenous injection of liposomes loaded with 2° antibody, and accumulation in liver was maximal at 2 hr and in spleen at 18 hr.

Similar experiments were performed in nude mice bearing xenografts of human colonic tumors. Two different tumor lines were used: P116, which is a poor secretor of CEA, and TAF, a good secretor. Again, injection of ^{125}I-labeled primary antibody was followed in the experimental group by liposomally entrapped secondary antibody, and in the controls by no further treatment. ^{125}I was determined in tissues including tumors. In all experiments the ^{125}I primary antibody

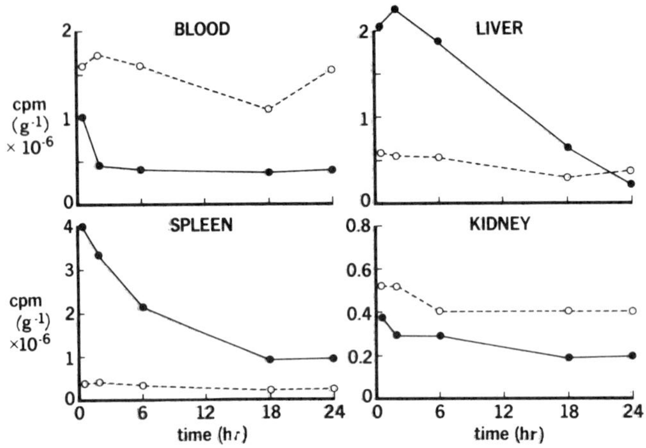

Figure 3 [^{125}I]anti-CEA distribution in normal mice after treatment with liposomes containing secondary antibody. All points are the mean of three animals. All animals were given intravenous injections of 15 μCi of [^{125}I] anti-CEA (primary antibody) 24 hr before the start of the experiment. Liposome-treated animals (o——o) were given sonicated, negatively charged liposomes containing secondary antibody (approximately 10 μmol of lipid per mouse) intravenously at 0 hr. Control mice (o----o) received no further treatment. (From B. E. Ryman, G. M. Barratt, H. M. Patel, and N. S. Tüzel, *Optimization of Drug Delivery, Alfred Benzon Symposium 17,* Munksgaard International Publishers, Ltd., Copenhagen, 1982.)

remaining in the blood of animals treated with liposomes containing secondary antibody was reduced compared to controls, and the reduction was related to the amount of lipid administered as liposomes (Table 2). Up to 6 hr after liposome injection the tumor radioactivity in treated animals was not different from the controls, as shown in Fig. 5. Twenty-four hours after liposome treatment tumor-associated ^{125}I-labeled primary antibody was reduced relative to controls; however, the tumor-to-blood ratio of primary antibody was still increased in treated animals (Table 2).

These results indicate that the liposomes containing secondary antibody cause a redistribution of blood-borne primary antibody to the liver and spleen. The fact that radioactivity in the tumors of liposome-secondary antibody-treated rats remained similar to the controls up to 6 hr after treatment and the clearance of primary antibody by the liposome-secondary antibody was rapid with a plateau after 2 hr adds support to the idea that these strategies may be useful in increasing the clarity of scans designed to seek out tumors, and we are currently planning such investigations in humans.

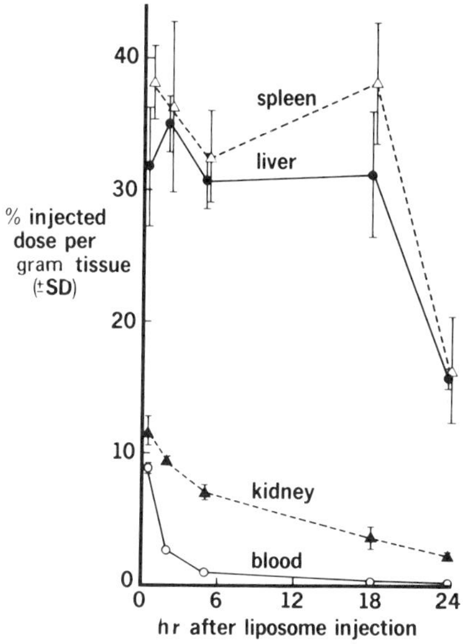

Figure 4 Distribution of ^{99m}Tc-labeled liposomes containing secondary antibody in normal mice pretreated with primary antibody. Each point is the mean of counts from three animals. Mice were given [^{125}I]primary antibody 24 hr prior to the start of the experiment and, at 0 hr, 9 μmol of lipids as liposomes containing entrapped secondary antibody externally labeled with ^{99m}Tc. [From B. E. Ryman and G. M. Barratt, in *Targetting of Drugs* (G. Gregoriadis, ed.), Plenum Press, New York, 1982, in press.]

USE OF LIPOSOMES IN THE INTRODUCTION OF DRUGS INTO THE LYMPHATIC CIRCULATION AND THEIR USE IN DETECTING LYMPH NODES INVOLVED IN METASTATIC SPREAD

In earlier work from our laboratory we reported animal studies which showed that ^{99m}Tc-labeled liposomes could be used for regional lymph node imaging [7,23] and that nodes involved in metastatic spread showed a suppression of uptake of labeled liposomes made from phosphatidylcholine and cholesterol [24]. It was also demonstrated that regional lymph nodes draining an area infected with irradiated tumor cells showed enhanced uptake of the labeled liposomes, whereas the presence of inflammation did not alter uptake patterns compared with those in normal animals [25].

This study was part of a larger project to assess the possibility of using lymphoscintigraphy of internal and axillary lymph node chains to

Table 2 [^{125}I]Anti-CEA Distribution in Nude Mice Bearing Human Tumor Xenografts After Treatment with Liposomally Entrapped Secondary Antibody[a]

Tumor line	Dose of liposomes (μmol lipids)	Time after injection (hr)	Tissue radioactivity as a percent of that in untreated controls		Ratio of tumor radioactivity to blood radioactivity	
			Blood	Tumor	Control	Liposomes
P116	3	6	30	122	0.30	1.22
		24	39	64	0.20	0.32
TAF	10	1/2	56	92	0.50	0.73
		2	34	140	0.40	1.69
		6	30	107	0.54	1.92
	27	24	5	51	0.53	5.57

[a]Values are means for two to three mice. All mice were given an intravenous injection of [^{125}I]primary antibody 24 hr prior to the start of the experiment. Treated mice were given liposomes (PC:CH:PA, 9:9:2, 10 min sonication) containing secondary antibody at 0 hr.

Source: B. E. Ryman and G. M. Barratt, in *Targetting of Drugs* (G. Gregoriadis, ed.), Plenum Press, New York, 1982, in press.

improve the preoperative staging of breast cancer, and 40 patients with breast cancer have now been assessed. Forty-five percent of these patients had abnormal scintigrams (suppression of uptake), suggesting the presence of lymph node metastases; 35% had normal images; and 20% were technically unsatisfactory, usually because of poor technetium-labeling efficiency. Twenty-two of the 32 interpretable images were correlated with the results of histopathological examinations of lymph node removed by radical mastectomy. Twelve of these had abnormal patterns, of which one had histologically normal nodes and constituted a false positive. Ten had normal patterns, of which two with enhanced uptake were found to have minimal lymph node metastases in the lower nodes with reactive hyperplasia of the nodes above [25].

These findings support our animal experiments and suggest that labeled liposomes may be a useful means of assessing in vivo activity of lymph nodes in response to the presence of a tumor and thus yield valuable information preoperatively on which lymph nodes have cancer deposits and may identify lymph nodes draining a tumor which has not yet metastasized. Work is continuing in this area [26].

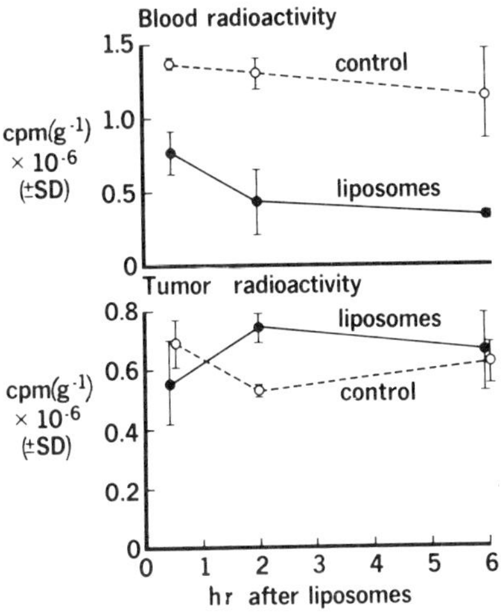

Figure 5 [^{125}I]Anti-CEA distribution in tumor-bearing mice after treatment with liposomes containing secondary antibody. Values are means for three nude mice bearing TAF tumor xenografts. All mice were given an intravenous injection of [^{125}I]primary antibody 24 hr prior to the start of the experiment. Treated mice were given 10 μmol of lipid as liposomes at 0 hr. (From B. E. Ryman, G. M. Barratt, H. M. Patel, and N. S. Tüzel, *Optimization of Drug Delivery, Alfred Benzon Symposium 17*, Munksgaard International Publishers, Ltd., Copenhagen, 1982.)

POSSIBLE PLACENTAL TRANSFER OF DRUGS ENTRAPPED IN LIPOSOMES

Placental transfer of materials of therapeutic interest is another aspect of liposome delivery that we are currently considering. Small (25-100 nm diameter) negatively charged fluid liposomes administered intravenously have been shown to be particularly effective in transferring labeled penicillin from the maternal circulation to placental tissue and uterus in pregnant rats and rabbits with a severalfold increase over the free drug. Penicillin was also found in the fetuses and amniotic fluid of these animals. Similar observations were made when [^{14}C]inulin was entrapped in liposomes and injected intravenously, although no accumulation of label was seen in the fetus and amniotic fluid, probably due to the impermanent nature of inulin in the placenta [27]. Intraperitoneal administration of labeled inulin entrapped in liposomes to rats has shown an increased uptake by placenta and uterus over the free drug; however, free and entrapped [^{14}C]penicillin injected by this route did not show such a marked difference. Since many drugs do not cross the placenta readily, there may be a potential use of liposomes as drug deliverers to uterus, placenta, and in certain instances to the fetus for the possible treatment of infections or tumors.

While liposomes present a very intriguing carrier system for targeting and drug delivery, it must be emphasized that the size of the liposomes (the smallest are 25 nm in diameter) almost certainly precludes their usefulness in targeting to a wide range of tissues. It appears that following intravenous injection, liposomes are able to cross fenestrated and discontinuous capillaries and can probably escape from the circulation into organs such as liver, spleen, and bone marrow where discontinuous capillaries exist.

The involvement of the elements of the reticuloendothelial system (RES) in liposome uptake has been exploited in several areas of targeting, which include the treatment with drug-loaded liposomes of certain tropical diseases (e.g., visceral leishmaniasis) in which the parasite invades the RES. Removal of unwanted materials into the RES utilizing liposomes has been discussed in this chapter in relation to drug overload and antibody clearance in tumor localization. Liposome uptake into lymph nodes (probably involving macrophages) appears a hopeful approach to drug delivery to the lymphatic system and the detection of metastases in lymph nodes. Enzyme replacement therapy in conditions where the defect is found within the RES (e.g., Gaucher's lipidosis) may also be amenable to treatment by enzyme delivery in liposomes, as may chelation therapy in heavy metal poisoning with chelator-carrying liposomes.

Not only do the fixed phagocytic cells of the RES take up liposomes, but the circulating monocytes do also, and this may have serious implications when liposome-encapsulated antitumor drugs are administered in attempted improved cancer chemotherapy, as has been suggested by Poste and Fidler [28]. Impairment of host RES occurs in the presence of the encapsulated drug compared with free drug, and this leads to an undesired enhanced metastatic spread of a number of mouse tumors examined.

On the other hand, this group of workers [28-33] have shown that both macrophage activating factor (MAF—a lymphokine-containing preparation) and muramyl dipeptide (MDP) delivered in liposomes and injected intravenously are engulfed by circulating monocytes which penetrate the alveolar space and become effective in the lung bed and are able to reduce lung metastases in both mice and dogs. The liposome system is therefore effective in introducing materials (MAF or MDP) which turn on the natural defense mechanism of body mediated through macrophages. In this exciting approach to the control of metastases it will be seen that the natural targeting of liposomes—to elements of the RES—is again being exploited.

Intravascular targeting of liposomes has also been considered by Poste and Fidler [28] and the possibility of introducing materials specifically to cells bathed by the liposomes following their intravenous administration and with appropriate ligands on their surface is under consideration. Thus endothelial cells of kidney or specific subsets of T lymphocytes may prove to be possible targets for modification by the liposome system.

ACKNOWLEDGMENTS

It is my pleasure to acknowledge the people who have been involved in liposome work in our laboratory over the last 12 years and whose contributions are quoted in our references, and the skilled abilities of Linda Readings in the preparation of the manuscript.

REFERENCES

1. D. A. Tyrrell, T. D. Heath, C. M. Colley, and B. E. Ryman, *Biochim. Biophys. Acta*, *457*:259 (1976).
2. B. E. Ryman and D. A. Tyrrell, Liposomes—methodology and applications, in *Lysosomes in Biology and Pathology*, Vol. 6: *Lysosomes in Applied Biology and Therapeutics* (J. T. Dingle, P. J. Jacques, and I. H. Shaw, eds.), Elsevier/North-Holland, Amsterdam, 1979, pp. 549-574.
3. B. E. Ryman and D. A. Tyrrell, Liposomes—bags of potential, in *Essays in Biochemistry*, Vol. 16 (P. N. Campbell and R. D. Marshall, eds.), Academic Press, London, 1980, pp. 49-98.
4. G. Gregoriadis, *Nature*, *265*:407 (1977).
5. G. Gregoriadis, Liposomes, in *Drug Carriers in Biology and Medicine* (G. Gregoriadis, ed.), Academic Press, London, 1979, pp. 287-341.
6. D. Papahadjopoulos, ed., *Ann. N.Y. Acad. Sci.*, *308*:1 (1978).
7. B. E. Ryman, R. F. Jewkes, K. Jeyasingh, M. P. Osborne, H. M. Patel, V. J. Richardson, M. H. N. Tattersall, and D. A. Tyrrell, *Ann. N.Y. Acad. Sci.*, *308*:281 (1978).
8. V. J. Richardson, K. Jeyasingh, R. F. Jewkes, B. E. Ryman, and M. H. N. Tattersall, *J. Nucl. Med.*, *19*:1049 (1978).
9. V. J. Richardson, B. E. Ryman, R. F. Jewkes, K. Jeyasingh, M. H. N. Tattersall, E. S. Newlands, and S. B. Kaye, *Br. J. Cancer*, *40*:35 (1979).
10. S. B. Kaye, J. A. Boden, and B. E. Ryman, *Eur. J. Cancer*, *17*:279 (1981).
11. H. S. Schwartz, J. E. Sodergren, S. S. Sternberg, and F. S. Philips, *Cancer Res.*, *26*:1873 (1966).
12. D. Papahadjopoulos, G. Poste, W. J. Vail, and J. L. Biedler, *Cancer Res.*, *36*:2988 (1976).
13. M. J. Kosloski, F. Rosen, R. J. Milholland, and D. Papahadjopoulos, *Cancer Res.*, *38*:2848 (1978).

14. Y. M. Rustum, C. Dave, E. Mayhew, and D. Papahadjopoulos, *Cancer Res.*, *39*:1390 (1979).
15. E. Mayhew, Experimental cancer treatment with liposome-entrapped anti-tumor drugs, in *Targetting of Drugs* (G. Gregoriadis, ed.), Plenum Press, New York, 1981, in press.
16. D. Layton and A. Trouet, *Eur. J. Cancer*, *16*:945 (1980).
17. G. Gregoriadis and B. E. Ryman, *Eur. J. Biochem.*, *24*:485 (1972).
18. G. Gregoriadis and B. E. Ryman, *Biochem. J.*, *129*:123 (1972).
19. P. I. Campbell, N. G. L. Harding, B. E. Ryman, and D. A. Tyrrell, *Eur. J. Biochem.*, *109*:87 (1980).
20. D. M. Goldenberg, F. Deland, E. Kim, S. Bennett, F. J. Primus, J. R. Van Nagell, N. Estes, P. De Simone, and P. Rayburn, *N. Engl. J. Med.*, *298*:1384 (1978).
21. R. H. Begent, G. Stanway, B. E. Jones, K. D. Bagshawe, F. Searle, R. F. Jewkes, and P. Vernon, *J. R. Soc. Med.*, *73*:624 (1980).
22. G. M. Barratt, B. E. Ryman, J. A. Boden, P. A. Keep, F. Searle, R. H. Begent, and K. D. Bagshawe, *Biochem. Soc. Trans.*, *9*: 564-565 (1981).
23. M. P. Osborne, V. J. Richardson, K. Jeyasingh, and B. E. Ryman, *Int. J. Nucl. Med. Biol.*, *6*:75 (1979).
24. V. J. Richardson, M. P. Osborne, K. Jeyasingh, B. E. Ryman, and J. I. Burn, *Br. J. Cancer*, *38*:177 (1978).
25. M. P. Osborne, B. E. Ryman, J. H. Payne, and V. R. McCready, The use of ^{99m}Tc-labelled neutral liposomes in lymphoscintigraphy: a comparison of scintigram interpretations with node histology in a series of breast cancer patients, in *Progress in Radiopharmacology*, Vol. 2 (P. H. Cox, ed.), Elsevier/North-Holland, Amsterdam, 1981, pp. 317-325.
26. M. P. Osborne, V. J. Richardson, K. Jeyasingh, and B. E. Ryman, *Int. J. Nucl. Med. Biol.*, *9*:47 (1982).
27. N. S. Tuzel, H. M. Patel, and B. E. Ryman, *Biochem. Soc. Trans.*, *8*:559 (1981).
28. G. Poste and I. J. Fidler, Modifications of host defence functions by liposome-encapsulated immunomodulators, in *Targetting of Drugs* G. Gregoriadis, ed.), Plenum, New York, 1982, in press.
29. I. J. Fidler, A. Raz, W. C. Fogler, L. C. Hoyer, and G. Poste, *Cancer Res.*, *41*:495 (1981).
30. W. E. Fogler, A. Raz, and I. J. Fidler, *Cell. Immunol.*, *53*:214 (1980).
31. A. Rax, C. Bucana, W. E. Fogler, G. Poste, and I. J. Fidler, *Cancer Res.*, *41*:487 (1981).
32. S. Sone and I. J. Fidler, *J. Immunol.*, *125*:2454 (1980).
33. S. Sone, G. Poste, and I. J. Fidler, *J. Immunol.*, *124*:2197 (1980).

Chapter 3

Controlled Release of Drugs: Prodrug Performance in Target Tissues

WILLIAM I. HIGUCHI,* AKIRA KUSAI,† JEFFREY L. FOX, NEAL A. GORDON, and NORMAN F. H. HO The University of Michigan College of Pharmacy, Ann Arbor, Michigan

CHUNG-CHIANG HSU Abbott Laboratories, North Chicago, Illinois

JUNG Y. PARK Boehringer Ingelheim, Ridgefield, Connecticut

DAVID C. BAKER The University of Alabama, University, Alabama

WILLIAM M. SHANNON Southern Research Institute, Birmingham, Alabama

The antiviral agent 9-β-D-arabinofuranosyladenine (vidarabine, ara-A) has been reported to possess highly significant antiviral activity against herpes viruses replicating in cell culture [1-4], in animals [3, 5-12], and in human patients [13-23]. The drug is now marketed as an aqueous suspension (Vira-A) for treatment of herpes keratitis of the eye. This drug has been shown to be effective against herpes encephalitis in humans, where in a controlled study, the mortality was dramatically lowered from 70% to 28% [24]. The U.S. Food and Drug Administration (FDA), based on the results of this study and other evidence, has recently approved this drug for intravenous use against these systemic, life-threatening diseases and, at present, vidarabine is the leading antiviral drug approved by the FDA for local and parenteral use in the treatment of herpesvirus infections in humans.

Although the effectiveness of vidarabine as an antiviral agent has been clearly established, there are numerous reports of the drug's lack of effectiveness in animals and in humans in certain therapeutic situations. Vidarabine has been shown to be effective against herpes simplex virus (HSV) type 2 encephalitis in mice inoculated intraperitoneally [25] or intracerebrally [9] with virus; other reports have indicated,

Present affiliations

*College of Pharmacy, University of Utah, Salt Lake City, Utah

†Sankyo Corporation, Tokyo, Japan

however, that the drug is ineffective against HSV type 2 infection in mice inoculated either intranasally or intravaginally with virus and treated either systemically [25-27] or topically [25] with the drug. In a recent prospective double-blind evaluation of topical vidarabine against herpes progenitalis in humans, no differences could be seen in the clinical or the virological responses between vidarabine-treated and the control (untreated) groups [28]. The investigators suggested that the problem is probably one of drug delivery, that is, one of relative insolubility and lack of ability to penetrate the lesions. In other studies [29], it was reported that topical treatment with 3% vidarabine did not influence the course of either primary or recurrent genital herpetic infection in either men or women. These negative findings suggest that the understanding of the target tissue and/or target cell pharmacokinetics and local metabolism factors would be essential to the successful development of a topical antiviral delivery system involving vidarabine.

It is also to be noted that vidarabine has several nonoptimal properties which present barriers to its effective delivery and which may be responsible for the examples of poor efficacy discussed above. Vidarabine has a low aqueous solubility (0.4 mg/ml) and at the same time the molecule is not very lipophilic (log P = -0.48 in pentanol-water). In addition, vidarabine lacks resistance to adenosine deaminase, the enzyme ubiquitous to body tissues that converts vidarabine to arahypoxanthine, a compound of much lower antiviral activity than vidarabine. The poor solubility and low lipophilicity are reflected in our recent studies [30-34] with the hairless mouse skin. Vidarabine has an extremely low permeability coefficient ($P = 3 \times 10^{-8}$ cm/sec) for the stratum corneum of this tissue. As a result of this, there could be a very large concentration drop from the surface of the stratum corneum to the basal layer of the epidermis when the drug is topically applied. Our analysis shows that even when vidarabine is applied at maximum strength (the saturated solution), the steady-state vidarabine levels in the epidermis may be 100 times below the minimum inhibitory concentration (MIC) for viral replication in tissue cultures.

Recently, a large number of vidarabine monoesters, diesters, and triesters were synthesized by Baker et al. [35,36]. These compounds offer a wide range of aqueous solubilities and lipophilicities. All of the straight-chain 5'-monoesters were found to be effective in antiviral plaque-reduction assays. Also, the 5'-monoesters were found not to be deaminated by adenosine deaminase. In recent studies in our laboratories [37] on the transport and metabolism of the 5'-valerate ester of vidarabine, it was found that this prodrug was capable of giving rise to cell concentrations of vidarabine in KB cell culture that were as high as those obtained in cells whose adenosine deaminase enzyme activity had been completely inhibited by treatment with 2'-deoxycoformycin (2'-dCF) [38]. Subsequent in vitro studies [39] with calf mucosal adenosine deaminse showed that the 5'-valerate was indeed a weak competitive inhibitor of the enzyme. Although this adenosine deaminase enzyme inhibitor activity in no way approaches that afforded by the potent inhibitor 2'-dCF, the results are dramatic in that these drugs, which are lipophilic, soluble, and resistant to adenosine deaminase, are acting at the target site to provide a mild suppression of adenosine deaminase activity and thus protect the vidarabine as it is liberated. Furthermore, the inhibitor action is self-limiting. It prolongs the activity of vidarabine and vanishes as the prodrug level diminishes, ultimately clearing the system of vidarabine.

The purpose of this presentation is to describe a method that combines in vitro experiments with biological membranes or tissues and theoretical techniques for predicting target site levels of a drug (vidarabine) delivered by a prodrug (vidarabine esters). It involves developing a physically meaningful model, then applying the model to calculate concentration profiles. As will be shown, this method can be used for the design of controlled release prodrugs in target tissues—the "control" being chemical and biochemical rather than physical (as are most controlled release systems).

Three 5'-monoesters (-acetate, -valerate, and the -octanoate) of vidarabine have now been investigated with hairless mouse skin and the mouse vaginal membrane. A three-layer model was employed in both cases (stratum corneum, epidermis, and dermis in the case of skin; a cornified layer, the epithelium, and the lamina propria in the case of the vaginal membrane). Thicknesses, diffusivities, and enzyme activities (both the activating enzyme, esterase, and the deactivating enzyme, deaminase) were assigned (based on independent experiments) or deduced from the permeation experiments with the membranes. Important effects of the estrous cycle on the transport parameters were also considered in the case of the vaginal membrane. Steady-state vidarabine levels were calculated for situations where the drug and the prodrugs are applied to the membrane under maximum thermodynamic conditions (i.e., as saturated solutions). The results were especially interesting with the mouse vaginal membrane studies, as the levels and the shapes of drug concentration profiles were found to be strongly dependent on enzyme saturation effects (Michaelis-Menten kinetics) and on the inhibition of the deaminase by the ester prodrug itself. These results show how the n-alkyl chain length at the 5'-position affects solubility, lipophilicity, esterase lability, and deaminase inhibition and how these, in turn, influence the steady-state vidarabine levels at the target site in topical chemotherapy.

MOUSE VAGINAL MEMBRANE SYSTEM

Figure 1 gives the chemical structures of the three ester prodrugs, ara-A (the drug), and ara-hypoxanthine, the much less active metabolite formed by the action of the enzyme adenosine deaminase upon

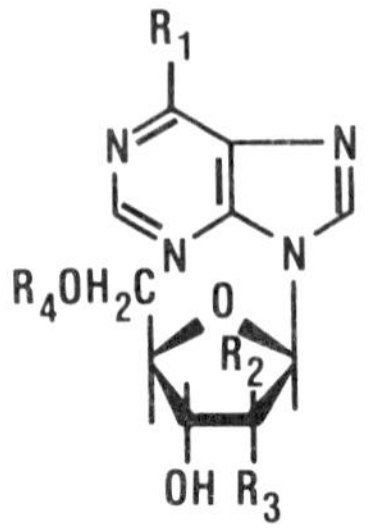

Figure 1 Chemical structures of ara-A, ara-H, and prodrug esters of ara-A.

Compound	R_1	R_2	R_3	R_4	Aqueous solubility (M)
Adenosine	NH_2	H	OH	H	
Ara-A	NH_2	OH	H	H	1.5×10^{-3}
-5'-acetate	NH_2	OH	H	CH_3CO	2.7×10^{-2}
-5'-valerate	NH_2	OH	H	$CH_3(CH_2)_3CO$	2.4×10^{-2}
-5'-octanoate	NH_2	OH	H	$CH_3(CH_2)_6CO$	5.8×10^{-4}
Ara-H	OH	OH	H	H	

[Reprinted from *Optimization of Drug Delivery, Alfred Benzon Symposium 17* (Hans Bundgaard, Anne Bagger Hanson, and Helmer Kofod, eds.), Munksgaard, Copenhagen, 1982.]

ara-A. In the biological membrane we have the following reaction scheme:

$$\text{A (prodrug)} \xrightarrow{\text{esterase}} \text{B (drug)} \xrightarrow{\text{deaminase}} \text{C (metabolite)}$$

In the quasi-steady state, we may write the following equations, which describe the (one-dimensional) simultaneous enzymatic reactions and diffusion:

$$D_{A,i} \frac{d^2[A]}{dX^2} - \frac{V_{m,i}[A]}{K_m + [A]} = 0 \qquad (1)$$

$$D_{B,i}\frac{d^2[B]}{dX^2} + \frac{V_{m,i}[A]}{K_m + [A]} - \frac{V'_{m,i}[B]}{(1 + [A]/k_I)K'_m + [B]} = 0 \tag{2}$$

$$D_{C,i}\frac{d^2[C]}{dX^2} + \frac{V'_{m,i}[B]}{(1 + [A]/k_I)K'_m + [B]} = 0 \tag{3}$$

The D's are the diffusivities. The subscripts A, B, and C refer to the three species and i refers to the ith component or stratum of the membrane. The coordinate X is the perpendicular depth in the membrane. V_m and K_m are the Michaelis-Menten kinetics parameters for the esterase and V'_m and K'_m are those for the deaminase. k_I is the deaminase inhibition constant for the prodrug [37]. For the general case, the D's, K_m's, V_m's, and the k_I's may all be functions of X. It is shown, however, that although the parameter values may be different for the different components of a membrane (e.g., cornified layer, epithelium, and lamina propria in the case of the vaginal membrane), they may be assumed to be constant within a particular membrane component [40,41].

At low concentrations of the prodrug, Eqs. (1)-(3) reduce to

$$D_{A,i}\frac{d^2[A]}{dX^2} - k_i[A] = 0 \tag{4}$$

$$D_{B,i}\frac{d^2[B]}{dX^2} + k_i[A] - k'_I[B] = 0 \tag{5}$$

$$D_{C,i}\frac{d^2[C]}{dX^2} + k'_i[B] = 0 \tag{6}$$

Much of the model development studies and model validation studies were conducted using tracer levels of substrates and Eqs. (4)-(6).

Figure 2 schematically illustrates the vaginal membrane model. The cornified layer is present during the early estrus and the estrus phases and is absent during the remainder of the estrous cycle. Thickness determinations of the cornified layer, epithelium, and the lamina propria were made using a combination of micrometer and microscope techniques [40] with excised membranes. Diffusion cell experiments [31,40] yielded permeability coefficients. The enormous effect of the estrous cycle (ca. 5 days) on the ara-A permeability coefficient for the whole membrane is shown in Fig. 3. The vaginal membrane thickness

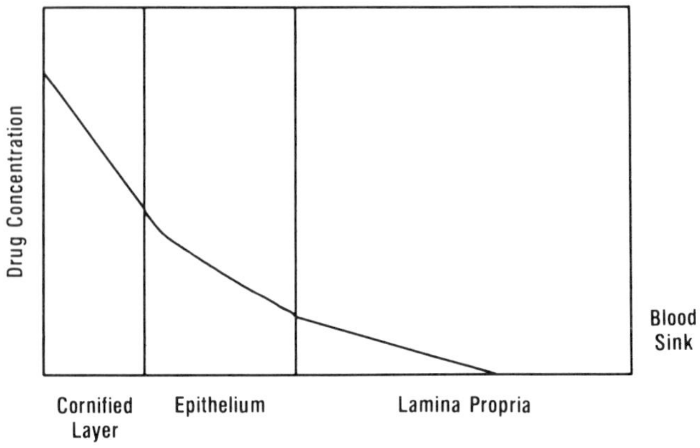

Figure 2 Multilayer model for simultaneous diffusion and metabolism of drug in the mouse vaginal membrane. [Reprinted from *Optimization of Drug Delivery, Alfred Benzon Symposium 17* (Hans Bundgaard, Anne Bagger Hanson, and Helmer Kofod, eds.), Munksgaard, Copenhagen, 1982.]

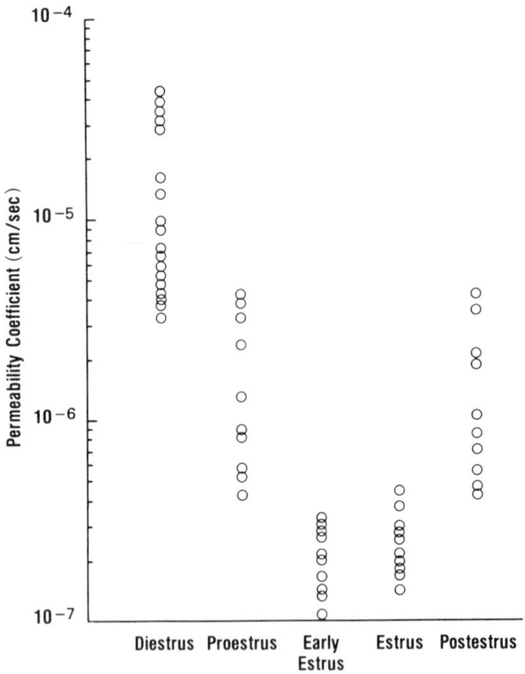

Figure 3 Enormous effect of the estrous cycle (ca. days) on the ara-A permeability coefficient for the whole membrane. [Reprinted from *Optimization of Drug Delivery, Alfred Benson Symposium 17* (Hans Bundgaard, Anne Bagger Hanson, and Helmer Kofod, eds.), Munksgaard, Copenhagen, 1982.]

changed only moderately (ca. <2 x) during the sex cycle. The D values may be calculated from the relation D = Ph, where P is the permeability coefficient and h is the thickness for the membrane component in question.

Model validation studies were conducted for all three ester prodrugs using Eqs. (4)-(6) for tracer levels and using Eqs. (1)-(3) when prodrug levels were near saturated solution concentrations. The following procedures were employed. Data were obtained in a two-chamber diffusion cell for simultaneous transport and bioconversion as described previously [34]. Equations (4)-(6) or (1)-(3) were solved numerically using experimental D values and thicknesses for each of the membrane components. Back-diffusion fluxes (drug and metabolite) and forward fluxes for prodrug, drug, and metabolite were best-fitted to the mathematics. In the tracer-level case [Eqs. (4)-(6)], the fitting involved deducing the best set of k_i and k_i' values. These were then compared to k_i and k_i' values obtained directly from homogenates of the epithelium layer and the lamina propria layer. The good agreement between the directly obtained experimental homogenate values and the model-deduced values is seen in Table 1.

Table 1 Comparisons of Specific Enzymatic Activities in Homogenates of the Epithelium and the Lamina Propria of the Mouse Vaginal Membrane and the Corresponding Model-Deduced Values

		Specific enzymatic activity × 10^2 (sec^{-1}/g tissue)			
		Deaminase	Esterase		
Mouse number	Fraction of the membrane	ara-A	A-ara-A	V-ara-A	O-ara-A
80437	Epithelium	4.5-5.6	--	2.7-3.4	--
	Lamina propria	1.0	--	0.5	--
80428	Epithelium	9.4-11.8	0.15-0.20	4.6-5.7	14-17
	Lamina propria	1.1	0.02	0.4	1.2
Model-deduced values	Epithelium	7.9-18.9	0.08	3.4-5.8	12.0
	Lamina propria	1.5	0.01	0.3-0.7	1.0

Source: Reprinted from *Optimization of Drug Delivery, Alfred Benzon Symposium 17* (Hans Bundgaard, Anne Bagger Hanson, and Helmer Kofod, eds.), Munksgaard, Copenhagen, 1982.

Model validation studies with high concentrations of the prodrugs entails first determining the K_m, K'_m, and k_I values for all three prodrugs with the homogenates. $V_{m,i}$ and $V'_{m,i}$ values were then calculated from $V_{m,i}/K_m = k_i$ and $V'_{m,i}/K'_m = k'_i$. These parameter values were then used in Eqs. (1)-(3) and fluxes were numerically calculated for the two-chamber diffusion cell experiments. Tables 2-4 show the reasonably good agreement obtained between experiments ("go-through" experiments in the two-chamber diffusion call with the epithelium side facing the donor chamber) and predictions for the ara-A-acetate, the ara-A-valerate, and the ara-A-octanoate cases. Further analysis of the data in Tables 2-4 showed that the esterase saturation effect (K_m), the daminase saturation (K'_m), and the deaminase inhibition by the prodrug (k_I) were all important when the prodrug concentration in the

Table 2 Fitting of Experimental Fluxes from Go-Through Experiment: Ara-A-Acetate in Mouse Vaginal Membrane (Diestrus)

	(Flux/initial donor conc.) × 10^6 (cm/sec)							
	Donor				Receiver			
	A-ara-A	ara-A + ara-H	ara-A	ara-H	A-ara-A	ara-A + ara-H	ara-A	ara-H
Expt. data	--	3.70	3.32	0.38	5.10	0.85	0.54	0.31
Calc. data[a]	--	3.76	3.33	0.43	5.00	0.88	0.59	0.29

[a]Parameters used in calculation:

$D_{epi} = 2.95 \times 10^{-8}$ cm^2/sec
$V_{m,epi}$ (esterase) $= 2.6 \times 10^{-5}$ mol/sec
$V'_{m,epi}$ (deaminase) $= 3.3 \times 10^{-5}$ mol/sec
$h_{epi} = 50 \times 10^{-4}$ cm
K_m (esterase) $= 3.3 \times 10^{-2}$ M
K'_m (deaminase) $= 3.3 \times 10^{-4}$ M
$D_{LP} = 1.5 \times 10^{-6}$ cm^2/sec
$h_{LP} = 150 \times 10^{-4}$ cm
$k_I = 2.2 \times 10^{-4}$ M
$V_{m,LP}$ (esterase) $= 3.3 \times 10^{-6}$ mol/sec
$V'_{m,LP}$ (deaminase) $= 3.3 \times 10^{-6}$ mol/sec

Source: Reprinted from *Optimization of Drug Delivery, Alfred Benzon Symposium 17* (Hans Bundgaard, Anne Bagger Hanson, and Helmer Kofod, eds.), Munksgaard, Copenhagen, 1982.

Table 3 Fitting of Experimental Fluxes from Go-Through Experiment: Ara-A-Valerate in Mouse Vaginal Membrane (Diestrus)

	(Flux/initial donor conc.) × 10^6 (cm/sec)							
	Donor				Receiver			
	V-ara-A	ara-A + ara-H	ara-A	ara-H	V-ara-A	ara-A + ara-H	ara-A	ara-H
Expt. data	--	2.98	2.67	0.31	0.14	0.62	0.15	0.47
Calc. data[a]	--	2.25	2.01	0.24	(1.2 × 10^{-9})	0.70	0.14	0.55

[a]Parameters used in calculation:

$D_{epi} = 3.75 \times 10^{-9}$ cm^2/sec
$V_{m,epi}$ (esterase) = 3.5×10^{-5} mol/sec
$V'_{m,epi}$ (deaminase) = 1.2×10^{-5} mol/sec
$h_{epi} = 50 \times 10^{-4}$ cm
K_m (esterase) = 1.0×10^{-3} M
K'_m (deaminase) = 3.3×10^{-4} M
$D_{LP} = 1.5 \times 10^{-6}$ cm^2/sec
$h_{LP} = 150 \times 10^{-4}$ cm
$k_I = 1.0 \times 10^{-5}$ M
$V_{m,LP}$ (esterase) = 3.0×10^{-6} mol/sec
$V'_{m,LP}$ (deaminase) = 1.2×10^{-6} mol/sec

Source: Reprinted from *Optimization of Drug Delivery, Alfred Benzon Symposium 17* (Hans Bundgaard, Anne Bagger Hanson, and Helmer Kofod, eds.), Munksgaard, Copenhagen, 1982.

donor chamber was near its solubility value; that is, fluxes differed up to around 10-fold when these results were compared to predictions based on $K_m = K'_m = k_I = \infty$.

The satisfactory agreement between the predictions based on the model using input data from homogenate experiments and the actual experimental results leads to the following important conclusion. The local access kinetics for both the esterase and the deaminase enzymes are quantitatively accounted for by the model with the diffusivities obtained in the permeability experiments. The effects of local barriers (e.g., the plasma membrane), if they are important, are believed to be already included in the diffusivity value. It follows from this argument that concentration profiles that are obtainable from Eqs. (1)-(3) or (4)-(6) with the appropriate transport and metabolism parameters

Table 4 Fitting of Experimental Fluxes from Go-Through Experiment: Ara-A-Octanoate in Mouse Vaginal Membrane (Diestrus)

	(Flux/initial donor conc.) $\times 10^6$ (cm/sec)							
	Donor				Receiver			
	O-ara-A	ara-A + ara-H	ara-A	ara-H	O-ara-A	ara-A + ara-H	ara-A	ara-H
Expt. data	--	39.9	33.5	6.43	0.10	7.74	1.24	6.50
Calc. data[a]	--	39.8	33.5	6.36	0.02	8.40	1.35	7.05

[a]Parameters used in calculations:

$D_{epi} = 4.0 \times 10^{-8}$ cm^2/sec
$V_{m,epi}$ (esterase) $= 2.3 \times 10^{-5}$ mol/sec
$V'_{m,epi}$ (deaminase) $= 3.3 \times 10^{-5}$ mol/sec
$h_{epi} = 50 \times 10^{-4}$ cm
K_m (esterase) $= 1.5 \times 10^{-4}$ M
K'_m (deaminase) $= 3.3 \times 10^{-4}$ M
$D_{LP} = 1.5 \times 10^{-6}$ cm^2/sec
$h_{LP} = 150 \times 10^{-4}$ cm
$k_I = 7.5 \times 10^{-7}$ M
$V_{m,LP}$ (esterase) $= 1.5 \times 10^{-6}$ mol/sec
$V'_{m,LP}$ (deaminase) $= 3.3 \times 10^{-6}$ mol/sec

Source: Reprinted from *Optimization of Drug Delivery, Alfred Benzon Symposium 17* (Hans Bundgaard, Anne Bagger Hanson, and Helmer Kofod, eds.), Munksgaard, Copenhagen, 1982.

should be physically meaningful; the calculated species concentrations are expected to be the actual aqueous steady-state concentrations and therefore may be directly considered in the drug efficacy predictions.

Figures 4 and 5 show plots from such concentration profiles based on calculations using Eqs. (1)-(3) and the best parameter values deduced from the model validation studies described above. These are for topically applied saturation solutions. Table 5 presents the calculations for all three prodrugs and for ara-A itself. These results may now be viewed in light of the pharmacotherapeutics involved in the treatment of vaginal herpes simplex virus (HSV) infections.

It is believed that the primary target sites are the parabasal cells and the intermediate epithelial cells [42] that are located at about the 50-75% level of depth in the epithelium. Furthermore, considering that

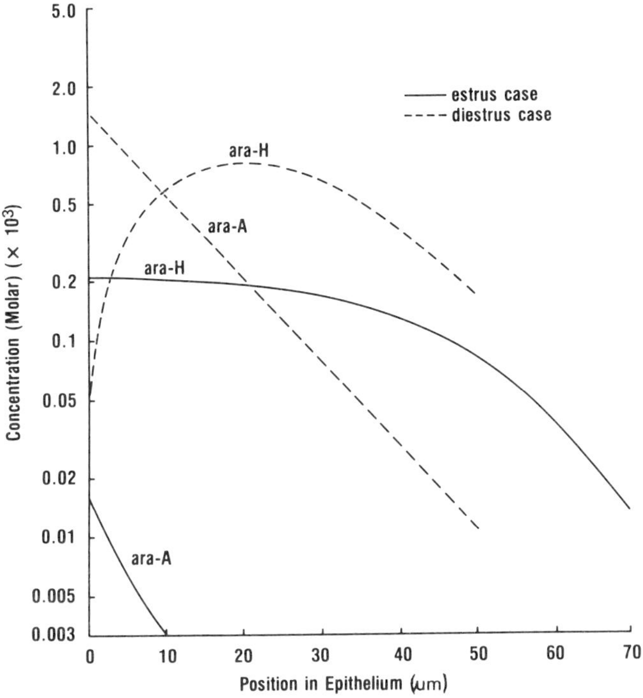

Figure 4 Semilog plot of epithelium concentration-distance profiles for topically applied saturated solutions of ara-A for the mouse vaginal membrane parameter values taken from model validation studies. [Reprinted from *Optimization of Drug Delivery, Alfred Benzon Symposium 17* (Hans Bundgaard, Anne Bagger Hanson, and Helmer Kofod, eds.), Munksgaard, Copenhagen, 1982.]

the minimum inhibitory concentration of ara-A for viral replication in vitro is of the order of 1×10^{-5} M [4], chemotherapeutic predictions may be made from the plots given in Figs. 4 and 5 and the results in Table 5. When ara-A itself or ara-A-octanoate is topically applied at maximum strength (i.e., as the saturated solution), the treatment in the mouse would be expected to be ineffective during the estrus and the late diestrus phases; during early diestrus, ara-A-octanoate or ara-A itself may be marginally effective. When ara-A-valerate is topically applied, it would be expected to be effective during early diestrus, marginally effective during late diestrus, and ineffective during estrus. Interestingly, ara-A-acetate is predicted to perform more evenly (during the estrous cycle) than ara-A-valerate. During diestrus, the former is predicted to sustain lower ara-A levels than the

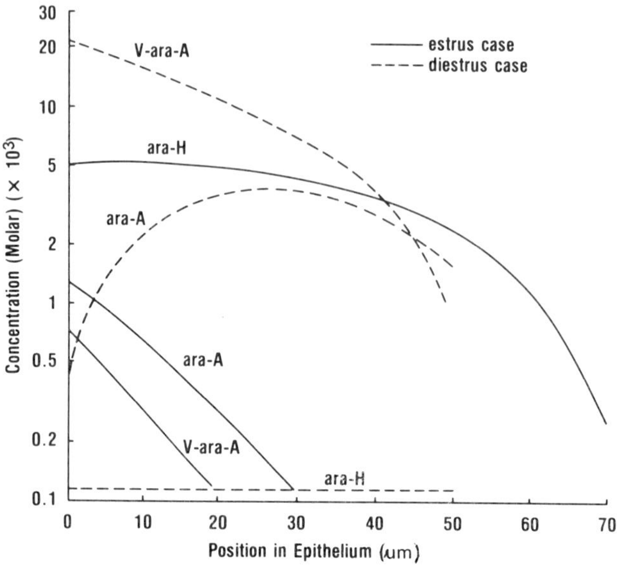

Figure 5 Semilog plot of epithelium concentration-distance profiles for topically applied saturated solutions of ara-A valerate for the mouse vaginal membrane. Parameter values taken from model validation studies. [Reprinted from *Optimization of Drug Delivery, Alfred Benzon Symposium 17* (Hans Bundgaard, Anne Bagger Hanson, and Helmer Kofod, eds.), Munksgaard, Copenhagen, 1982.]

latter, but these are still far above the MIC levels. During late diestrus and during estrus, ara-A-acetate is expected to perform better than ara-A-valerate. The primary reason for the difference in behavior between ara-A-valerate and ara-A-acetate is that the latter has a much smaller esterase deacylation rate; as a result there is a "sustained release" effect as ara-A-acetate diffuses across the epithelium. The valerate ester, on the other hand, is deacylated much more rapidly. Consequently, during the estrus phase and to some extent during the late diestrus phase, most of the valerate is rapidly converted to ara-A, which is also rapidly converted to ara-H via the deaminase before much of the valerate and ara-A reaches the deeper recesses of the epithelium.

Limited experiments (unpublished) by Dr. Earl Kern (University of Utah) on the topical therapy of vaginal HSV infections in mice are consistent with the predictions given above for ara-A-valerate and for ara-A itself. Both of these compounds were marginally effective in mice and more strongly effective in the vaginal HSV infections of the guinea pig. Our preliminary work with guinea pig vaginal membranes

Table 5 Concentration of Ara-A from Different Prodrugs at Different Depths in the Epithelium of the Mouse Vaginal Membrane[a]

Phase of estrous cycle	Prodrug used	Ara-A concentration (M)				
		Position in the epithelium[b]				
		0%	25%	50%	75%	100%
Early	A-ara-A	2.26×10^{-5}	5.12×10^{-4}	6.30×10^{-4}	4.74×10^{-4}	1.56×10^{-4}
diestrus,	V-ara-A	1.13×10^{-4}	2.80×10^{-3}	3.82×10^{-3}	3.24×10^{-3}	1.26×10^{-3}
$P = 8 \times 10^{-6}$	O-ara-A	1.83×10^{-5}	2.87×10^{-4}	2.00×10^{-4}	7.16×10^{-5}	9.14×10^{-6}
and	ara-A	1.46×10^{-3}	4.87×10^{-4}	1.14×10^{-4}	2.11×10^{-5}	2.22×10^{-6}
$h = 50\ \mu m$						
Late	A-ara-A	1.82×10^{-5}	2.43×10^{-3}	2.12×10^{-3}	9.29×10^{-4}	2.23×10^{-5}
diestrus,	V-ara-A	7.39×10^{-4}	9.27×10^{-3}	4.39×10^{-3}	2.40×10^{-4}	$\times 10^{-7}$
$P = 1.0 \times$	O-ara-A	7.83×10^{-6}	4.69×10^{-4}	1.50×10^{-7}	0	0
10^{-6} and	ara-A	1.48×10^{-5}	1.21×10^{-5}	3.30×10^{-8}	9.05×10^{-11}	0
$h = 70\ \mu m$						
Estrus,	A-ara-A	2.80×10^{-4}	2.05×10^{-4}	9.43×10^{-5}	2.76×10^{-5}	1.00×10^{-6}
$P = 2.5 \times$	V-ara-A	1.29×10^{-3}	3.85×10^{-4}	1.23×10^{-5}	3.74×10^{-8}	0
10^{-7} and	O-ara-A	1.81×10^{-5}	7.39×10^{-7}	8.49×10^{-9}	9.52×10^{-11}	6.42×10^{-11}
$h = 70\ \mu m$	ara-A	1.46×10^{-5}	1.62×10^{-7}	1.77×10^{-9}	2.13×10^{-11}	4.97×10^{-11}

[a]Prodrugs and ara-A are topically applied as saturated solutions.
[b]Expressed as distance to the surface of the epithelium/total epithelial thickness × 100%.
Source: Reprinted from *Optimization of Drug Delivery, Alfred Benzon Symposium 17* (Hans Bundgaard, Anne Bagger Hanson, and Helmer Kofod, eds.), Munksgaard, Copenhagen, 1982.

suggest that compared to the mouse, the estrous cycle-averaged permeability coefficient is significantly greater for the guinea pig and the esterase activities are lower in the guinea pig. Both of these factors would tend to make the valerate prodrug more effective in the guinea pig. More complete studies are under way in our laboratories with the guinea pig vaginal membranes so that an analysis for the guinea pig similar to that presented above for the mouse can be given.

HAIRLESS MOUSE SKIN

Validation Studies

An investigation similar to that for the mouse vaginal membrane and involving all three ester prodrugs of ara-A was recently completed for the hairless mouse skin [34,43]. Figure 6 schematically illustrates the hairless mouse skin model, which is comprised of stratum corneum ($h \cong 40\text{-}50\ \mu m$), epidermis ($h \cong 10\text{-}20\ \mu m$), and dermis ($h \cong 250\ \mu m$). Diffusion cell experiments [34,43] using full-thickness hairless mouse skin, stripped skin (Scotch tape removal of stratum corneum), and dermis skin yielded permeability coefficients. Table 6 shows the permeability coefficients of ara-A and its three monoesters for full-thickness skin. Moderate increases in permeability coefficients are seen with increases in lipophilicity of the prodrug. Stripped skin permeabilities are listed in Table 7. Permeability coefficients are about 100 times larger when the stratum corneum is removed. The moderate influence of lipophilicity on the permeability coefficient is still present when the stratum corneum is removed. The diffusivity (D) values may be calculated from the relation $D = Ph$, where P is the permeability coefficient and h is the thickness for the membrane component in question.

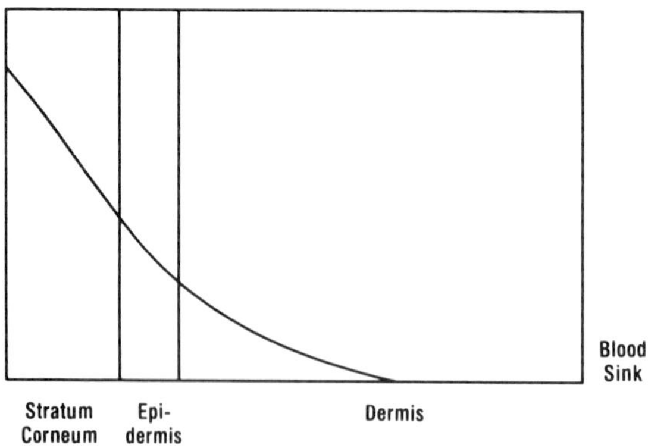

Figure 6 Multilayer model for simultaneous diffusion and metabolism of drug in the skin.

Table 6 Permeability Coefficients of Ara-A, A-ara-A, V-ara-A, and O-ara-A Through Whole Skin

Mouse number	Permeability coefficient × 10^8 (cm/sec)				Ester/ara-A
	ara-A	A-ara-A	V-ara-A	O-ara-A	
0621797	0.74	0.90	--	--	1.21
0621798	0.93	1.18	--	--	1.26
0714802	0.81	0.97	--	--	1.20
0714803	0.65	0.84	--	--	1.30
0621797	0.74	--	1.39	--	1.87
0621798	0.93	--	1.92	--	2.06
0714802	0.81	--	1.47	--	1.81
0714803	0.65	--	1.34	--	2.07
0621797	0.74	--	--	3.22	4.33
0621798	0.93	--	--	3.37	3.61
0714802	0.81	--	--	3.42	4.22
0714803	0.65	--	--	3.01	4.65

Table 7 Permeability Coefficients of Ara-A, A-ara-A, V-ara-A, and O-ara-A in Stripped Skin

Mouse number	Permeability coefficient × 10^6 (cm/sec)				Ester/ara-A
	ara-A	A-ara-A	V-ara-A	O-ara-A	
0405802	1.25	1.90	--	--	1.52
0417802	1.19	0.82	--	--	1.53
0405802	1.25		3.78	--	3.02
0417802	1.19	--	3.67	--	3.08
0405802	1.25	--	--	8.11	6.49
0417802	1.19	--	--	7.98	6.71

Model validation studies were conducted for tracer levels of all three ester prodrugs. Equations (4)-(6) were solved numerically using experimental D values and thicknesses for each of the membrane components. Data were obtained in a two-chamber diffusion cell for the simultaneous transport and bioconversion as described previously [34, 43]. Tables 8 and 9 give the back-diffusion fluxes and forward fluxes of prodrug and drug for ara-A-acetate, ara-A-valerate, and ara-A-octanoate. Tables 10-12 show the best fit of the calculated data to the experimental fluxes for ara-A-acetate, ara-A-valerate, and ara-A-

Table 8 Observed Fluxes in Go-Through Experiment with A-ara-A → V-ara-A → O-ara-A Using Stripped Skin from a 12-Week-Old Mouse[a]

			(Flux/initial donor conc.) × 10^6 (cm/sec)			
			Donor		Receiver	
Order of run[b]	Direction[c]	Prodrug	Prodrug	ara-A	Prodrug	ara-A
1	Epidermis → dermis	A-ara-A	—	1.12	1.37	0.77
2	Epidermis → dermis	V-ara-A	—	3.64	1.24	2.26
3	Epidermis → dermis	O-ara-A	—	16.70	1.55	6.86

[a]Number 0417804A; skin was soaked and rinsed for 2 hr before the first run.
[b]Indicates the first, second, or third run with the given skin preparation.
[c]Indicates the permeation direction: the donor side to the receiver side.

Table 9 Observed Fluxes in Go-Through Experiment with A-ara-A → V-ara-A → O-ara-A Using Stripped Skin from a 12-Week-Old Mouse[a]

			(Flux/initial donor conc.) × 10^6 (cm/sec)			
			Donor		Receiver	
Order of run[b]	Direction[c]	Prodrug	Prodrug	ara-A	Prodrug	ara-A
1	Dermis → epidermis	A-ara-A	—	7.05	1.17	0.69
2	Dermis → epidermis	V-ara-A	—	22.30	1.16	2.15
3	Dermis → epidermis	O-ara-A	—	59.00	1.14	5.03

[a]Number 0417804B; skin was soaked and rinsed for 2 hr before the first run.
[b]Indicates the first, second, or third run with the given skin preparation.
[c]Indicates the permeation direction: the donor side to the receiver side.

Table 10 Least-Squares Fitting of the Calculated Fluxes to the Experimental Data for the Determination of the Esterase Rate Constants

	(Flux/initial donor conc.) × 10^6 (cm/sec)							
	Epidermis → dermis[a] (first run)				Dermis → epidermis[a] (second run)			
	Donor		Receiver		Donor		Receiver	
	A-ara-A	ara-A	A-ara-A	ara-A	A-ara-A	ara-A	A-ara-A	ara-A
Expt. data	—	1.12	1.37	0.77	—	7.05	1.17	0.69
Best fit[b]	—	0.98	1.39	0.67	—	6.95	1.27	0.68

[a]Indicates the permeation direction: the donor side to the receiver side.
[b]Iteration parameters:

$k_{epi} = 2.52 \times 10^{-3}\ sec^{-1}$
$D_{PDepi} = 3.22 \times 10^{-9}\ cm^2/sec$
$h_{epi} = 1.0 \times 10^{-3}\ cm$
$D_{dermis} = 5.3 \times 10^{-7}\ cm^2/sec$
$k_{dermis} = 2.96 \times 10^{-4}\ sec^{-1}$
$D_{Depi} = 2.61 \times 10^{-9}\ cm^2/sec$
$h_{dermis} = 2.5 \times 10^{-2}\ cm$

Source: Based on data in Tables 8 and 9.

Table 11 Least-Squares Fitting of the Calculated Fluxes to the Experimental Data for the Determination of the Esterase Rate Constants

	(Flux/initial donor conc.) × 10^6 (cm/sec)							
	Epidermis → dermis[a] (first run)				Dermis → epidermis[a] (second run)			
	Donor		Receiver		Donor		Receiver	
	V-ara-A	ara-A	V-ara-A	ara-A	V-ara-A	ara-A	V-ara-A	ara-A
Expt. data	—	3.64	1.24	2.26	—	22.3	1.16	2.15
Best fit[b]	—	3.96	1.18	2.63	—	23.7	1.18	2.21

[a]Indicates the permeation direction: the donor side to the receiver side.
[b]Iteration parameters:
$k_{epi} = 1.21 \times 10^{-2}\ sec^{-1}$
$D_{PDepi} = 4.90 \times 10^{-9}\ cm^2/sec$
$h_{epi} = 1.0 \times 10^{-3}\ cm$
$D_{dermis} = 5.3 \times 10^{-7}\ cm^2/sec$
$k_{dermis} = 1.63 \times 10^{-3}\ sec^{-1}$
$D_{Depi} = 3.10 \times 10^{-9}\ cm^2/sec$
$h_{dermis} = 2.5 \times 10^{-2}\ cm$
Source: Based on the data in Tables 8 and 9.

Table 12 Least-Squares Fitting of the Calculated Fluxes to the Experimental Data for the Determination of the Esterase Rate Constants

	(Flux/initial donor conc.) × 10^6 (cm/sec)							
	Epidermis → dermis[a] (first run)				Dermis → epidermis[a] (second run)			
	Donor		Receiver		Donor		Receiver	
	O-ara-A	ara-A	O-ara-A	ara-A	O-ara-A	ara-A	O-ara-A	ara-A
Expt. data	—	16.7	1.55	6.86	—	59.0	1.14	5.03
Best fit[b]	—	14.8	1.43	8.02	—	49.8	1.16	5.18

[a]Indicates the permeation direction: the donor side to the receiver side.

[b]Iteration parameters:

$k_{epi} = 5.03 \times 10^{-2}$ sec $^{-1}$
$D_{PDepi} = 1.61 \times 10^{-8}$ cm^2/sec
$h_{epi} = 1.0 \times 10^{-3}$ cm
$D_{dermis} = 5.3 \times 10^{-7}$ cm^2/sec
$k_{dermis} = 4.87 \times 10^{-3}$ sec^{-1}
$D_{Depi} = 3.79 \times 10^{-9}$ cm^2/sec
$h_{dermis} = 2.5 \times 10^{-2}$ cm

Source: Based on data in Tables 8 and 9.

octanoate, respectively. The fitting involved deducing the best set of k_i and k_i' values.

Direct experimental values for k_i and k_i' in the epidermis and dermis were obtained by the use of trypsin to separate the dermis from the epidermis. Tissue homogenization of the separated components yielded k_i and k_i' in the epidermis and dermis for ara-A and its three monoesters (Table 13). Examining Table 14, it can be seen that for all three monoesters the rate constants in the epidermis are 8-10 times higher than in the dermis. This is in agreement with the results previously obtained by Yu et al. [34] for ara-A-valerate.

The good agreement between the directly obtained experimental homogenate values and the model-deduced values in the epidermis is seen in Table 14. Table 15 shows the good agreement between experimental and model-deduced enzyme constants in the dermis.

After completing the model validation studies for tracer levels [Eqs. (4)-(6)], the validity of the model when prodrug levels were near saturation solution concentrations [Eqs. (1)-(3)] was established. The results of saturated go-through experiments are presented in Tables 16-18 for ara-A-acetate, ara-A-valerate, and ara-A-octanoate, respectively. In these experiments the first and third runs were always tracer levels, with the second run having saturated or near-saturated drug concentrations. The foregoing sequence of runs allowed for direct comparison of the effect, if any, of using saturated drug concentrations.

Table 13 Comparison of Esterase and Adenosine Deaminase Activities in the Epidermis and Dermis of the Hairless Mouse Skin

		Specific enzymatic activity × 10^3 (sec^{-1}/g tissue)			
		Deaminase	Esterase		
Mouse number	Fraction of membrane	ara-A	A-ara-A	V-ara-A	O-ara-A
1027806	Epidermis	9.62	2.33	13.30	43.10
	Dermis	1.54	0.25	1.41	5.20
1201802	Epidermis	7.75	2.60	11.20	47.00
	Dermis	1.20	0.32	1.51	5.90
1201804	Epidermis	7.62	2.71	15.50	56.60
	Dermis	1.41	0.31	1.71	4.15

Table 14 Comparison of Epidermis Esterase Rate Constant Obtained from Model Fitting to Those Obtained from Trypsin Treatment

Prodrug	Trypsin × 10^3 ($K_{sec}{}^{-1}$/g tissue)	Model × 10^3 ($K_{sec}{}^{-1}$/g tissue)	$\frac{K_{trypsin}}{K_{e\ acetate}}$	$\frac{K_{model}}{K_{e\ acetate}}$
A-ara-A	2.3-2.7	2.5-3.5	1	1
V-ara-A	11.2-15.5	10.6-13.5	4.3-5.7	3.8-4.3
O-ara-A	43.1-56.6	46.3-56.8	17.1-20.8	16.1-18.6
Ara-A	7.6-9.6	6.5-9.3	—	—

Table 15 Comparison of Dermis Esterase Rate Constant Obtained from Model Fitting to Those Obtained from Trypsin Treatment

Prodrug	Trypsin × 10^4 ($K_{sec}{}^{-1}$/g tissue)	Model × 10^4 ($K_{sec}{}^{-1}$/g tissue)	$\frac{K_{trypsin}}{K_{d\ acetate}}$	$\frac{K_{model}}{K_{d\ acetate}}$
A-ara-A	2.5-3.1	2.8-3.1	1	1
V-ara-A	14.1-17.7	11.3-15.2	4.5-7.0	4.8-5.4
O-ara-A	41.5-59.0	41.9-45.7	13.2-23.4	13.3-16.4
Ara-A	1.2-1.5	1.4-1.6	—	—

Table 16 Go-Through Experiment with Saturated A-ara-A Solution (Number 0418811)

	(Flux/initial donor conc.) × 10^6 (cm/sec)					
	Donor			Receiver		
Order of runs[a]	A-ara-A	ara-A	ara-H	A-ara-A	ara-A	ara-H
First[b]	—	0.82	0.24	1.72	0.19	0.57
Second[c]	—	0.59	0.08	1.55	0.37	0.23
Third[b]	—	0.82	0.25	1.77	0.19	0.58

[a]All runs were conducted with epidermis facing the donor chamber.
[b]Only trace amounts of [^{3}H]A-ara-A were used in these two runs.
[c]Saturated A-ara-A solution (2.69 × 10^2 M) spiked with trace amount of [^{3}H]A-ara-A was used in this run.

Table 17 Go-Through Experiment with Saturated V-ara-A Solution (Number 0418812)

Order of runs[a]	(Flux/initial donor conc.) × 10^6 (cm/sec)					
	Donor			Receiver		
	V-ara-A	ara-A	ara-H	V-ara-A	ara-A	ara-H
First[b]	—	2.28	0.87	1.13	0.54	1.62
Second[c]	—	0.84	0.21	1.19	0.59	0.83
Third[b]	—	2.31	0.87	1.12	0.55	1.66

[a]All runs were conducted with epidermis facing the donor chamber.
[b]Only trace amounts of [^{3}H]V-ara-A were used in these two runs.
[c]Saturated V-ara-A solution (2.39×10^{-2} M) spiked with trace amount of [^{3}H]V-ara-A was used in this run.

Table 18 Go-Through Experiment with Saturated O-ara-A Solution (Number 0418813)

Order of runs[a]	(Flux/initial donor conc.) × 10^6 (cm/sec)					
	Donor			Receiver		
	O-ara-A	ara-A	ara-H	O-ara-A	ara-A	ara-H
First[b]	—	6.68	10.20	1.08	1.15	4.65
Second[c]	—	10.20	5.88	1.18	1.77	3.37
Third[b]		6.70	10.20	1.13	1.17	4.71

[a]All runs were conducted with epidermis facing the donor chamber.
[b]Only trace amounts of ^{3}H-O-ara-A were used in these two runs.
[c]Saturated A-ara-A solution (2.69×10^{-2} M) spiked with trace amounts of ^{3}H-A-ara-A was used in this run.

Model validation studies with high concentrations of the prodrugs entailed determining the K_m, k'_m, and k_I values for all three prodrugs with the homogenates. $V_{m,i}$ and $V'_{m,i}$ values were then calculated from $V_{m,i}/K_m = k_i$ and $V'_{m,i}/K'_m = k'_i$. These parameter values were then used in Eqs. (1)-(3) and fluxes were numerically calculated for the two-chamber diffusion cell experiments. It should be noted that all variables except diffusivities were determined independently, the diffusivities being obtained directly from permeability experiments. Tables 19-21 show the reasonably good agreement obtained between the calculated and experimentally determined fluxes for ara-A-acetate, ara-A-valerate, and ara-A-octanoate.

Table 19 Fitting of Experimental Fluxes from Go-Through Experiment Using the Modified Physical Model (Number 0418811)

	(Flux/initial donor conc.) × 10^6 (cm/sec)							
	Donor				Receiver			
	A-ara-A	ara-A + ara-H	ara-A	ara-H	A-ara-A	ara-A + ara-H	ara-A	ara-H
Expt. data	—	0.67	0.59	0.08	1.55	0.60	0.37	0.23
Calc. data[a]	—	0.71	0.62	0.09	1.54	0.63	0.39	0.24

[a]Parameters used in the calculations:

$D_{epi} = 1.1 \times 10^{-9}$ cm^2/sec
$V_{m,epi}$ (esterase) $= 3.5 \times 10^{-5}$ mol/sec
$V_{m,dermis}$ (esterase) $= 5.0 \times 10^{-6}$ mol/sec
$h_{epi} = 1.0 \times 10^{-3}$ cm
K_m (esterase) $= 3.3 \times 10^{-2}$ M
$k_I = 2.3 \times 10^{-4}$ M
$D_{dermis} = 5.0 \times 10^{-7}$ cm^2/sec
$V'_{m,epi}$ (deaminase) $= 1.0 \times 10^{-5}$ mol/sec
$V'_{m,dermis}$ (deaminase) $= 1.5 \times 10^{-6}$ mol/sec
$h_{dermis} = 2.5 \times 10^{-2}$ cm
K'_m (deaminase) $= 3.3 \times 10^{-4}$ M

Table 20 Fitting of Experimental Fluxes from Go-Through Experiment Using the Modified Physical Model (Number 0418812)

	(Flux/initial donor conc.) $\times 10^6$ (cm/sec)							
	Donor				Receiver			
	V-ara-A	ara-A + ara-H	ara-A	ara-H	V-ara-A	ara-A + ara-H	ara-A	ara-H
Expt. data	—	1.05	0.34	0.21	1.19	1.42	0.59	0.83
Calc. data[a]	—	1.02	0.83	0.19	1.16	1.37	0.57	0.79

[a]Parameters used in the calculations:

$D_{epi} = 2.2 \times 10^{-9}$ cm^2/sec
$V_{m,epi}$ (esterase) $= 2.9 \times 10^{-5}$ mol/sec
$V_{m,dermis}$ (esterase) $= 2.6 \times 10^{-6}$ mol/sec
$h_{epi} = 1.0 \times 10^{-3}$ cm
K_m (esterase) $= 1.08 \times 10^{-3}$ M
$k_I = 1.2 \times 10^{-5}$ M
$D_{dermis} = 5.0 \times 10^{-7}$ cm^2/sec
$V'_{m,epi}$ (deaminase) $= 1.0 \times 10^{-5}$ mol/sec
$V'_{m,dermis}$ (deaminase) $= 1.5 \times 10^{-3}$ mol/sec
$h_{dermis} = 2.5 \times 10^{-2}$ cm
K'_m (deaminase) $= 3.3 \times 10^{-4}$ M

Table 21 Fitting of Experimental Fluxes from Go-Through Experiment Using the Modified Physical Model (Number 0418813)

	(Flux/initial donor conc.) × 10^6 (cm/sec)							
	Donor				Receiver			
	O-ara-A	ara-A + ara-H	ara-A	ara-H	O-ara-A	ara-A + ara-H	ara-A	ara-H
Expt. data	—	16.0	10.2	5.88	1.18	5.14	1.77	3.37
Calc. data[a]	—	16.1	10.1	6.03	1.15	5.05	1.72	3.33

[a]Parameters used in the calculations:

$D_{epi} = 5.8 \times 10^{-9}$ cm^2/sec
$V_{m,epi}$ (esterase) = 1.3×10^{-5} mol/sec
$V_{m,dermis}$ (esterase) = 1.0×10^{-6} mol/sec
$h_{epi} = 1.0 \times 10^{-3}$ cm
K_m (esterase) = 1.51×10^{-4} M
$k_I = 8.8 \times 10^{-7}$ M
$D_{dermis} = 5.0 \times 10^{-7}$ cm^2/sec
$V'_{m,epi}$ (deaminase) = 1.0×10^{-5} mol/sec
$V'_{m,dermis}$ (deaminase) = 1.5×10^{-6} mol/sec
$h_{dermis} = 2.5 \times 10^{-2}$ cm
K'_m (deaminase) = 3.3×10^{-4} M

It can be concluded that both esterase and deaminase enzymes are quantitatively accounted for by the model with the diffusivities obtained in the permeability experiments.

Concentration-Distance Profiles

Having validated the model and having obtained the appropriate transport and metabolism parameters for ara-A, ara-A-acetate, ara-A-valerate, and ara-A-octanoate, concentration-distance profiles can now be obtained from Eqs. (1)-(3) or (4)-(6). These calculated species concentrations are expected to be the actual aqueous steady-state concentrations and therefore may be directly considered in the drug efficacy predictions.

The plots in Figs. 7 and 8 represent the epidermal concentration-distance profiles for ara-A-valerate in whole skin and stripped skin,

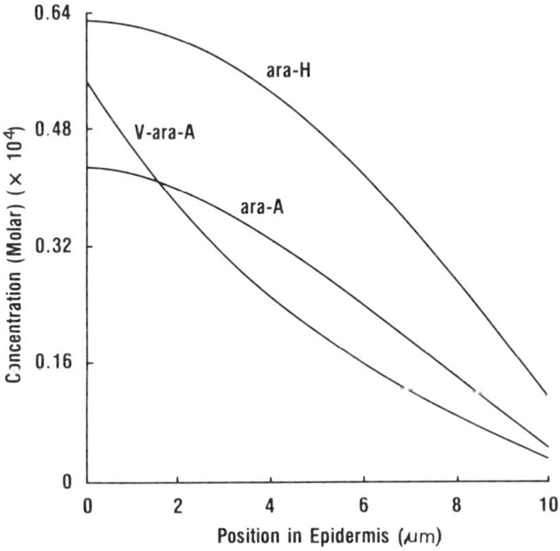

Figure 7 Concentration-distance profile for ara-A-valerate in the epidermis of whole skin based on the modified model. The following parameters were used to generate the plot (values are listed in order of stratum corneum, epidermis, and dermis for each parameter):

Diffusivity of ara-A-valerate: 6.8×10^{-11}, 3.9×10^{-9}, and 5.0×10^{-7} cm^2/sec

Diffusivity of ara-A and ara-H: 6.8×10^{-11}, 2.2×10^{-9}, and 5.0×10^{-7} cm^2/sec

Thickness: 40, 10, and 250 μm

k_e: 0, 1.18×10^{-2} and 1.12×10^{-3} sec^{-1}

k_d: 0, 7.4×10^{-3} and 1.5×10^{-3} sec^{-1}

$K_{m,e}$: 1.1×10^{-3} M; $K_{m,d}$: 3.3×10^{-4} M; k_I: 1.2×10^{-5} M

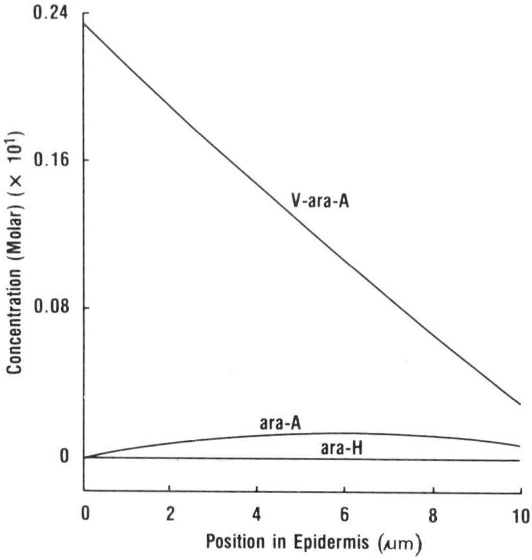

Figure 8 Concentration-distance profile for ara-A-valerate in the epidermis of stripped skin based on the modified model. The following parameters were used to generate the plot (values are listed in order of epidermis and dermis for each parameter):

Diffusivity of ara-A-valerate: 3.9×10^{-9} and 5.0×10^{-7} cm^2/sec
Diffusivity of ara-A and ara-H: 2.2×10^{-9} and 5.0×10^{-7} cm^2/sec
Thickness: 10 and 250 μm
k_e: 1.2×10^{-2} and 1.1×10^{-3} sec^{-1}
k_d: 7.4×10^{-3} and 1.5×10^{-3} sec^{-1}
$K_{m,e}$: 1.1×10^{-3} M; $K_{m,d}$: 3.3×10^{-4} M; k_I: 1.2×10^{-5} M

respectively, when saturated solutions are topically applied. Similar plots for ara-A-acetate and ara-A-octanoate have also been obtained [43]. The fifth and eighth rows in Table 22 give the steady-state drug and metabolite concentrations for ara-A and its three monoesters in whole skin and stripped skin when saturated solutions are topically applied. It can be seen (upper-half of Table 22) that for whole skin the incorporation of Michaelis-Menten kinetics and/or the prodrug-inhibition consideration have only small effects. With saturated prodrug or drug concentrations, the low permeabilities of ara-A and its three monoesters through the stratum corneum preclude the buildup of high-enough prodrug and drug concentrations for saturation of esterase or deaminase to be important in the epidermis. It can be concluded that for whole skin the enzymatic reactions can be well approximated with first-order kinetics even when saturated drug solutions are

Table 22 Calculated Steady-State Drug and Metabolite Concentrations in Whole Skin and Stripped Skin

Compound	Interface	Steady-state concentrations: Drug, First-order kinetics	Drug, Enzyme saturation only	Drug, Enzyme saturation and prodrug inhibition	Metabolite, First-order kinetics	Metabolite, Enzyme saturation only	Metabolite, Enzyme saturation and prodrug inhibition
Whole skin							
Ara-A	Sc/epi[a]	2.0×10^{-6}	2.0×10^{-6}	—	2.7×10^{-6}	2.7×10^{-6}	—
	Epi/dermis[b]	6.5×10^{-8}	6.5×10^{-8}	—	4.0×10^{-7}	4.0×10^{-7}	—
Ara-A-acetate	Sc/epi	1.4×10^{-5}	1.4×10^{-5}	1.6×10^{-5}	2.3×10^{-5}	2.3×10^{-5}	2.1×10^{-5}
	Epi/dermis	1.7×10^{-6}	1.7×10^{-6}	1.9×10^{-6}	4.4×10^{-6}	4.4×10^{-6}	4.2×10^{-6}
Ara-A-valerate	Sc/epi	3.9×10^{-5}	4.2×10^{-5}	3.9×10^{-5}	6.4×10^{-5}	6.1×10^{-5}	6.3×10^{-5}
	Epi/dermis	4.2×10^{-6}	4.4×10^{-6}	4.4×10^{-6}	1.2×10^{-5}	1.2×10^{-5}	1.2×10^{-5}
Ara-A-octanoate	Sc/epi	1.9×10^{-6}	$1.9 \quad 10^{-6}$	2.0×10^{-6}	3.1×10^{-6}	3.0×10^{-6}	3.1×10^{-6}
	Epi/dermis	2.9×10^{-7}	$2.9 \quad 10^{-7}$	1.9×10^{-7}	5.6×10^{-7}	5.5×10^{-7}	5.7×10^{-7}
Stripped skin							
Ara-A	Sc/epi	1.3×10^{-3}	1.3×10^{-3}	—	3.3×10^{-9}	1.2×10^{-9}	—
	Epi/dermis	4.0×10^{-5}	6.1×10^{-5}	—	6.1×10^{-5}	6.3×10^{-5}	—
Ara-A-acetate	Sc/epi	1.9×10^{-8}	1.5×10^{-8}	1.6×10^{-8}	5.1×10^{-9}	1.3×10^{-9}	1.6×10^{-10}
	Epi/dermis	3.8×10^{-4}	4.7×10^{-4}	6.0×10^{-4}	4.0×10^{-4}	1.8×10^{-4}	4.5×10^{-5}
Ara-A-valerate	Sc/epi	7.0×10^{-8}	8.7×10^{-9}	9.9×10^{-9}	1.7×10^{-8}	1.2×10^{-9}	1.1×10^{-11}
	Epi/dermis	1.2×10^{-3}	6.4×10^{-4}	8.3×10^{-4}	1.3×10^{-3}	2.0×10^{-4}	3.7×10^{-6}
Ara-A-octanoate	Sc/epi	6.4×10^{-9}	2.3×10^{-9}	2.8×10^{-9}	1.5×10^{-8}	5.4×10^{-10}	8.4×10^{-12}
	Epi/dermis	9.7×10^{-5}	9.3×10^{-5}	1.6×10^{-4}	1.1×10^{-4}	6.5×10^{-5}	2.6×10^{-6}

[a]Stratum corneum-epidermis boundary.
[b]Epidermis-dermis boundary.

applied on the surface of the membrane. The bottom half of Table 22 similarly examines the cases for stripped skin. It can be seen that the effects of enzyme saturation and prodrug inhibition of deaminase are roughly of the same order of magnitude (ca. ± a factor of 2) for all three prodrugs. By examining Table 22, the reader may evaluate more critically the relative importances of esterase saturation, deaminase saturation, and the prodrug inhibition of deaminase for each of the prodrugs.

Figures 9 and 10 present plots of the steady-state ara-A concentrations based on these calculations for the saturated solution cases. From these results and those in Table 22, one may predict that these prodrugs are either marginal (ara-A-valerate) or less than marginal (ara-A-acetate and ara-A-octanoate) in the case of whole skin, and that, in traumatized skin, all three prodrugs may be effective, with -acetate ≅ -valerate > -octanoate. It is seen that ara-A-acetate gains on ara-A-valerate when one goes from whole skin to stripped skin. This is primarily because of the much smaller K_m for the valerate ester.

The most significant outcome of these concentration profile calculations may be that, at best, these topically applied prodrugs of ara-A

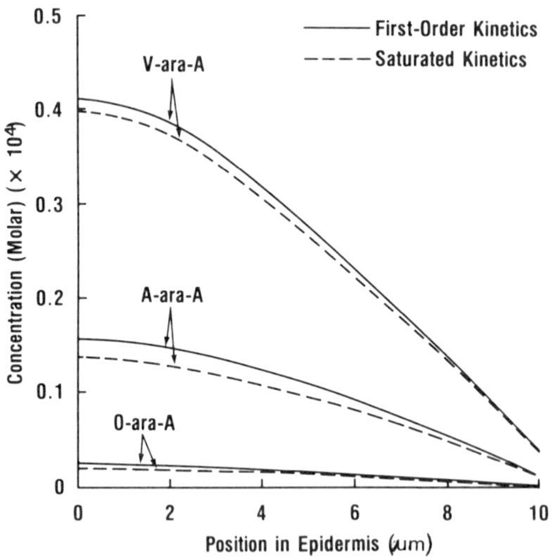

Figure 9 Concentration-distance profiles of ara-A from topically applied saturated solutions of ara-A-acetate, ara-A-valerate, and ara-A-octanoate in hairless mouse full thickness skin. Parameter values taken from model validation studies.

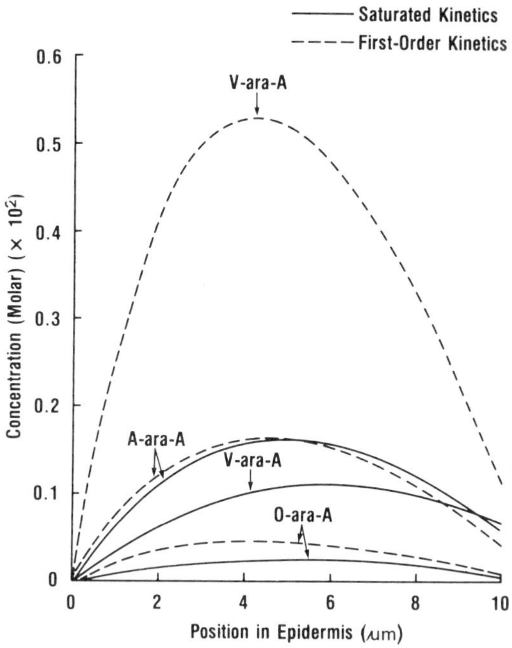

Figure 10 Concentration-distance profiles of ara-A from topically applied saturated solutions of ara-A-acetate, ara-A-valerate, and ara-A-octanoate in hairless mouse stripped skin. Parameter values taken from model validation studies.

would be only marginally effective in intact hairless mouse skin. This arises mainly because of the extremely great barrier nature of the stratum corneum ($P \cong 3 \times 10^{-8}$ cm/sec) and the consequent extremely large concentration gradient that is established across this membrane component during transport.

Ara-A-valerate is predicted to be the best among all three prodrugs when the prodrugs are topically applied to whole skin as their saturated solutions. This contrasts with the predicted behavior of these compounds in the mouse vaginal membrane during the estrus phase (see Table 5), where ara-A-acetate was predicted to be better than ara-A-valerate in delivering ara-A into the deeper regions of the epithelium. The main reasons for the predicted difference between the hairless mouse skin and the mouse vaginal membrane during estrus is the lower permeability coefficient for the stratum corneum ($P \cong 3 \times 10^{-8}$ cm/sec) of the skin and the somewhat lower esterase activity for the skin.

ACKNOWLEDGMENT

This research has been supported by NIH Grants AI-14987 and AI-17456.

REFERENCES

1. M. Privat de Garilhe and J. De Rudder, *C.R. Acad. Sci. D (Paris)*, *259*:2725 (1964).
2. F. A. Miller, G. J. Dixon, J. Ehrlich, B. J. Sloan, and I. W. McLean, Jr., *Antimicrob. Agents Chemother.--1968*, p. 136 (1969).
3. F. M. Schabel, Jr., *Chemotherapy*, *13*:321 (1968).
4. W. M. Shannon, in *Adenine Arabinoside: An Antiviral Agent* (D. Pavan-Langston, R. A. Buchanan, and C. A. Alford, Jr., eds.), Raven Press, New York, 1975, p. 1.
5. R. W. Sidwell, G. J. Dixon, F. M. Schabel, Jr., and D. H. Kaump, *Antimicrob. Agents Chemother.--1968*, p. 148 (1969).
6. B. J. Sloan, F. A. Miller, J. Ehrlich, I. W. McLean, Jr., and H. E. Machamer, *Antimicrob. Agents Chemother.--1968*, p. 161 (1969).
7. H. E. Kaufman, E. D. Ellison, and W. M. Townsend, *Arch. Ophthalmol.*, *84*:783 (1970).
8. L. B. Allen and R. W. Sidwell, *Antimicrob. Agents Chemother.*, *2*:229 (1972).
9. B. J. Sloan, F. A. Miller, and I. W. McLean, Jr., *Antimicrob. Agents Chemother.*, *3*:74 (1973).
10. B. J. Sloan, in *Adenine Arabinoside: An Antiviral Agent* (D. Pavan-Langston, R. A. Buchanan, and C. A. Alford, Jr., eds.), Raven Press, New York, 1975, p. 45.
11. J. F. Griffith, J. F. Fitzwilliam, S. Casagrande, and S. R. Butler, *J. Infect. Dis.*, *132*:506 (1975).
12. E. Lefkowtiz, M. Worthington, M. A. Conliffe, and S. Baron, *Proc. Soc. Exp. Biol. Med.*, *152*:337 (1976).
13. L. T. Ch'ien, F. M. Schabel, Jr., and C. A. Alford, Jr., in *Selective Inhibitors of Viral Function* (W. A. Carter, ed.), CRC Press, Cleveland, Ohio, 1973, p. 227.
14. L. T. Ch'ien, N. J. Cannon, L. J. Charamella, W. E. Dismukes, R. J. Whitley, R. A. Buchanan, and C. A. Alford, Jr., *J. Infect. Dis.*, *128*:658 (1973).
15. L. R. Ch'ien, R. J. Whitley, L. J. Charamella, R. A. Buchanan, N. J. Cannon, W. E. Dismukes, and C. A. Alford, Jr., in *Adenine Arabinoside: An Antiviral Agent* (D. Pavan-Langston, R. A. Buchanan, and C. A. Alford, Jr., eds.), Raven Press, New York, 1975, p. 205.
16. R. J. Whitley, L. T. Ch'ien, A. J. Nahmias, R. A. Buchanan, and C. A. Alford, Jr., in *Adenine Arabinoside: An Antiviral Agent*

(D. Pavan-Langston, R. A. Buchanan, and C. A. Alford, Jr., eds.), Raven Press, New York, 1975, p. 225.
17. D. Pavan-Langston and C. H. Dohlman, *Am. J. Ophthalmol.*, *74*: 81 (1972).
18. R. A. Hyndiuk, R. O. Schultz, and D. S. Hull, in *Adenine Arabinoside: An Antiviral Agent* (D. Pavan-Langston, R. A. Buchanan, and C. A. Alford, Jr., eds.), Raven Press, New York, 1975, p. 331.
19. D. Pavan-Langston, in *Adenine Arabinoside: An Antiviral Agent* D. Pavan-Langston, R. A. Buchanan, and C. A. Alford, Jr., Eds.), Raven Press, New York, 1975, p. 345.
20. R. Abel, Jr., H. E. Kaufman, and J. Sugar, in *Adenine Arabinoside: An Antiviral Agent* (D. Pavan-Langston, R. A. Buchanan, and C. A. Alford, Jr., eds.), Raven Press, New Yrok, 1975, p. 393.
21. J. R. McKinnon, J. I. McGill, and B. R. Jones, in *Adenine Arabinoside: An Antiviral Agent* (D. Pavan-Langston, R. A. Buchanan, and C. A. Alford, Jr., eds.), Raven Press, New York, 1975, p. 401.
22. C. A. Alford, Jr. and R. J. Whitley, *J. Infect. Dis.*, *133*(Suppl.): A101 (1976).
23. M. D. Aronson, C. F. Philips, D. W. Gump, R. J. Albertini, and C. A. Phillips, *JAMA 235*:1339 (1976).
24. R. J. Whitley, S. J. Soong, R. Dolin, G. Gallasso, L. T. Ch'ien, and C. A. Alford, Jr., *N. Engl. J. Med.*, *297*:289 (1977).
25. E. R. Kern, J. C. Overall, and L. A. Glasgow, *Abstr. Ann. Mtg. Am. Soc. Microbiol.*, 1975, Abstr. No. A26, p. 5.
26. J. C. Overall, E. R. Kern, and L. A. Glasgow, in *Adenine Arabinoside: An Antiviral Agent* (D. Pavan-Langston, R. A. Buchanan, and C. A. Alford, Jr., eds.), Raven Press, New York, 1975, p. 95.
27. E. R. Kern, J. C. Overall, Jr., and L. A. Glasgow, *Antimicrob. Agents Chemother.*, *7*:587 (1975).
28. E. L. Goodman, J. P. Luby, and M. T. Johnson, *Antimicrob. Agents Chemother.*, *8*:693 (1975).
29. H. G. Adams, E. A. Benson, E. R. Alexander, L. A. Vontver, M. A. Remington, and K. K. Holmes, *J. Infect. Dis.*, *133*(Suppl.): A151 (1976).
30. J. L. Fox, C. D. Yu, W. I. Higuchi, and N. F. H. Ho, *Int. J. Pharmaceut.*, *2*:41 (1979).
31. C. D. Yu, J. L. Fox, N.F. H. Ho, and W. I. Higuchi, *J. Pharm. Sci.*, *68*:1341 (1979).
32. C. D. Yu, W. I. Higuchi, N. F. H. Ho, J. L. Fox, and G. L. Flynn, *J. Pharm. Sci.*, *69*:770 (1980).
33. C. D. Yu, J. L. Fox, W. I. Higuchi, and N. F. H. Ho, *J. Pharm. Sci.*, *69*:772 (1980).

34. C. D. Yu, N. A. Gordon, J. L. Fox, W. I. Higuchi, and N. F.H. Ho, *J. Pharm. Sci.*, *69*:775 (1980).
35. D. C. Baker, T. H. Haskell, and S. R. Putt, *J. Med. Chem.*, *21*: 1218 (1978).
36. D. C. Baker, T. H. Haskell, S. R. Putt, and B. J. Sloan, *J. Med. Chem.*, *22*:273 (1979).
37. R. A. Lipper, S. M. Machkovech, J. C. Drach, and W. K. Higuchi, *Mol. Pharmacol.*, *14*:366 (1978).
38. P. W. K. Woo, H. W. Dion, S. M. Lange, L. F. Dahl, and L. J. Durham, *J. Heterocycl. Chem.*, *11*:641 (1974).
39. S. M. Machkovech, R. A. Lipper, W. I. Higuchi, J. C. Drach, and D. C. Baker, *125th Meet. APhA* (Academy of Pharmaceutical Sciences), Montreal, 1978, Abstr. No. 69.
40. C. C. Hsu, J. Y. Park, N. F. H. Ho, W. I. Higuchi, and J. L. Fox, *J. Pharm. Sci.*, accepted (1981).
41. C. C. Hsu, A. Kusai, N. F. H. Ho, J. L. Fox, and W. I. Higuchi, *Meet. APhA* (Academy of Pharmaceutical Sciences), Orlando, Fla., 1981.
42. C. C. Hsu, Ph.D. thesis, Univerity of Michigan, 1980.
43. N. A. Gordon, Ph.D. thesis, University of Michigan, 1981.

Chapter 4

Macromolecular and Modeling Aspects of Swelling-Controlled Systems

RICHARD W. KORSMEYER and NIKOLAOS A. PEPPAS
Purdue University, West Lafayette, Indiana

One of the most important research problems in controlled release technology is the development of monolithic (matrix type) polymeric formulations, which can release drugs at a constant rate over a period of time. These systems are commonly known as zero-order release systems. Recent reviews [1-3] analyze the need for and applications of zero-order release systems of bioactive agents, and describe specific formulations which exhibit this type of kinetic behavior.

Although membrane-type controlled release polymeric formulations are widely used to achieve drug release at constant rate [1], it is rather difficult to achieve similar release kinetics with conventional monolithic nonporous systems. To understand the reasons for this behavior, one needs to consider the transient Fickian diffusion behavior of a solute through a polymer, as described by Eq. (1), and to examine mathematical solutions of this equation with appropriate boundary conditions.

$$\frac{\partial c_i}{\partial t} = D_i \frac{\partial^2 c_i}{\partial x^2} \qquad (1)$$

Here c_i is the concentration of the diffusing solute, D_i the concentration-independent diffusion coefficient of the solute, and t and x the release time and position in the medium, respectively. Isothermal, one-dimensional Fickian diffusion is assumed.

Mathematical solutions of Eq. (1) under simple boundary conditions, which describe frequently used experimental conditions of release in water or biological fluids, and for simple geometrical shapes, such as slabs, cylinders, and spheres, can be found in standard references [4,5]. They show that the solute release rate per surface area, $dM_i/A \cdot dt$, is proportional to $t^{-1/2}$, where M_i is the amount of drug released at time t, and A is the surface area of release. Therefore, one may come to the superficial conclusion that a constant drug release rate cannot be achieved with matrix-type systems.

However, in recent years there have been reports of interesting new methods of preparation of matrix-type systems which may exhibit zero-order release kinetics under specific experimental conditions. Three of the most successful methods are modification of the geometry of the monolithic device, use of porous polymers, and use of swelling-controlled release systems. For example, Langer and his collaborators [6] designed hemispherical monolithic devices which exhibit release behavior closely approximating zero-order kinetics. Our research group [7-9] examined hydrophobic porous polymeric systems which can release various water-soluble drugs at constant rate. Finally, Hopfenberg and his collaborators [10,11], and our research group [12-14] introduced swelling-controlled polymeric formulations which may exhibit release approximating zero-order kinetics.

Swelling-controlled release systems are the new member of a family of controlled release devices which have great potential for applications in pharmaceutical technology, and which have been inadequately described up to now. It is our intention in this chapter to describe the physics of controlled release of solutes under dynamic swelling of the matrix, and to establish preparative and experimental conditions under which swelling-controlled drug release polymeric formulations can be used to achieve zero-order release kinetics.

MECHANISMS OF SWELLING-CONTROLLED RELEASE BEHAVIOR

Release of bioactive agents by swelling-controlled mechanisms is related to the diffusion of a solute (drug) from and through an originally glassy polymer, under countercurrent diffusion of water or biological fluid into the polymer.

In swelling-controlled polymeric systems the drug is originally dissolved or dispersed in a dilute or concentrated polymer solution. As the solvent is evaporated, a solvent-free glassy polymeric matrix is obtained, with drug dispersed in it. This system constitutes a typical swellable pharmaceutical formulation.

In a release experiment there is no drug diffusion through the solid phase. However, as the dissolution medium (e.g., water, saline, biological fluid) penetrates the matrix, the solvent-free polymer starts swelling. If the thermodynamic compatibility of the dissolution medium with the polymer is favorable, the glass transition temperature of the polymer is lowered below the temperature of the release experiment. Under these conditions the swollen polymer is in its rubbery state, and it allows the drug to diffuse outward. A simple graphical description of this phenomenon is shown in Fig. 1.

Thermodynamic Considerations

Further analysis of the dynamic swelling behavior of the polymer and its effect on solute diffusion requires understanding of the thermodynamics of the binary (polymer/dissolution medium) and tertiary (drug/polymer/dissolution medium) systems involved in this type of drug release.

As noted before, solvent penetration in a glassy polymer leads to a considerable increase in macromolecular mobility, which is observed as a continuous decrease of the glass transition temperature T_g, as shown in Fig. 2. From a thermodynamic point of view the compatibility of a dissolution medium for a polymer may be expressed in terms of the solubility parameters of the two components, δ, or the Flory interaction parameter of the pair, χ.

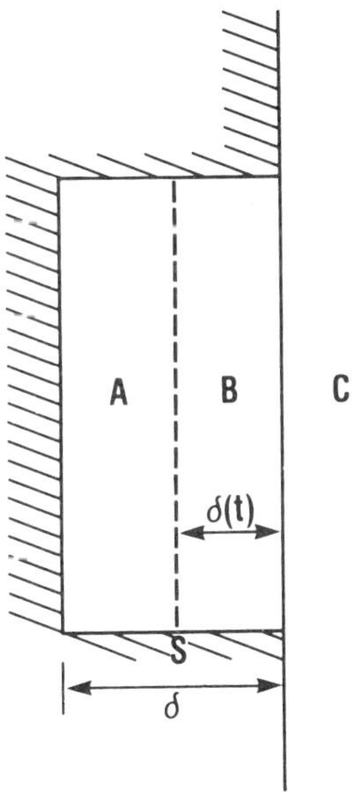

Figure 1 Swelling-controlled release system without volume change; A, glassy polymer with drug; B, continuously swelling polymer with drug diffusing outward; C, dissolution medium; S, swelling interface.

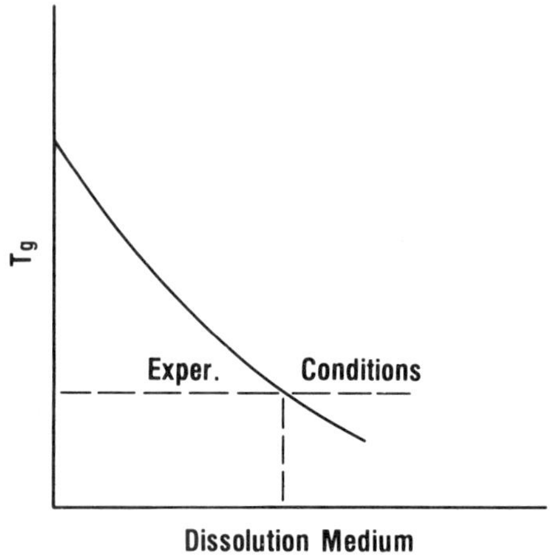

Figure 2 Effect of dissolution medium on glass transition temperature of polymer.

If the dissolution medium is poorly compatible with the polymer, it may not be able to lower the T_g enough to lead to the rubbery state. Consequently, at thermodynamic equilibrium one may observe a polymer which is still glassy under experimental conditions. Drug diffusion through such systems is still very slow, and practical pharmaceutical applications are limited.

However, when in contact with thermodynamically good solvents, a glassy polymer is almost sure to transform to its rubbery state. This dynamic swelling phenomenon may lead to considerable volume expansion of the original formulation.

Two fronts (interfaces) are characteristic of this swelling behavior: a front separating the glassy from the rubbery state (swelling interface) which moves toward the glassy state with velocity v; and a front separating the rubbery polymer from the pure dissolution medium (polymer interface) which moves outward, as shown in Fig. 3.

In the absence of physical or molecular restrictions to swelling, the polymer will eventually dissolve. Dissolution of the polymer may be avoided if one works with semicrystalline, uncrosslinked, or amorphous, slightly crosslinked polymers. In this case, the crystallites and crosslinks act as permanent junctions, preventing dissolution. These systems are called swellable, nonerodible release systems. Despite the existence of permanent junctions, dissolution of the polymer may occur due to chemical degradation (such as hydrolysis), in which case the system is classified as a swellable, erodible release system, or due to biodegradation (due to naturally occurring enzymes), in which case the system is classified as a swellable, bioerodible release system.

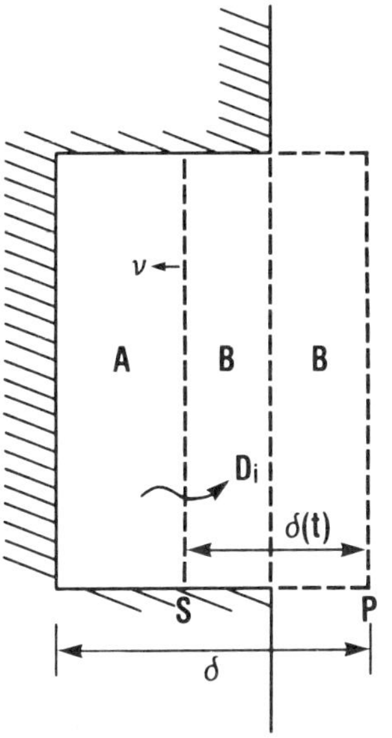

Figure 3 Moving fronts during dynamic swelling of a glassy polymer. A, glassy state; B, rubbery state; C, dissolution medium; S, swelling interface; P, polymer interface.

Although many pharmaceutical formulations can be classified as swellable systems, the term *swelling-controlled systems* is used to describe those formulations where the solute release is actually controlled by the swelling phenomenon, namely by the relative position and velocity of the swelling interface.

Diffusive Mechanisms: Dissolution Medium

The mechanism of drug diffusion in swelling-controlled polymeric formulations is dependent on the thermodynamic state of the polymer during release. Fickian or non-Fickian drug diffusion mechanisms may be observed depending on the dynamics of polymer swelling, and on the relative mobility of drug and dissolution medium.

In general, as swelling of the polymer proceeds, macromolecular relaxations become important at the glassy/rubbery polymer front [15]. These relaxations may, in turn, control the mode of diffusion and release of the drug. Although diffusion in rubbery polymers obtained after swelling up to thermodynamic equilibrium with the dissolution medium is Fickian, diffusion in a rubbery state which is not "at equilibrium" (due to continuous swelling) may be Fickian or non-Fickian (anomalous).

For the penetration of the dissolution medium in the polymer (swelling), a convenient method of analysis is in terms of the dimensionless Deborah number De. The Deborah number is defined according to Eq. (2), where λ is the characteristic stress-relaxation time of the polymer/dissolution medium system, and θ is the characteristic time for diffusion of the dissolution medium in the polymer.

$$De = \frac{\lambda}{\theta} \tag{2}$$

with

$$\lambda = \frac{\int_0^\infty sG(s)\, ds}{\int_0^\infty G(s)\, ds} \tag{3}$$

and

$$\theta = \frac{\delta^2}{D_s} \tag{4}$$

The parameters involved in this definition are the shear relaxation modulus G(s), the thickness of the sample δ, and the dissolution medium diffusion coefficient D_s.

Vrentas and his collaborators [16,17] have attempted to define regions of Fickian and non-Fickian (anomalous) diffusion of the dissolution medium in the polymer by calculating the value of De. Fickian diffusion is observed for $De \gg 1$ or for $De \ll 1$. Anomalous diffusive behavior occurs when the Deborah number is of the order of 1. A special case of anomalous diffusion, known also as case II transport, is observed when the glassy/rubbery front moves at a constant velocity.

Diffusive Mechanisms: Drug

The relative mobility of the diffusing solute (drug) with respect to the penetrating dissolution medium is the controlling factor in the mechanism of drug release. For this purpose, it is convenient to define a dimensionless number, the swelling interface number Sw, according to

$$Sw = \frac{v\delta(t)}{D_i} \tag{5}$$

The number Sw compares the velocity of the swelling interface v to the diffusion coefficient of the drug. The parameter $\delta(t)$ is the time-dependent thickness of the rubbery (gel-like) layer.

The importance of this number in drug release was independently recognized by Hopfenberg and his associates [11] and by our group [13], although it was Hopfenberg who published it first. Indeed, Hopfenberg et al. [11] used the reciprocal of the swelling number Sw to establish regions of zero-order release. We prefer the definition of Eq. (5) because it shows the similarity of this dimensionless number to the Peclet number used in diffusive/convective problems.

When the rate of solute transport through the solvated region is faster than the rate at which the glassy/rubbery front advances, the swelling interface number Sw is much smaller than 1, and zero-order release kinetics of the drug is observed. Values of $Sw \gg 1$ designate the case where the swelling front advances faster than the release of the drug. In this case, diffusion occurs through a "quasi-equilibrium"-swollen gel, and Fickian release is observed. For values of $Sw \approx 1$, non-Fickian, non-zero-order release is observed.

MATHEMATICAL ANALYSIS OF SWELLABLE SYSTEMS

Complete mathematical analysis of solute (drug) release from initially glassy swellable polymeric systems is not yet available. The main reasons for the lack of rigorous mathematical analysis are that (1) modeling problems related to this phenomenon are problems of simple or multicomponent diffusion with moving boundaries, (2) the diffusion coefficients are coupled and concentration dependent, and (3) the continuous relaxation of the macromolecular chains during diffusion must be expressed in terms of appropriate constitutive equations.

Scientific and engineering problems of diffusion accompanied by a change of phase are commonly known as *Stefan problems* or *moving* (or *free*) *boundary problems*. An essential feature of these problems is the existence of moving surfaces separating the phases of the material. The position of these interfaces is not known a priori. Numerous studies of Stefan and Stefan-Neumann problems have been discussed in excellent reviews, which also present many applications [18,19]. The only known exact solutions are those of Neuman, which of course do not treat polymer relaxations. Some of the problems related to rigorous modeling of swellable polymers have been discussed recently by Peppas and Korsmeyer [20,21].

Models for Pharmaceutical Systems

Attempts at rigorous mathematical modeling of drug release from swellable polymeric systems have been expertly presented by Lee [22]. Lee solved certain moving boundary problems encountered during the diffusional release of a solute from a polymeric matrix, and he presented approximate and exact (where possible) analytical solutions. He drew attention to the importance of the mobility of the swelling interface in establishing conditions of zero-order release. An interesting aspect of Lee's work is his effort to describe erodible and swelling-controlled systems by the same type of diffusion equations and boundary conditions, since swelling ("phase erosion" in Lee's terminology) and mass erosion are physically similar situations.

Peppas et al. [23] developed pseudo-steady-state models for drug diffusion from swellable polymers exhibiting significant volume expansion, but with constant diffusion coefficients. Good [24] offered a mathematical model employing time-dependent drug diffusion coefficient with continuous swelling, but at constant total volume. Some approximate and simplified solutions for swellable polymers with volume expansion were also described recently by Puisieux, Carstensen, and their collaborators [25,26].

Owing to the implicit assumption of steady state, the models of Peppas [23] and Carstensen [25,26] predict a $t^{-1/2}$-dependent drug release rate. Good's model [24] predicts release rates which are dependent on an exponential expression of time. Only Lee's approximate models [22] have the capability of predicting constant release rates from swellable systems under certain experimental conditions.

Other Relevant Models

As pointed out before [21], new insight into the modeling of swellable controlled release systems can be obtained from similar modeling already published in other areas of polymer science. In many polymer applications, an originally glassy polymer containing a solute is placed in contact with a penetrant* and swelling is observed. Such systems are important in the description of additive migration, dyeing processes, and so on.

Rudolph and Figge [27,28] developed a mathematical model of solute diffusion in a multicomponent inhomogeneous system with moving internal fronts, but at constant total volume. This model assumes constant diffusion coefficients for the solute in the penetrant-free polymer and for the penetrant in the polymer, and concentration-dependent diffusion coefficient of the solute in the "gel-like" polymer/penetrant layer. Prediction of sharp changes in concentration at the glassy/rubbery and rubbery/penetrant interfaces is achieved by using predetermined, Nernst-type, thermodynamic partition coefficients. A

---

*In swelling-controlled drug release systems the term *penetrant* is synonymous with *dissolution medium*. In most of the models mentioned here, the *solute* is a low molecular weight organic liquid, originally incorporated in the polymer in small quantities.

similar approach without a glassy/rubbery interface but with various boundary conditions and mass transfer limitations at the polymer/penetrant interface was presented by Reid et al. [29]. In both cases the release rate, dM_i/dt, is dependent on $t^{-1/2}$ over most of the period of solute release.

Coupled-diffusion problems with concentration-independent diffusion coefficients of solute and penetrant, volume expansion, but no internal fronts were solved by Wang et al. [30]. Analytical solutions were presented for the initial stage of the diffusion process, whereas numerical solutions using finite differences were presented for the complete release problem.

Frisch [31] solved a class of boundary value problems, assuming simultaneous nonlinear Fickian diffusion of a solute and a penetrant at constant total volume. This treatment is more complete from a polymer point of view, since it describes diffusion coefficients dependent on concentration, according to a Fujita-like free-volume theory.

Finally, some interesting exact solutions of penetrant diffusion into a glassy polymer with moving boundaries have been recently presented by Peterlin [32] for case II transport behavior, and by Tu [33] for Fickian diffusion with concentration-dependent diffusion coefficients and associated dissolution of the polymers. Although this work does not address the problem of simultaneous release of a solute, it may be a good starting point for further rigorous mathematical modeling.

Treatment of Drug Release Data

Drug release data from a glassy polymeric slab under countercurrent simultaneous diffusion of a swelling agent may be fitted to Eq. (6):

$$\frac{M_i}{M_\infty} = kt^n \tag{6}$$

where M_i/M_∞ is the fraction of a drug released at time t, and k and n are constants characteristic of the slab/dissolution medium system. Release rates can be fitted to the corresponding equation (7), which is readily obtained from Eq. (6) upon differentiation.

$$\frac{dM_i}{A\ dt} = nc_d kt^{n-1} \tag{7}$$

Here c_d is the initial loading of drug in the polymer.

Equations (6) and (7) may describe the release kinetics of drugs which diffuse by Fickian mechanisms in non-moving-boundary problems. In this case, n = 0.5 and k can be expressed by

$$k = 4\left(\frac{D_i}{\pi\delta^2}\right)^{1/2} \tag{8}$$

This solution is the well-known short-time approximation of the solution of the Fickian diffusion equation (1) with constant surface concentration [5].

Moving boundaries and non-Fickian (anomalous) mechanisms are characterized by $n > 0.5$. A case of special interest is when the drug release is described by Eq. (7) with $n = 1$. This limiting case of non-Fickian transport may be called case II transport of the drug; it is associated with zero-order release.

Swellable Zero-Order-Release Systems

As discussed before, the necessary and sufficient condition for observing zero-order-release kinetics when using swelling-controlled systems is that the swelling interface number Sw be much smaller than 1. Simple case II transport of the dissolution medium is only a necessary but not sufficient condition.

Recently, we examined experimental conditions under which case II penetration of the dissolution medium does not lead to zero-order release. Consider the one-dimensional case of a glassy polymer containing an initially uniformly distributed drug, which is then placed in a dissolution medium. After a short release time, the situation may be described by Fig. 1.

Since for many systems of interest the diffusion coefficient of the drug in the glassy region of the polymer is virtually zero, the drug concentration in the glassy region remains at its initial value, and a concentration gradient develops in the solvated region. Using Fickian diffusion, the surface flux of drug may be calculated as

$$\frac{dM_i}{A\,dt} = -D_i\left(\frac{\partial c_i(x,t)}{\partial x}\right)_{x=0} \tag{9}$$

where D_i is the drug diffusion coefficient in the solvated polymer and in the vicinity of $x = 0$. Then the total amount of drug released at time t, M_i, is given by

$$M_i = AD_i \int_0^t \left(\frac{\partial c_i(x,t)}{\partial x}\right)_{x=0} dt \tag{10}$$

Zero-order release is obtained when the gradient of the concentration is independent of t at $x = 0$. In order to use this approach to determine release rates, the drug concentration profile must be known. In general, this means solving the following boundary value problem:

$$\frac{\partial c_i}{\partial t} = \frac{\partial}{\partial x}\left(D_i \frac{\partial c_i}{\partial x}\right) \tag{11}$$

with

$$c_i(x,0) = c_{i0}$$

$$c_i(0,t) = 0$$

and

$$c_i(x,t) = C_{i0} \qquad \text{for } x \geq \delta(t)$$

where $\delta(t) = vt$ for case II penetration of the dissolution medium.

For the purpose of illustration, assume a pseudo-steady state in the solvated region with constant D_i. Then the problem is simplified to

$$\frac{\partial^2 c_i}{\partial x^2} = 0 \tag{12}$$

which is readily solved to give

$$c_i = \frac{c_{i0} x}{\delta(t)} \tag{13}$$

Therefore, the release rate can be calculated as

$$\frac{dM_i}{A\ dt} = -D_i \frac{c_{i0}}{\delta(t)} \tag{14}$$

It is interesting that Eq. (14) predicts infinite release rate at the beginning of the release experiment where $\delta(t) = 0$. This mathematical conclusion is only a result of the pseudo-steady-state approximation.

APPLICATIONS

Although the previous sections addressed problems related to the physics and mathematics of swellable systems in general, here we concentrate on the few experimental attempts that have been reported of the use of swelling-controlled release systems for achievement of zero-order release kinetics.

In one of the earliest investigations of this type of monolithic controlled release formulations, Good [24] studied the release of tripelennamine-hydrochloride from initially dry (glassy) sheets of poly(2-hydroxyethyl methacrylate) (PHEMA) over a period of 10 hr. The release data show that a significant portion of the release curve (between 1 and 5 hr, depending on the initial drug loading) can be fitted with a straight line. Good noted no major change of the thickness of the slabs used in these experiments, although PHEMA was swollen by the water. He attributed this dimensional stability to the fact that the volume of drug removed was approximately equal to the volume of water absorbed. In view of the rather low equilibrium swelling of PHEMA, which is known to swell only up to 40% of its original weight, and the lack of data on the velocity of the swelling front v, one is led to believe that Sw was of the order of 1. Drug release was controlled by macromolecular relaxations and diffusion mechanisms, and release approximating zero-order kinetics was observed.

Unequivocal demonstration of the potential of swelling-controlled systems to yield zero-order-release kinetic behavior was offered by Hopfenberg and Hsu [10]. They used a system consisting of Sudan Red dye IV dispersed in polystyrene and placed in n-hexane, and they observed constant release rate from 0 to 60 hr, depending on the thickness and temperature of release; the initial loading of the dye was kept constant.

In a subsequent contribution Hopfenberg et al. [11] investigated the release of sodium chloride and Malachite Green from three copolymers of ethylene-vinyl alcohol (EVA) of different vinyl alcohol content. It was determined that by varying the vinyl alcohol content, the hydrophilicity and dynamic swelling behavior of the EVA copolymers could be controlled, so that favorable conditions of zero-order release of the solute could be obtained. For EVA copolymers with 70% vinyl alcohol content, a swelling number of Sw = 0.05 was determined for NaCl diffusion, whereas a swelling number of 1.0 characterized Malachite Green diffusion. As expected, diffusion of the dye could not be achieved by zero-order release. However, although diffusion of NaCl was expected to be according to zero-order-release kinetics (in view of the value of the swelling number and the previous discussion), rather complex kinetics were observed, which were attributed to possible osmotic phenomena occurring during this process.

In an effort to design swelling-controlled release systems for pharmaceutical applications, we investigated the release of theophylline from glassy, poly(vinyl alcohol) (PVA) slabs under different experimental conditions [13]. Since PVA is considerably more hydrophilic than PHEMA, which had been previously studied by Good [24], we attempted to control the swelling interface number by crosslinking and/or crystallizing the polymer prior to the release experiments. Even the "best" formulation, showing release kinetics that could be modeled by Eq. (6) with n = 0.76, could not exhibit zero-order-release behavior. Possible modifications of the solubility of the polymer may lead to a desirable swelling-controlled formulation.

CONCLUSIONS

The purpose of this chapter was to analyze the physical conditions and mathematical implications of the development of zero-order-release polymeric systems for pharmaceutical applications, by employing the glassy/rubbery transition and dynamic swelling behavior of polymers. Despite the great promise of these "swelling-controlled" release systems, no successful pharmaceutical formulation of this type is yet known in the literature.

Prerequisites for zero-order-release kinetics by swellable polymeric systems are (1) that the candidate-polymer exhibit a glassy/rubbery transition in a desired temperature range in the presence of a dissolution medium, and (2) that the swelling interface number be smaller than 1. Methods to achieve these criteria include modification of the swelling behavior of the polymer by chemical or physical methods and change of the drug diffusion coefficient by physical methods (crosslinking or crystallization).

ACKNOWLEDGMENTS

A portion of this work was completed while one of us (R.W.K.) was performing part of his Ph.D. Thesis at the University of Geneva, Switzerland, in the spring of 1981. The financial support provided by Prof. P. Buri of this university is gratefully acknowledged.

REFERENCES

1. R. Langer, *Chem. Eng. Commun.*, *6*:1 (1980).
2. S. W. Kim, R. V. Petersen, and J. Feijen, in *Drug Design*, Vol. 10 (E. J. Ariens, ed.), Academic Press, New York, 1980, p. 193.
3. R. Langer and N. A. Peppas, *Biomaterials*, *2*:201 (1981).
4. J. Crank, *The Mathematics of Diffusion*, Clarendon Press, Oxford, 1975.
5. N. A. Peppas, in *Bioavailability and the Pharmacokinetic Control of Drug Response* (V. F. Smolen, ed.), Wiley, New York, in press.
6. W. Rhine, V. Sukhatme, D. Hsieh, and R. Langer, in *Controlled Release of Bioactive Materials* (R. Baker, ed.), Academic Press, New York, 1980, p. 83.
7. R. Gurny, E. Doelker, and N. A. Peppas, *Biomaterials*, *3*:27 (1982).

8. E. A. Swan and N. A. Peppas, *Proc. Int. Symp. Controlled Release Bioact. Mater.*, *8*:18 (1981).
9. R. Gurny, E. Doelker, J. L. Solomon, R. W. Korsmeyer, and N. A. Peppas, manuscript 3c, Summer AIChE Nat. Meet., August 1981.
10. H. B. Hopfenberg and K. C. Hsu, *Polym. Eng. Sci.*, *18*:1186 (1978).
11. H. B. Hopfenberg, A. Apicella, and D. E. Saleeby, *J. Membr. Sci.*, *8*:273 (1981).
12. R. W. Korsmeyer and N. A. Peppas, *Proc. Int. Symp. Controlled Release Bioact. Mater.*, *8*:85 (1981).
13. R. W. Korsmeyer and N. A. Peppas, *J. Membr. Sci.*, *9*:211 (1981).
14. C. T. Reinhart, R. W. Korsmeyer, and N. A. Peppas, *Int. J. Pharm. Technol.*, *2*:9 (1981).
15. H. Hopfenberg and H. L. Frisch, *J. Polym. Sci.*, *B7*:405 (1969).
16. J. S. Vrentas, C. M. Jarzebski, and J. L. Duda, *AIChE J.*, *21*: 894 (1975).
17. J. S. Vrentas, C. M. Jarzebski, and J. L. Duda, *J. Polym. Sci., Polym. Phys.*, *15*:441 (1977).
18. L. I. Rubinstein, *The Stefan Problem*, American Mathematical Society, New York, 1971.
19. S. G. Bankoff, *Adv. Chem. Eng.*, *5*:75 (1964).
20. N. A. Peppas and R. W. Korsmeyer, *Polym. News*, *6*:149 (1980).
21. N. A. Peppas, *Polym. News*, *6*:221 (1980).
22. P. I. Lee, *J. Membr. Sci.*, *7*:255 (1980).
23. N. A. Peppas, R. Gurny, E. Doelker, and P. Buri, *J. Membr. Sci.*, *7*:241 (1980).
24. W. R. Good, in *Polymeric Delivery Systems* (R. Kostelnik, ed.), Gordon and Breach, New York, 1976, p. 139.
25. M. Bamba, F. Puisieux, J. P. Marty, and J. T. Carstensen, *Int. J. Pharmaceut.*, *2*:307 (1979).
26. M. Bamba, F. Puisieux, J. P. Marty, and J. T. Carstensen, *Proc. Int. Congr. Pharmaceut. Technol.*, *2*:127 (1980).
27. F. B. Rudolph, *J. Polym. Sci., Polym. Phys.*, *17*:1709 (1979).
28. K. Figge and F. B. Rudolph, *Angew. Makromol. Chem.*, *78*:157 (1979).
29. R. C. Reid, K. R. Sidman, A. D. Schwope, and D. E. Till, *Ind. Eng. Chem., Prod. Res. Dev.*, *19*:580 (1980).
30. F. H. L. Wang, J. L. Duda, and J. S. Vrentas, *Polym. Eng. Sci.*, *20*:120 (1980).
31. H. L. Frisch, *J. Poly. Sci., Polym. Phys. Ed.*, *16*:1651 (1978).
32. A. Peterlin, *J. Polym. Sci., Polym. Phys. Ed.*, *17*:1741 (1979).
33. Y. O. Tu, *Q. Appl. Math.*, 269 (1977).

Chapter 5

Controlled Release of Norethindrone from Poly (Ortho Esters)

JORGE HELLER, D. W. H. PENHALE, ROBERT F. HELWING,* and BRUCE K. FRITZINGER SRI International, Menlo Park, California

The objective of this chapter is to describe the development of a bioerodible polymer implant that would release an incorporated drug by zero-order kinetics for at least 6 months. A further objective is the development of a system where drug release and polymer erosion take place concomitantly so that no polymer remains when the drug is depleted.

To meet these objectives, it is necessary to confine polymer bioerosion to the surface of a solid device, and as previously discussed [1,2], one approach to the development of such a system is to choose a pH-sensitive polymer hydrolysis reaction and to buffer the interior of the matrix to prevent bulk erosion.

Because poly(ortho esters) are stable in base and become progressively more labile as the pH of the surrounding medium decreases, our original approach emphasized devices containing dispersed drug and the basic salt sodium carbonate. With these devices we expected that the polymer would hydrolyze and concomitantly release its incorporated drug only at the outer surface of the device, where the basic salt is neutralized by the external buffer.

Earlier studies [3] have shown that the incorporation of a basic water-soluble salt into a hydrophobic polymer leads to an osmotic imbibing of water, and because the matrix is stable in an alkaline medium, extensive swelling without polymer erosion was noted.

Nevertheless, drug was released in a reasonably linear manner by what we assumed to be a moving, swelling front analogous to that described by Hopfenberg and Hsu [4]. That is, we assumed that the

*Present affiliation: Memorex Corporation, Santa Clara, California

drug was completely immobilized in the hydrophobic rigid polymer and was released by the swelling-induced relaxation of the matrix. Because drug is released from a solid device as a consequence of the uniform movement of a swelling front, the drug release rate should be directly proportional to drug loading, and this was, indeed, observed [3].

In a subsequent study [5], we described the use of water-soluble salts that would release incorporated drugs by osmotically driving water into a hydrophobic matrix, but by not creating an alkaline environment within the polymer would not prevent polymer erosion.

These studies have been continued, and in this chapter we present additional details of the mechanism of drug release and polymer erosion.

EXPERIMENTAL

The polymers were prepared as described previously [6] by the condensation of equimolar amounts of 3,9-bis(methylene)-2,4,8,10-tetraoxaspiro[5,5]undecane and 1,6-hexanediol in tetrahydrofuran using iodine in pyridine catalysis.

Circular disks about 6.3 mm in diameter and either 0.6 or 1.2 mm in thickness were punched from a sheet fabricated by first blending polymer, drug, and salt in a Teflon-coated pan, in a dry box, at temperatures between 135 and 180°C, then pressing in a Carver press at the same temperatures and 10,000 psi. Before the disks were punched, the sheets were warmed to 50 to 60°C. Rods were prepared by using a simple screw-activated extruder with a 0.125-in. dye and were cut to 10-mm lengths. Detailed procedures have been published [3,5]. The drug release rate was measured using a method described previously [5,7]. However, two changes were made in the polymer erosion and drug release studies: (1) the polypropylene mesh bags used previously to enclose the devices were replaced by stainless steel bags, and (2) drug concentration in the aqueous solution was followed by high-pressure liquid chromatography rather than by the ultraviolet absorption at 240 nm.

RESULTS

In this work we describe the erosion and kinetics of norethindrone release from disks or rods containing 10 wt % norethindrone and 10 wt % of one of the following three salts: sodium carbonate, sodium sulfate, or sodium chloride.

Figure 1 shows a comparison of rate of norethindrone release from devices 1.2 mm thick containing 10 wt % sodium carbonate and 10 wt % sodium sulfate. The rate of drug release from the sodium sulfate devices (shown in Fig. 1) was measured in a previous study and

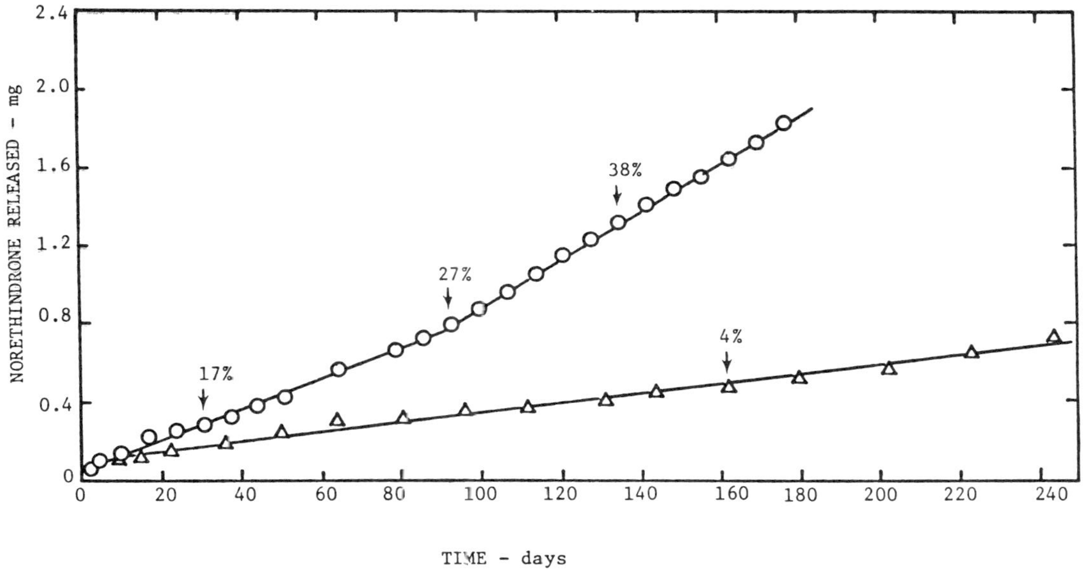

Figure 1 Norethindrone release from 3,9-bis(methylene)-2,4,8,10-tetraoxaspiro[5,5]undecane/1,6-hexanediol poly(ortho ester) disks loaded with 10 wt % norethindrone and various salts at pH 7.4 and 37°C. Thickness of both devices, 1.2 mm. (Arrows indicate weight loss.) o[o 10 wt % Na_2SO_4 (4.0 mg drug)]; △[△ 10 wt % Na_2CO_3 (4.0 mg of drug)].

published in an analogous figure [5]. However, the previously published rate of drug release from the sodium carbonate devices continued a cumulative error and was high by an approximate factor of 2. The correct rate of drug release from the sodium carbonate devices shown in Fig. 1 was obtained in the current study.

Although the rates of drug release from the sodium carbonate and sodium sulfate devices are not the same, weight loss data (shown above the arrows in Fig. 1) confirmed our expectation that neutral salts would osmotically drive water into the polymer and release the drug but would not inhibit polymer erosion.

Release of norethindrone from devices 0.6 mm thick containing sodium sulfate carried out in this study is shown in Fig. 2. The data show good linear drug release for about 80 days, after which time the drug delivery rate begins to accelerate up to drug depletion, which occurs at about 190 days.

It is interesting and gratifying that the kinetics of norethindrone release from sodium sulfate devices shown in Fig. 1 and 2 are quite similar even though the experiments were carried out at different times and that slightly different experimental techniques were used. Furthermore, even though both experiments utilized the same polymer/drug/salt composite, circular devices were pressed to 0.6 and 1.2 mm thickness, and as shown in Fig. 1 and 2, the 0.6-mm devices were drug depleted in 190 days, while the 1.2-mm devices were only half depleted after that time interval. These data indicate that the swelling front moves at a more or less uniform rate through the matrix, and the rate of movement of the swelling front is not affected by device thickness. Furthermore, the time interval after which deviation from linearity occurs is also about the same. It is also interesting that the polymer erosion rate is about the same for both systems and is also not affected by device thickness.

Release of norethindrone from disk-shaped devices containing sodium chloride is shown in Fig. 3, and release from rod-shaped devices also containing sodium chloride is shown in Fig. 4. Both sets of data again show a good linear drug release for 80 and 110 days, followed by an acceleration in drug release rate.

The release of norethindrone from disk-shaped devices containing sodium carbonate is shown in Fig. 5. Even though the experiment was discontinued after only 18% of the drug was depleted, it is clear that despite some scatter in the experimental points, the rate of drug release is linear with no acceleration in release rate evident up to 240 days. Also significant is that the rate of drug release is only one-half that noted in the linear portions of the sodium sulfate or sodium chloride devices (0.0025 mg/day versus 0.005 mg/day).

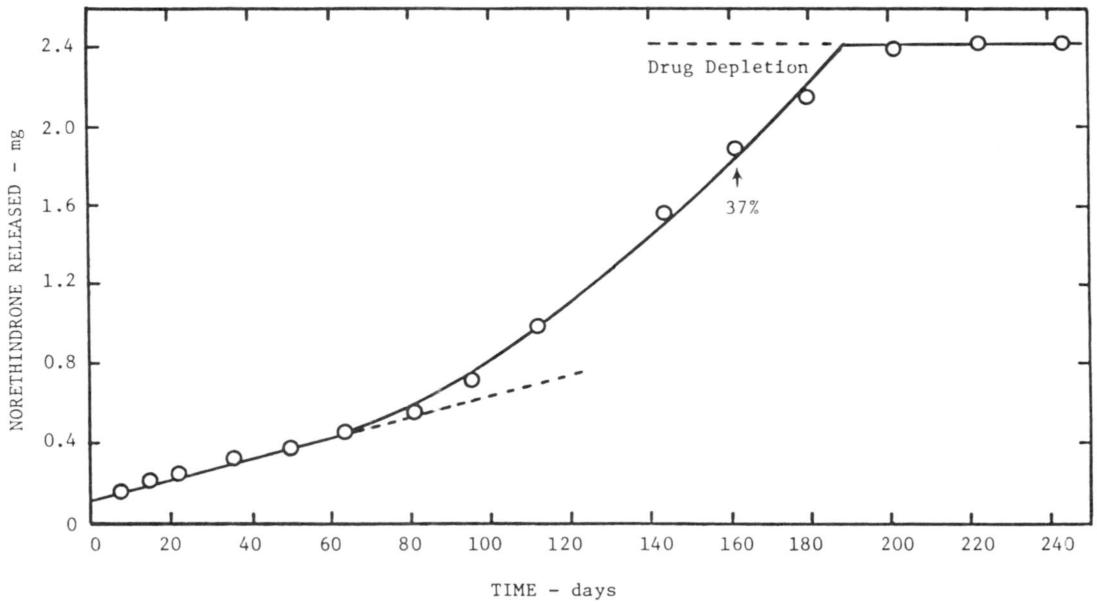

Figure 2 Norethindrone release from 3,9-bis(methylene)-2,4,8,10-tetraoxaspiro[5,5]undecane/1,6-hexanediol poly(ortho ester) disks loaded with 10 wt % norethindrone (2.4 mg of drug) and 10 wt % Na_2SO_4 at pH 7.4 and 37°C. Device thickness 0.6 mm. (Arrow indicates weight loss.)

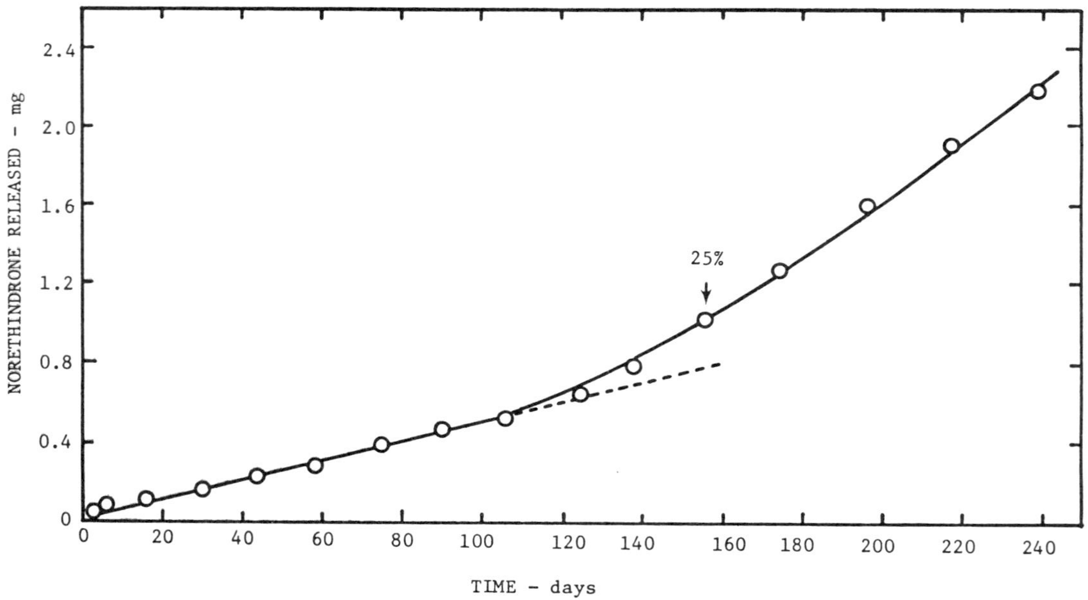

Figure 3 Norethindrone release from 3,9-bis(methylene)-2,4,8,10-tetraoxaspiro[5,5]undecane/1,6-hexanediol poly(ortho ester) disks loaded with 10 wt % norethindrone (2.5 mg drug) and 10 wt % NaCl, at pH 7.4 and 37°C. Device thickness 0.6 mm. (Arrow indicates weight loss.)

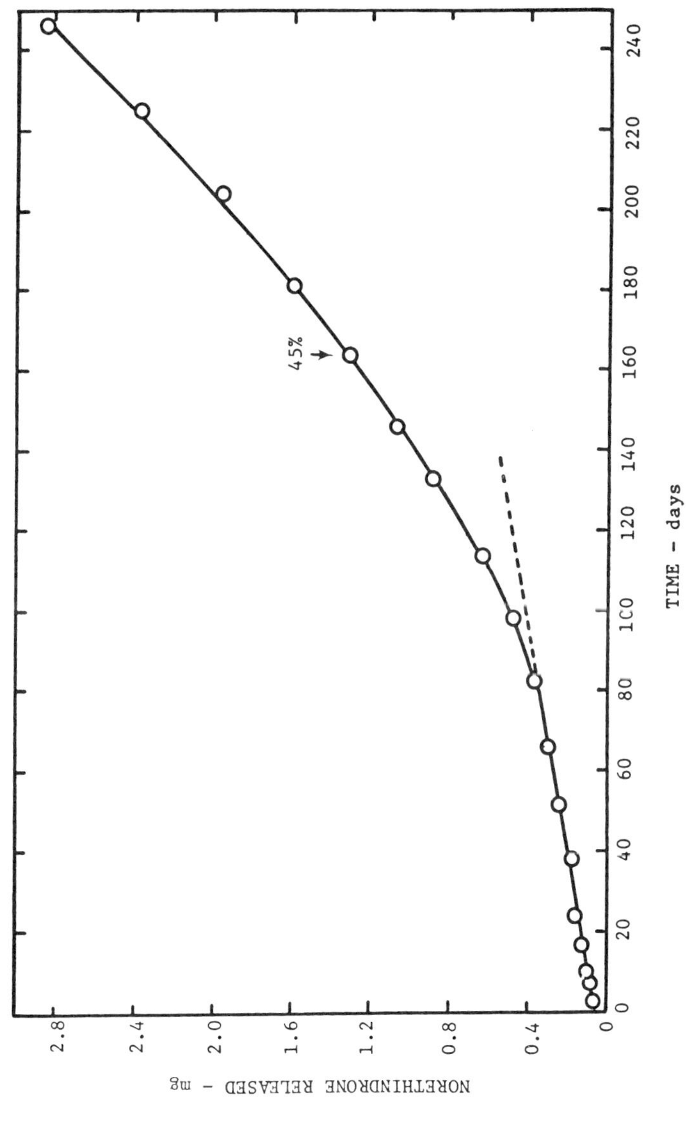

Figure 4 Norethindrone release from 3,9-bis(methylene)-2,4,8,10-tetraoxaspiro[5,5]undecane/1,6-hexanediol poly(ortho ester) rods loaded with 10 wt % norethindrone (4.5 mg of drug) and 10 wt % NaCl at pH 7.4 and 37°C. (Arrow indicates weight loss.)

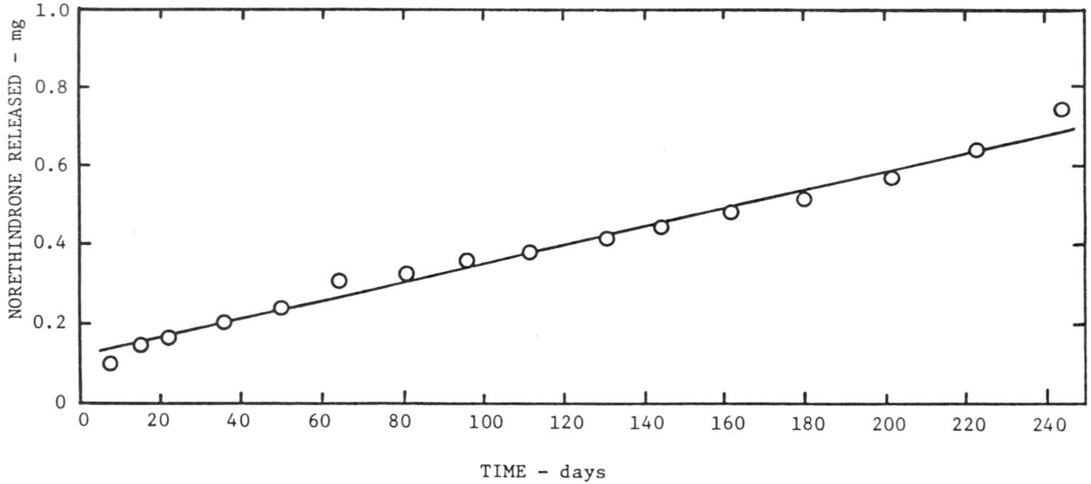

Figure 5 Norethindrone release from 3,9-bis(methylene)-2,4,8,10-tetraoxaspiro[5,5]undecane/1,6-hexanediol poly(ortho ester) disks loaded with 10 wt % norethindrone (4.0 mg of drug) and 10 wt % Na_2CO_3 at pH 7.4 and 37°C. Device thickness 1.2 mm.

DISCUSSION

The observed drug release behavior for the sodium sulfate and sodium chloride devices is clearly not consistent with that expected from a simple surface erosion process where the drug release rate should gradually decrease as the total surface area of the device decreases because of the erosion process. However, the observed release rates are consistent with a process in which the total area of the device increases with time.

This increase in device size has been verified. Figure 6 shows a photograph of an original device before exposure to the erosion medium and a sodium chloride and sodium sulfate device after 162 days in the erosion medium. All photographs are at 7 x magnification and show a substantial size increase. The diameter of the sodium chloride disk increased by a factor of 1.3, and the diameter of the sodium sulfate disk increased by a factor of 1.6. Note that the original circular shape was preserved. A similar increase in size was also noted for the rods, which also retained their original length-to-diameter ratios.

Additional insight into the behavior of these devices can be obtained by scanning electron microscope examination as shown in Fig. 7. The original device is dense with a smooth surface, whereas the sodium sulfate device is spongelike with heavy surface cratering. An examination of disks and rods containing sodium chloride revealed identical topological features.

As before [3,5], these data are consistent with the osmotic water imbibition mechanism described by Fedors [8]. According to this mechanism, when a hydrophobic polymer containing water-soluble

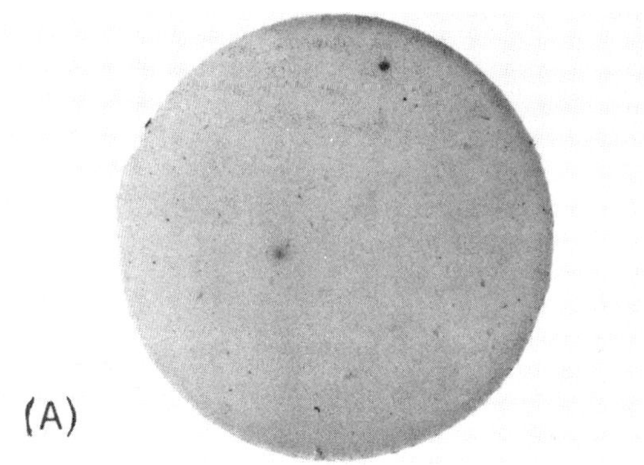

Figure 6 Photographs of devices at 7 x magnification. (A) Original device. (B) NaCl device after 162 days in erosion bath. (C) Na_2SO_4 device after 162 days in erosion bath.

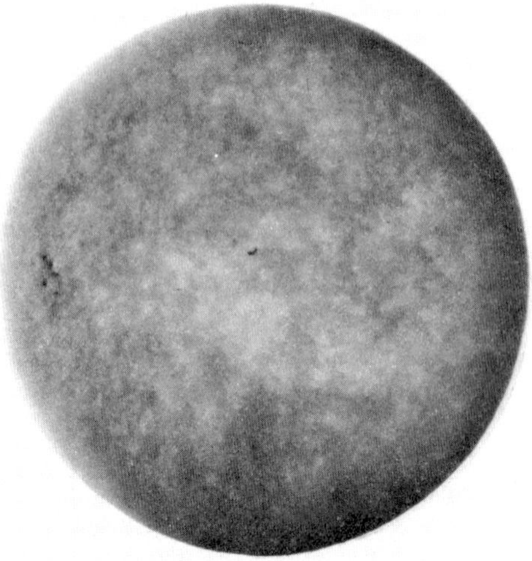

(B)

(C)

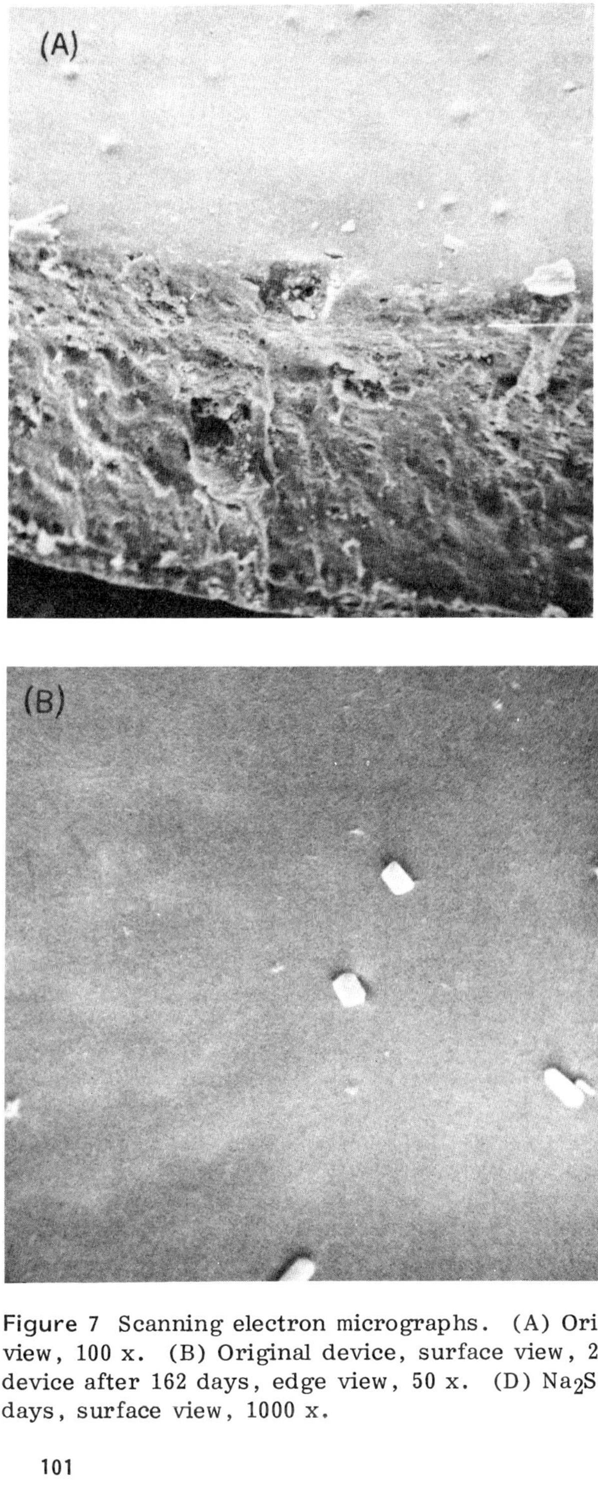

Figure 7 Scanning electron micrographs. (A) Original device, edge view, 100 x. (B) Original device, surface view, 2000 x. (C) Na_2SO_4 device after 162 days, edge view, 50 x. (D) Na_2SO_4 device after 162 days, surface view, 1000 x.

(C)

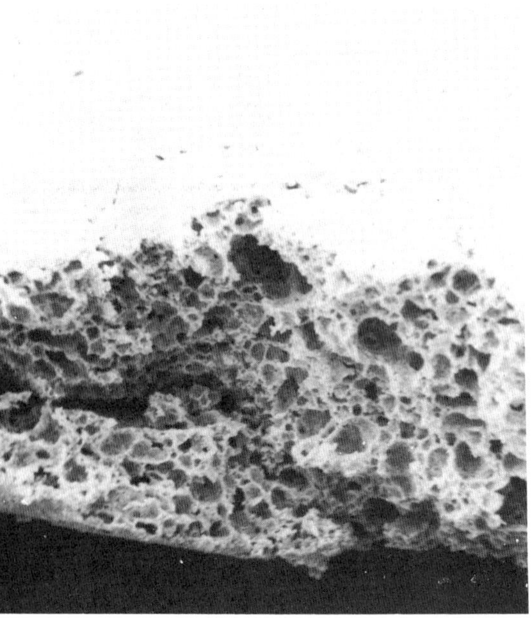

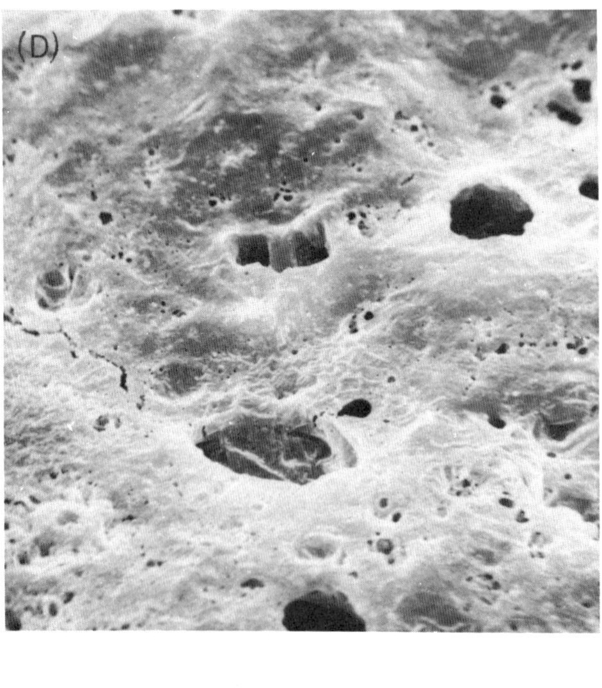

inclusions is placed in an aqueous environment, water will begin to diffuse into the polymer until it comes into contact with an included salt particle, which will then begin to dissolve. Because the polymer acts as a semipermeable membrane, an osmotic pressure will begin to act radially outward as a result of the increasing volume of water drawn into the inclusion. The overall size increase of the devices is due to the osmotic expansion and consequent polymer chain slippage, which results in a permanent increase in size.

Because the erosion rate of poly(ortho esters) at pH 7.4 is low, osmotic water imbibition is much faster than polymer erosion, and as a consequence, the predominant process is one where cells filled with concentrated salt solution form within the polymer matrix [9]. Due to a combination of osmotic pressure and polymer erosion that weakens the polymer, rupture of the cell walls takes place and an open cell foam is formed. Continuing polymer erosion gradually enlarges the cells. The acceleration of drug release can then be rationalized in terms of a gradually increasing surface area caused by the overall expansion of the device and conversion to an open cell structure, which facilitates water penetration deeper into the matrix.

Two major differences are apparent when the behavior of sodium carbonate devices is compared with that of sodium chloride or sodium sulfate. First, drug release (Fig. 5) is linear for 240 days with no apparent acceleration, and the rate of drug release is about one-half that of the sodium chloride or sodium sulfate devices. Second, even though the sodium carbonate devices show a considerable size increase, the circular shape was not retained, and electron scanning micrographs shown in Fig. 8 reveal a much smoother surface with no evidence of foaming and only occasional surface cratering.

Because the principal difference between the sodium carbonate and the sodium chloride or sodium sulfate devices is the basicity of sodium carbonate, the unique behavior of the sodium carbonate devices is due to a lack of polymer erosion. Consequently, in these devices drug release is determined exclusively by the movement of a swelling front into the device, liberating the drug immobilized in the hydrophobic matrix. The linearity of the release rate indicates that at least in the early stages the rate-limiting process is the movement of the swelling front and not diffusion through the continuously increasing swollen polymer layer. The faster rate of a drug release from sodium chloride or sodium sulfate devices is probably due to erosion-aided water penetration into the matrix.

Current studies are aimed at the development of systems in which polymer erosion does not lag drug release, and a better understanding of the mechanism of polymer erosion and its relationship to drug release.

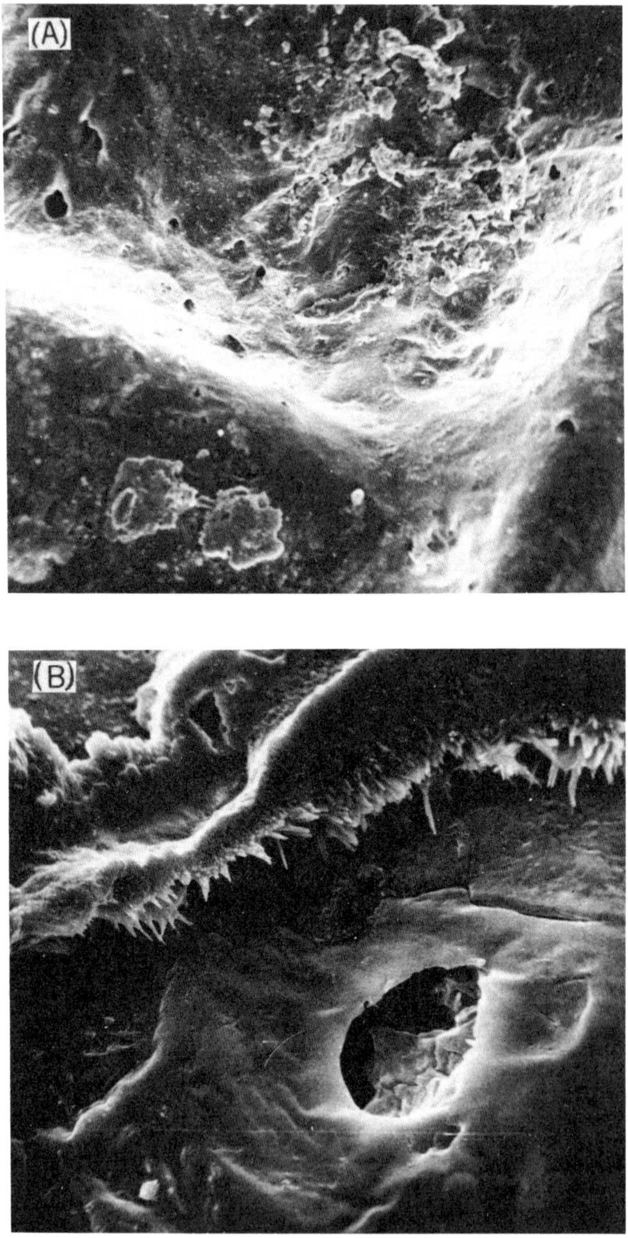

Figure 8 Scanning electron micrographs. (A) Na_2CO_3 device after 162 days, 100 x. (B) Na_2CO_3 device after 162 days, 1000 x.

ACKNOWLEDGMENT

This work was supported by the Contraceptive Development Branch, Center for Population Research, National Institute of Child Health and Human Development, NIH, under Contract NO1-HD-7-2826.

REFERENCES

1. J. Heller, *Biomaterials, 1*:51 (1980).
2. J. Heller and R. W. Baker, in *Controlled Release of Bioactive Materials* (R. W. Baker, ed.), Academic Press, New York, 1980, pp. 1-17.
3. J. Heller, D. W. H. Penhale, R. F. Helwing, B. K. Fritzinger, and R. W. Baker, in *Controlled Release Systems* (S. K. Chandrasekaran, ed.), AIChE Symp. Ser. No. 206, Vol. 77, New York, 1981, p. 28.
4. H. B. Hopfenberg and K. C. Hsu, *Polym. Eng. Sci., 18*:1186 (1978).
5. J. Heller, D. W. H. Penhale, R. F. Helwing, and B. K. Fritzinger, *Polym. Eng. Sci., 21*:727 (1981).
6. J. Heller, D. W. H. Penhale, and R. F. Helwing, *Polym. Lett. 18*: 619 (1980).
7. J. Heller, R. W. Baker, R. M. Gale, and J. O. Rodin, *J. Appl. Polym. Sci., 22*:1991 (1978).
8. R. F. Fedors, *Polymer, 21*:207 (1980).
9. N. Narkis and M. Narkis, *J. Appl. Polym. Sci., 20*:3431 (1976).

Chapter 6

Controlled Release from Glycosaminoglycan Drug Complexes

RANDALL V. SPARER, NNOCHIRI EKWURIBE, and ALAN G. WALTON*
Case Western Reserve University, Cleveland, Ohio

The concept of controlled release of pharmaceuticals can be described as either prolonging the action of drug over time by allowing continual release from a "depot" device [1-5], or increasing the bioavailability of the pharmacon through the formation of a prodrug [6,7] or targeting the drug to a given tissue with the use of a macromolecular carrier system [8,9].

There have been, however, studies where polymer-drug complexes have been synthesized, the major objective of which was to provide a controlled or prolonged action of the drug by the natural hydrolysis or biological scission of the covalent polymer-drug bond. The general assumption of this chemical approach to controlled release was that the polymer and the polymer-drug complex were pharmacologically inactive and the released drug was active over prolonged periods. In this way, mescaline [10], insulin [11], salicylic acid [12], D-isoproterenol [13], naloxone [14], plant cytokinins [15], 2,4-dichlorophenoxyacetic acid [16], norethindrone [17], and cortisol-21-acetate [18] have been attached to and released from various synthetic and natural polymers through covalent bonds such as amide [10,11], ester [12,16], azo [13], carbomate [15], carbonate [17], oxime ester [18], and hydrazone [14].

In this study we have chosen for the macromolecular carrier a class of natural polymers known as the glycosaminoglycans (GAG). They are water-soluble polysaccharides found in the ground substance of human and other animal connective tissues [19-21] and are highly charged linear polyanions having the general formula $(AB)_n$, where A

Present affiliation: University Genetics Company, Norwalk, Connecticut

is a uronic acid residue and B is a hexosamine (Fig. 1). The most abundant isomers are the chondroitin sulfates.

Glycosaminoglycans offer favorable attributes as drug carriers. These molecules are biocompatible. Subcutaneous injections of up to 1400 mg/kg in rats have proved to be nontoxic with no inflammatory response detected [22]. Since they are species-independent [23], they are nonimmunogenic. GAGs are biodegradable by enzymatic means normal to the host. It has been estimated that in humans, the GAGs are recycled in a period ranging from days to weeks [24]. Because they possess a variety of functional groups, different types of GAG-drug bonds may be formed.

We have taken advantage of the various types of functional groups available on the GAG backbone (carboxyl, primary and secondary hydroxyl, and sulfate) in preparing and testing a series of complexes

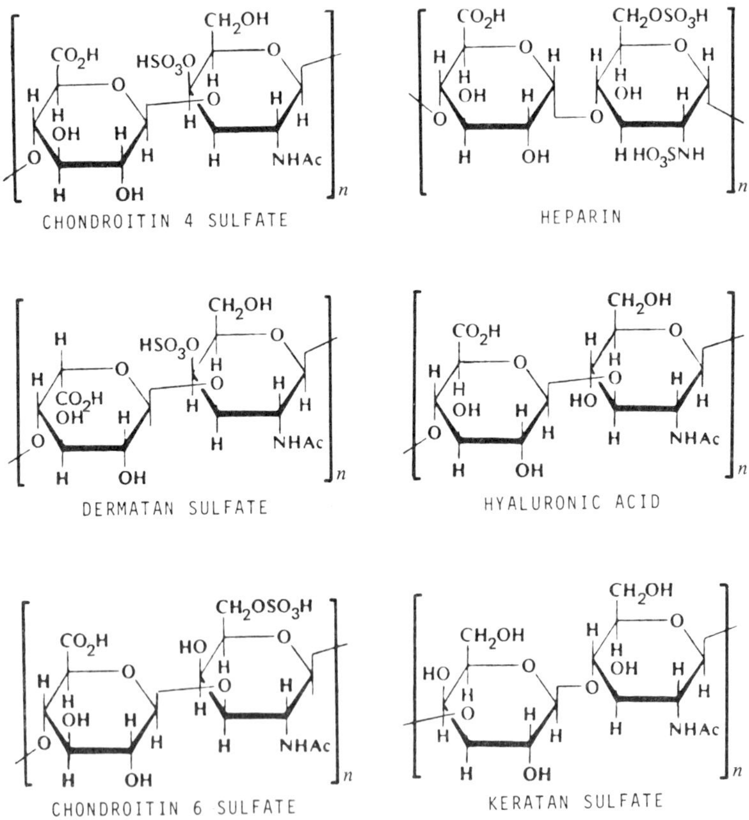

Figure 1 Glycosaminoglycan structures.

in which the drug was bound directly to the polymer or via an intermediate linking group such as an amino acid or other such bioacceptable entity.

This report describes the performance of amide- and ester-linked GAG drug complexes. Current work with other drugs bound to the GAG backbone by the same and different bond types (i.e., carbomate, ionic) will be reported in the near future.

EXPERIMENTAL

The GAGs chondroitin-4-sulfate (C4S), chondroitin-6-sulfate (C6S), and hyaluronic acid (HA) were purchased from Sigma Chemical Co. as the sodium salt. Dicyclohexylcarbodiimide (DCC), cysteine (Cys), and alanine (Ala) were obtained from Fisher Scientific Company. Carbobenzoxychloride and 4-pyrrolidinopyridine were obtained from Aldrich Chemical Company. Chloramphenicol (Cpl) and 1-ethyl-3,3-dimethylaminopropyl carbodiimide (EDC) were supplied by Sigma Chemical Co. Radiolabeled [^{14}C]chloramphenicol and [^{35}S]cystine were purchased from New England Nuclear.

Synthesis of [^{14}C]chloramphenicol-glycosaminoglycan (Cpl-GAG) ester complexes were carried out by linking a bioacceptable intermediate spacer group, alanine, between the drug (ester) and the polymer (amide). N-carbobenzoxy-L-alanine was made from L-alanine by the method of Bergmann and Zervas [25]. The Ala-Cpl ester was synthesized by dissolving ^{14}C-Cpl (12.906 g), N-carbobenzoxy-L-Ala (10.003 g), and 4-pyrrolidinopyridine (0.597 g) in anhydrous tetrahydrofuran (THF, 30 ml). A solution of dicyclohexylcarbodiimide (DCC, 8.660 g) in THF (15 ml) was added dropwise to the above with stirring at room temperature. After 17 hr, the insoluble dicyclohexylurea by-product was filtered off and the solvent stripped off in vacuo at 40°C to yield a yellow oil. The oil was taken up in dichloromethane (300 ml) and extracted three times with 200-ml portions each of water, 5% acetic acid, saturated sodium bicarbonate, and finally water. The organic layer was dried over magnesium sulfate and concentrated to about 20 ml. Addition of 30% HBr in acetic acid (40 ml) to this solution under anhydrous conditions at room temperature over a period of 2 hr cleaved the protecting group from the amino function of the alanine. Addition of a large excess (450 ml) of anhydrous ethyl ether precipitated the hydrobromide salt of the Ala-Cpl ester. Recrystallization from anhydrous DMF/ether yielded 18.693 g as a hygroscopic white powder (nuclear magnetic resonance in d_6-DMSO δ: 2.52, d, ester CH_2; infrared (KBr): 1735 cm^{-1}, ester C=O).

The salt of the ester-linked drug spacer (Ala-Cpl) produced above was amide-linked to GAGs as follows. The sodium salt of C6S (3.024 g) and [^{14}C]Cpl-Ala hydrobromide (5.173 g) was dissolved in 2:1 DMF/water (55 ml) and the pH was adjusted to 4.75. To this solution was added a solution of 1-ethyl-3,3-dimethylaminopropyl carbodiimide (EDC, 2.075 g) in 2:1 DMF/water (10 ml) slowly over a period of 1.5 hr, maintaining the pH at 4.75. After an additional 2 hr of stirring at room temperature, the solution was neutralized with dilute sodium hydroxide and then dialyzed extensively against water and lyophilized. The yield of C6S-Ala[^{14}C]Cpl prodrug was 3.890 g. Similar reactions were run with C4S (3.016 g) and [^{14}C]Cpl-Ala (5.133 g) in 55 ml 2:1 DMF/water, EDC (2.074 g) in 10 ml 2:1 DMF/water; and HA (650 mg) and [^{14}C]Cpl-Ala (1.260 g) in 80 ml 2:1 DMF/water, EDC (490 mg) in 5 ml 2:1 DMF/water, to yield 3.894 g of C4S-Ala[^{14}C]Cpl complex and 727 mg of HA-Ala[^{14}C]Cpl. Analysis by FTIR (KBr) showed the ester C=O at about 1735 cm^{-1} and a new amide C=O at about 1695 cm^{-1}. Scintillation counting showed 18.6% by weight chloramphenicol in the C6S prodrug, 19.4% in the C4S prodrug, and 6.7% in the HA prodrug.

In vitro hydrolysis of Cpl-GAG prodrugs prepared in this way were performed in a "physiological" solution containing 0.2 M NaCl and 0.05 M tris buffer (pH 7.4) at 37°C. Samples were dissolved in the solvent (5 ml) and placed in dialysis tubing to be "dialyzed" against 80 ml of the solvent. The ultraviolet (UV) absorbance of the dialysate was monitored at 274 nm.

Tests were carried out on the GAG[^{14}C]Cpl prodrugs by injecting the same as a solution in sterile saline (145 mg/ml) subcutaneously into the flanks of 350-g Sprague-Dawley female rats. The dosage of these and of a control group which received injections of chloramphenicol in 50% aqueous propyleneglycol was equivalent to 200 mg of chloramphenicol per kilogram of rat body weight. Urine and feces were assayed by standard liquid scintillation techniques. Small (2-ml) blood samples were drawn once via intraorbital bleeding for radiolabel counting and to assay for active chloramphenicol against *Sarcina lutea* (ATCC 9341) by standard methods [37].

The synthesis of amide-linked GAG-cysteine materials followed in general the procedure of Danishefsky and Siskovic [29]. S-Ethylthiocysteine methyl ester was made from known procedures [26,27] from [^{35}S]cystine. To a solution of the sodium salt of C4S (180.0 mg) in water (5 ml) was added radiolabeled S-ethylthiocysteine methyl ester (108.0 mg) and EDC (151.6 mg). The pH was kept at 4.75 for 7 hr by the addition of 0.1 M HCl. The pH was then brought to 8 with dilute NaOH and dithiothreitol (89.2 mg) was added to cleave the S-protecting group of cysteine. After 12 hr the solution was neutralized, dialyzed extensively, and lyophilized, yielding 157.0 mg of pure C4S-Cys. Scintillation counting showed 31% of the carboxyls of C4S to be derivatized with cysteine. FTIR analysis detected a new amide band at 1696 cm^{-1}, and no methyl ester. Crosslinking of this material through the sulfhydryl groups of cysteine was typically accomplished by dissolving the C4S-Cys material in a pH 8 buffer at a concentration of about 350 mg/ml; after sitting overnight at 10°C in an atmosphere of oxygen, the solution gelled.

The in vivo release of cysteine from the aforementioned gelled material was tested in 200-g Sprague-Dawley male cats. Gel pieces were crushed and injected subcutaneously into the rat flank as a slurry in sterile saline. Urine and feces were assayed by standard liquid scintillation techniques. Autoradiographic analysis of one of the rats was performed by Arthur D. Little, Inc., Cambridge, Massachusetts, 53 days after the injection.

In vitro enzymatic digestion of derivatized GAG-Cys materials (gelled and ungelled) followed essentially the procedure of Yamagata et al. [28]. Approximately 1 mg of C4S-Cys was either dissolved or suspended in 1 ml of a tris pH 7.4 buffer at 37°C containing 0.01 unit of chondroitinase ABC (NCTC 4636, Miles Biochemical). The course of the reaction was followed by the increase in UV absorbance at 232 nm and standardized against pure C4S.

RESULTS AND DISCUSSION

The amino acid cysteine and the antibiotic chloramphenicol were utilized in forming amide- and ester-linked GAG complexes, respectively. The in vitro and/or in vivo release of cysteine or chloramphenicol was monitored in order to assess the effect of the chemical bond type on the kinetics of release. Amide and ester bond types were chosen because both are susceptible to chemical hydrolysis and both are prevalent naturally and thus are potentially dependable by enzymes.

Chloramphenicol has been attached to various GAGs via an ester linkage to the spacer group alanine, which was itself amide-linked to the GAG; the drug has also been directly bonded to the GAG by an ester bond (Fig. 2). Ester derivatization of the carboxyl groups of GAGs was possible by most classical methods (acid halide, mixed anhydride, carbodiimide, etc.) in polar organic (DMF, DMSO) or aqueous solvents, but we have determined that amide formation in H_2O/DMF with a carbodiimide was a particularly facile method of derivatizing the carboxyl groups of GAGs. Even though chloramphenicol could be ester linked directly to the polymer, somewhat higher loadings of chloramphenicol were obtained by using the alanine spacer; thus our attention has focused on this type of linking system for this drug complex.

Danishefsky and Siskovic have shown that certain amino acids, such as glycine, phenylalanine, and glycylphenylalanine, can be amide-linked to a GAG with a water-soluble carbodiimide [29]. We have expanded on this mild, facile procedure to include drugs and spacer groups (i.e., amino acids and other difunctional amine-carrying molecules). As a model of an amide-linked GAG complex, the amino acid cysteine was chosen as the agent to be released. The reasons for this were threefold: (1) attachment of cysteine facilitates the synthesis of a natural disulfide crosslink, which may affect the release rate; (2) cysteine as an intermediate spacer provides a sulfhydryl group for

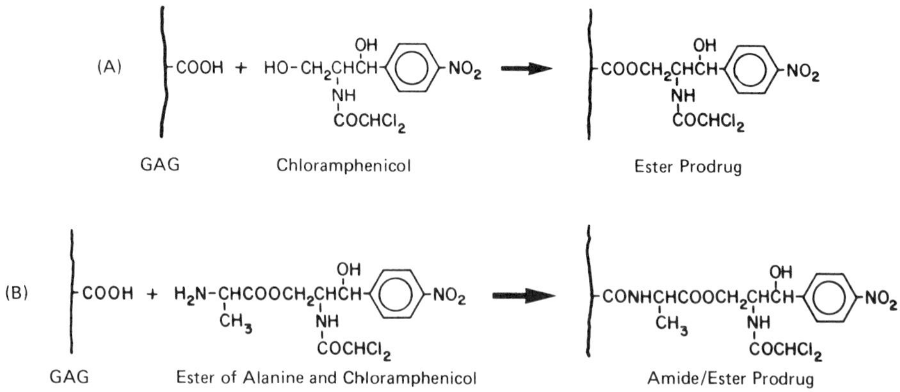

Figure 2 Covalent attachment of chloramphenicol: (A) directly to the GAG backbone, or (B) through the intermediate linking group alanine. The ester bond is formed through the primary hydroxyl of the chloramphenicol.

thioester or disulfide linkages to drugs; and (3) the GAG-Cys system, which has no inherent therapeutic value, acts as a model for amide-linked GAG-anticancer agent prodrugs. Based on these results, we are now studying such amide-linked GAG complexes of adriamycin and methotrexate.

The chemistry of attachment of cysteine to a GAG is outlined in Fig. 3. Cysteine-derivatized GAGs have been synthesized with loading values ranging from 5 to 87% of the GAG carboxyls substituted, and the mild and reversible oxidation of these to form crosslinked GAG hydrogels with various physical properties has been investigated [30]. Further studies have shown these materials to be biocompatible and biodegradable.

The in vitro release profile of C6S-Ala-Cpl prodrug in a "physiological" buffer appears in Fig. 4. The release was pseudo-first order

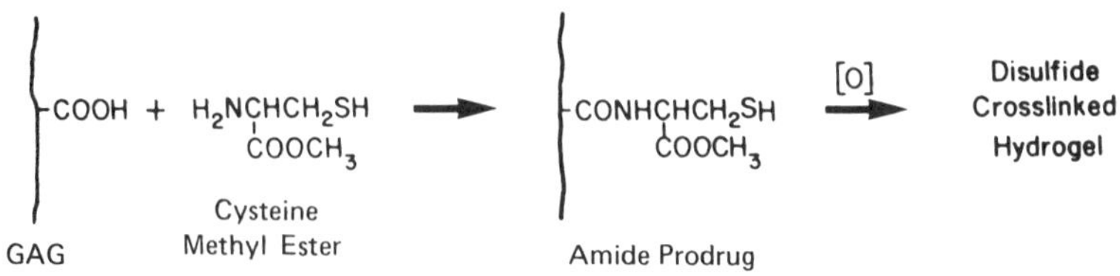

Figure 3 Covalent attachment of cysteine to a GAG backbone. Disulfide-crosslinked hydrogels can be formed from concentrated solutions of GAG-Cys complexes under mild oxidizing conditions.

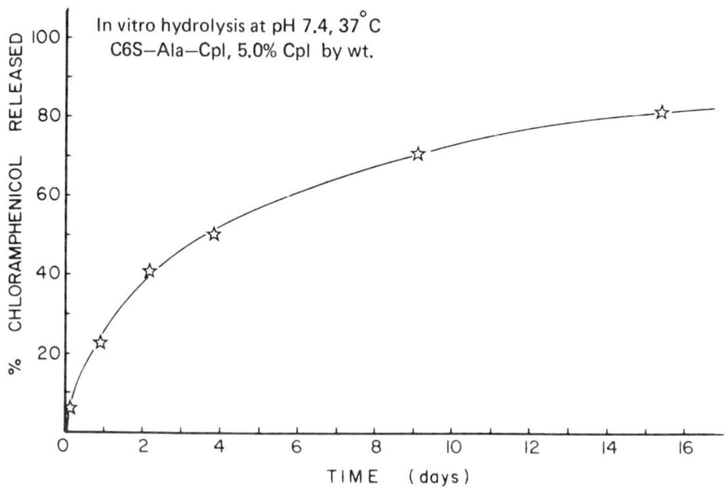

Figure 4 In vitro release of [^{14}C]chloramphenicol from a C6S-Ala-Cpl complex. The drug was released into a 0.05 M sodium phosphate buffer (containing 0.2 M sodium chloride) at pH 7.4 and 37°C.

with a release rate constant of 0.10 day^{-1} and a half-life of 3.8 days. This is what one would expect if the rate-determining step for release is the chemical hydrolysis of the ester bond in the prodrug. The amide bond between the GAG and alanine is expected to hydrolyze much more slowly than the ester under these conditions. Actually, cysteine-GAG complexes hydrolyzed only slightly during 4 days under the same conditions.

The rate of release of [^{14}C]chloramphenicol from various GAG-Ala-Cpl complexes as injected subcutaneously into rats is shown in Table 1. Whereas the polymer formulations prolonged the release over a period of days, the unconjugated drug administered in the same way was cleared within 24 hr, as expected [31]. The rate of release from the C4S and C6S complexes was similar, but release from the HA complex was faster. This could be due to the fact that hyaluronic acid is architecturally somewhat different from the chondroitin sulfates and thus provided a different microenvironment for hydrolysis of the complex. HA is not sulfated and therefore is not as highly charged as C4S or C6S. HA also has a higher molecular weight than the chondroitin sulfates [21]. Reactions on polymers, such as the hydrolytic cleavage of GAG-drug bonds, has been shown to be affected by polymer chain length and conformation, steric isolation, and neighboring group effects [32]. Furthermore, since more of the carboxyl groups on the HA formulation were left underivatized, the free acidic

Table 1 In Vivo Appearance of Chloramphenicol (%) in the Rat

Day	C4S	C6S	HA	Control
0.5	22	23	43	80
1	52	57	69	100
2	80	83	84	
3	87	89	88	
5	92	94	92	
7	94	96	94	
14	97	98	97	

functions contributed by carboxyl groups may have had an autocatalyzing effect on these prodrugs. Autocatalysis of the hydrolysis of poly(acrylate esters) has been observed by Plate [33] and by Harris et al. [16]. The effect of loading on in vitro release rate is presently being investigated with GAG-Cpl drug complexes.

In vivo release rates were found to be somewhat quicker than those in vitro. The in vivo half-lives for the formulations were as follows: C4S and C6S complexes, 24 hr; HA complex, 14 hr; free Cpl, 3 hr. Comparison to the in vitro hydrolysis of a C6S complex (Fig. 4) shows that the half-life of the ester bond is expected to be 3.8 days. Therefore, there must have been enzymatic processing of the GAG-Cpl complex in the rat. This is not surprising, since the rat possesses an esterase capable of hydrolyzing chloramphenicol palmitate to free chloramphenicol [34].

Microbiological assays of blood samples taken from the same group of rats after the injections of free drug or complex showed efficacious levels of active chloramphenicol. Radiolabel counting of the blood samples gave an estimate of the total amount of drug in the blood. These data appear in Table 2. It is not surprising that only a small part of the total chloramphenicol in the blood was active since chloramphenicol is readily inactivated in the rat [35]. The presence of active Cpl in the complex-injected rats' blood indicates that hydrolysis of the ester bond occurred, since the ester-linked complexes before hydrolysis exhibited only very low levels of antibiotic activity.

In contrast to the chloramphenicol ester complexes, the cysteine amide complexes released much more slowly in vivo. Figure 5 shows the release profile of a subcutaneously injected C4S[^{35}S]Cys cross-linked material in the rat. The radiolabel appeared in the urine at a rate of approximately 0.2% per day and was relatively constant over a period of 5 months.

Table 2 Microbiological Assay for Active Chloramphenicol Levels and Radiolabel Counting for Total Chloramphenicol Levels in Rat Blood

Sample injected	Time after injection (hr)	Chloramphenicol plasma concentration (g/ml)	
		Active	Total
Cpl	5	37.5	325
C6S-Ala-Cpl	23	17.5	390
C4S-Ala-Cpl	22.5	22.5	485

Even though the amide bond between the drug and the polymer may hydrolyze slowly over this period and release cysteine, the rate-determining step for release was probably enzymatic breakdown of the complex. Since chondroitinases and other endoglycosidases are present at the injection site, a normal constant turnover of the complex is to be expected if such complexes can act as substrates for the enzymes.

To test this hypothesis, we have examined the interaction of chondroitinase ABC with C4S-Cys materials [36]. What was determined was that (1) the enzyme partially degraded the backbone of the C4S-Cys, (2) the degree of digestion by the enzyme was directly proportional to the degree of derivatization of C4S by Cys, (3) there was a limiting, average "space" between two derivatized disaccharide units needed for endoglycosidase activity (five underivatized consecutive repeat units), and (4) crosslinked C4S-Cys gels were also degraded, but at somewhat slower rates than uncrosslinked C4S-Cys solutions. What was not as yet examined was possible proteolytic cleavage of the GAG-Cys amide bond.

Thus, in general, amide-linked GAG complexes may be broken down by native glycosidases or proteases in vivo, producing a nearly constant rate of release which is governed by the host's steady-state GAG turnover rate. An initial burst period, as in Fig. 5, may have been due to increased concentrations of phagocytic enzymes and cells associated with the normal wound-healing process.

A large advantage of using glycosaminoglycans as drug carriers is that they are biocompatible and biodegradable. There is sufficient evidence to show that no unwanted toxic side effects or inflammatory effects have been evoked by these complexes, much unlike many other synthetic or natural polymer-based drug release systems. In fact, histologic evaluation of the implant sites of the rats injected with either cysteine or chloramphenicol complexes has shown no difference in the inflammatory response when compared with a sham wound.

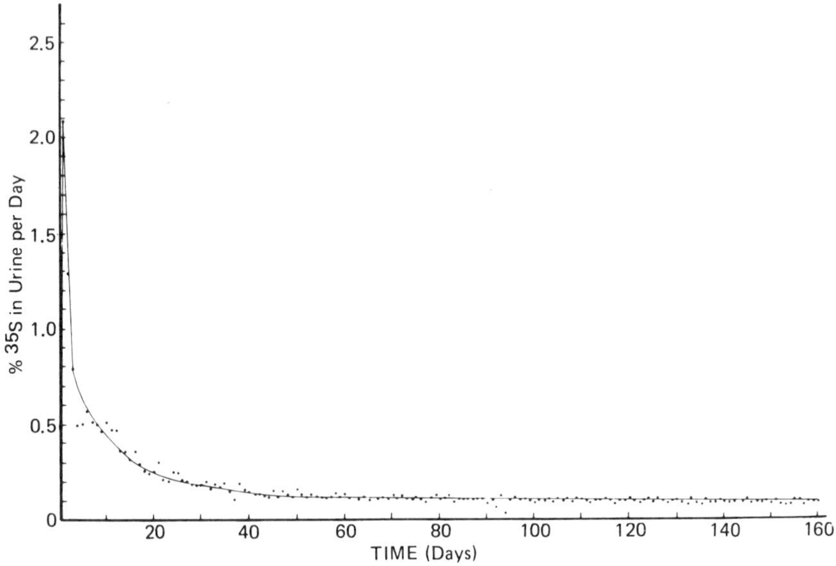

Figure 5 In vivo release of [^{35}S]cysteine from a subcutaneous injection of a C4S-Cys model amide complex in the rat.

Autoradiographic analysis of rats containing GAG[^{35}S]Cys indicated that the complex was resorbable but was not retained in the tissues or organs, with the exception of a small amount in the kidneys. Examination of the implant site of the rats containing GAG[^{14}C]Cpl 14 days after subcutaneous administration showed that the complex had been resorbed. Indeed, rats injected with the same dosage of free chloramphenicol were initially lethargic and exhibited some of the signs of chloramphenicol overdose (low white cell counts), but the rats injected with complex appeared healthy throughout the duration of the experiment. We are investigating this phenomenon, with the hope of using GAG complexes to allow larger doses of Cpl to be given without eliciting toxic responses.

SUMMARY AND CONCLUSIONS

It is fairly clear that release rates and mechanisms for the amide and ester complexes outlined above differed, although detailed studies of GAG-drug metabolism have not been performed. Chloramphenicol-GAG ester complexes released Cpl quickly by scission of the ester bond. Cysteine-GAG amide complexes degraded much more slowly and probably through enzymatic hydrolysis of the polymer or polymer-drug bond.

It has been demonstrated that the ester complexes regenerated active drug; however, the nature of the entity released from amide complexes was not entirely clear. From studies with chondroitinase ABC the initial cleavage produces an oligomeric GAG-Cys complex, the oligomers containing about five disaccharide residues on the average. Further enzymatic degradation of this complex may either reduce the size of the oligomer by glycosidic hydrolysis, or release the Cys by proteolytic hydrolysis. Thus free drug or drug-GAG oligomers, or both, are expected to be the metabolic products from this form of release. If the oligomeric GAG-drug complex cannot be degraded further before clearance, it is desired to have the drug remain active while still attached to the GAG oligomer. In fact, we have synthesized penicillin (from 6-aminopenicillanic acid), methotrexate, and adriamycin amide-linked GAGs and have found that these drugs retain their activity while linked to the polymer.

In contrast to ester complexes, which were released quickly (rates of release approximating first-order kinetic hydrolysis of the ester bond), the release rate from amide complexes was much slower and gave a prolonged constant rate of release. It would be ideal to obtain zero-order release in all cases, and still be able to vary the rate of release to fit the required dosage regimen. It has been shown that the release rate can be varied with GAG complexes by selecting a given polymer-drug bond but that zero-order release is not yet possible with all formulations. Nevertheless, this concept provides an interesting base from which to design a drug release system; the rate of release may in principle be engineered by the judicious choice of drug-GAG bond based on the hydrolytic stability of the bond.

ACKNOWLEDGMENT

The authors wish to express their gratitude to Valcor Scientific Ltd. for support throughout this work.

REFERENCES

1. A. C. Tanquary and R. E. Lacey, eds., *Controlled Release of Biologically Active Agents*, Adv. Exp. Med. Biol., Vol. 47, Plenum Press, New York, 1974.
2. D. R. Paul and F. W. Harris, eds., *Controlled Release Polymeric Formulations*, ACS Symp. Ser. No. 33, American Chemical Society, Washington, D.C., 1976.
3. R. J. Kostelnik, ed., *Polymeric Delivery Systems*, Midland Macromolecular Monographs, Vol. 5, Gordon and Breach, New York, 1978.
4. J. R. Robinson, ed., *Sustained and Controlled Release Drug Delivery Systems*, Marcel Dekker, New York, 1978.

5. R. L. Juliano, ed., *Drug Delivery Systems*, Oxford University Press, New York, 1980.
6. A. A. Sinkula, in *Sustained and Controlled Release Drug Delivery Systems* (J. R. Robinson, ed.), Marcel Dekker, New York, 1978, pp. 411-555.
7. T. Higuchi and V. Stella, eds., *Pro-drugs as Novel Delivery Systems*, ACS Symp. Ser. No. 14, American Chemical Society, Washington, D.C., 1975.
8. G. Gregoriadis, ed., *Drug Carriers in Biology and Medicine*, Academic Press, New York, 1979.
9. M. J. Poznansky and L. G. Cleland, in *Drug Delivery Systems* (R. L. Juliano, ed.), Oxford University Press, New York, 1980, p. 253.
10. H. Jatzkewitz, *Z. Naturforsch.*, *10*:27 (1955).
11. D. M. Kramer and K. Lehmann, *FEBS Lett.*, *22*:49 (1972).
12. B. Weiner and A. Zilkha, *Isr. J. Chem.*, *11*:567 (1973).
13. J. C. Venter, M. S. Verlander, N. O. Kaplan, M. Goodman, J. Ross, Jr., and S. Sesayama, in *Polymeric Delivery Systems* (R. J. Kostelnik, ed.), Gordon and Breach, New York, 1978, p. 237.
14. G. W. Pasternak, S. C. March, et al., *Life Sci.*, *18*:977 (1976).
15. S. Bittner, I. Perry, and Y. Knobler, *Phytochemistry*, *16*:305 (1977).
16. F. W. Harris, M. R. Dykes, et al., in *Controlled Release Pesticides* (H. B. Scher, ed.), ACS Symp. Ser. No. 53, American Chemical Society, Washington, D.C., 1977, p. 102.
17. D. Gregonis, J. Feijen, J. M. Anderson, and R. V. Peterson, *Polym. Prepr., Am. Chem. Soc., Div. Copolym. Chem.*, *21*:612 (1979).
18. N. Tani, M. Van Dress, and J. M. Anderson, *Controlled Release of Pesticides and Pharmaceuticals* (D. H. Lewis, ed.), Plenum, New York, 1980, p. 79.
19. R. W. Jeanloz, in *The Carbohydrates, Chemistry and Biochemistry* (W. Pigman and D. Horton, eds.), Academic Press, New York, 1970, pp. 589-625.
20. S. I. Lamberg and A. C. Stoolmiller, *J. Invest. Dermatol.*, *63*: 433 (1974).
21. A. Serafini-Francansini and J. Smith, eds., *The Structure and Biochemistry of Cartilage*, Churchill Livingstone, London, 1974, pp. 64-112.
22. R. V. Sparer, unpublished.
23. O. M. S. Toledo and C. P. Dietrich, *Biochim. Biophys. Acta*, *498*:114 (1977).
24. A. Wasteson, U. Lindahl, and A. Hallen, *Biochim. J.*, *130*:729 (1972).
25. M. Bergmann and L. Zervas, *Ber. Deutsch. Chem. Ges.*, *65*:1192 (1932).

26. J. R. Rachele, *J. Org. Chem.*, *28*:2898 (1963).
27. L. D. Small, J. H. Bailey, and C. J. Cavallito, *J. Am. Chem. Soc.*, *69*:1710 (1947).
28. T. Yamagata, H. Saito, O. Habuchi, and S. Suzuki, *J. Biol. Chem.*, *243*:1523 (1968).
29. I. Danishefsky and E. Siskovic, *Carbohyd. Res.*, *16*:199 (1971).
30. R. V. Sparer, M.S. thesis, Case Western Reserve University, 1980.
31. A. J. Glazko, L. M. Wolf, W. A. Dill, and A. C. Bratton, Jr., *J. Pharmacol. Exp. Ther.*, *96*:455 (1949).
32. E. M. Fettes, ed., *Chemical Reactions of Polymers*, Wiley-Interscience, New York, 1964.
33. N. A. Plate, *Pure Appl. Chem.*, *46*:49 (1976).
34. A. J. Glazko, W. H. Edgerton, W. A. Dill, and W. R. Lenz, *Antibiot. Chemother.*, *2*:234 (1952).
35. A. J. Glazko, W. A. Dill, and L. M. Wolf, *J. Pharmacol. Exp. Ther.*, *104*:452 (1952).
36. R. V. Sparer, D. Telford, and F. Wilcox, unpublished.
37. Code 21 of Federal Regulations, Subpart D, paragraphs 436.100 to 436.105 inclusive, revised April 1, 1976.

Chapter 7

Zero-Order Drug Delivery Systems with Magnetic Control

DEAN S. T. HSIEH* Harvard Medical School and Children's Hospital Medical Center, Boston, Massachusetts

ROBERT LANGER Massachusetts Institute of Technology, Cambridge, Massachusetts

Many physiological relevant agents such as insulin and other hormones from endocrine organs are released in a *modulated* fashion upon feeding, stimulus, or stress. For example, insulin is released from the pancreas of normal subjects 30-60 min after a meal is ingested. Evidently, a rising glucose level is accompanied by a prompt rise in insulin. This explains why in most humans, blood sugar after meals rarely rises above normal, whereas in diabetics, blood sugar levels become very high because the secretion of insulin from the pancreas is dysfunctional [1]. The prevalent way to control blood glucose is the use of subcutaneous insulin injections daily by diabetics. However, this approach often leads to poor control of blood glucose, which in turn may cause secondary complications such as retinopathy, neuropathy, nephropathy, and heart disease [2]. Because of these problems, as well as the inconvenience of daily shots, much effort has been devoted to improving insulin treatment regimens, such as the development of mechanical insulin infusion pumps [3-13].

While these infusion systems offer considerable promise as a practical alternative to daily shots, they also result in difficulties such as (1) thrombosis formation at the catheter area, necessitating frequent change of catheter sites; (2) possible infection at the catheter area; (3) bulkiness and expense; and (4) relatively short periods of insulin delivery (although this problem is often compensated for by the fact that some of these systems are refillable).

**Present affiliation:* College of Pharmacy of Rutgers, The State University of New Jersey, Piscataway, New Jersey

Initial studies in our laboratory have demonstrated effective blood glucose control in rats by means of small polymer pellets impregnated with insulin implanted subcutaneously [14]. Blood sugar levels fell from 400 mg/dl in diabetic rats to the normal 100 mg/dl in treated rats. Urine sugar was also eliminated. Body weight increased normally in the treated rats. A single polymer pellet maintained blood sugar levels stable for 1 month. Contrary to mechanical insulin infusion pumps, the major advantages of implantable polymers are: (1) a small volume of polymer can be impregnated with a large quantity of powdered insulin (e.g., a 0.03-cm^3 polymer can contain over 5000 units of insulin); (2) the cost of polymer material is inexpensive; and (3) the fabrication method is simple. However, the development of these polymer systems is at a much earlier stage and much work must be done before their use as a practical alternative can be evaluated. One major problem has been that all approaches thus far developed for implantable diffusion-controlled polymeric delivery systems result in systems which display either constant or decreasing release rates with increasing time [15-19]. There has been no way to change or modulate the release rate *on demand*, once release has been commenced. It may be desirable to have a drug delivery system in which release rates can be rhythmatically controlled *on demand* by those who suffer from the dysfunction of endocrine systems. In an earlier report, we demonstrated that by embedding small magnetic steel beads in a polymer matrix together with the drug, release rates can be increased when desired by an oscillating external bar magnet [20].

In that report, controlled release systems were made by incorporating bovine serum albumin (aggregate size ranged from 150 to 180 μm) and magnetic steel beads (1.4 mm in diameter) in an ethylene-vinyl acetate copolymer matrix in the form of a slab. When exposed to aqueous medium the polymer matrix released the albumin slowly and continuously. Application of an oscillating magnetic field increased the release rate by as much as 100%. It was speculated that the oscillating magnetic field caused alternating compression and expansion of small pores containing the drugs, thereby "squeezing" the drug out of the matrix. However, the precise mechanism of magnetic action is currently under investigation. Intervals of 6-hr periods of magnetic exposure and nonexposure were alternated over a 5-day period, resulting in corresponding increases and decreases in release and establishing a pattern of modulated sustained release. The problems associated with this system were: (1) the release decreased with time because the polymer matrix was fabricated in the shape of a slab, and (2) the release rates occurring during triggering periods were at most only threefold larger than those occurring during nontriggering periods.

To achieve constant release from diffusion-controlled matrix devices, we have previously proposed that optimal results can be obtained with a hemisphere-shaped system that is laminated with an impermeable coating except for a small cavity in the center face [17]. Since the release rate is inversely proportional to the drug diffusion distance from the release surface, the principle of altering matrix geometry is to increase the available area of drug so as to compensate for the increase in the drug diffusion distance [21]. Experiments were further designed to prove the theoretical analysis [19] and to develop simple fabrication procedures for releasing high molecular weight drugs at a constant rate [21]. Recently, we have shown that a hemisphere-shaped device made of ethylene-vinyl acetate copolymer and bovine serum albumin (BSA) can deliver BSA at a constant rate of 0.5 mg/day for 60 days [21].

In the present study, we have investigated a hemispheric magnetic system (Fig. 1) which combines an appropriate geometric design to achieve a constant baseline level release rate with the magnetically modulated system to obtain a burst of release upon triggering. We report here the fabrication procedures for constructing such a hemispheric magnetic device and also discuss results which further demonstrate the principle of modulated release of drugs controlled by magnetism.

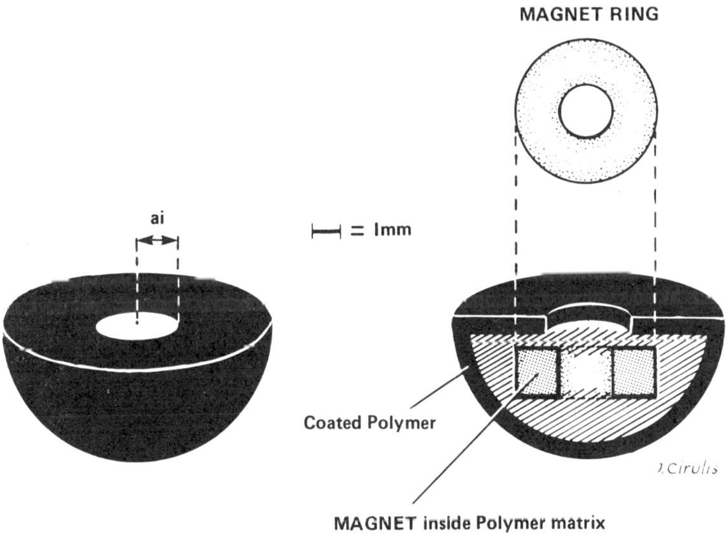

Figure 1 Schematic diagram of a hemispheric magnetic pellet. The polymer matrix was made of ethylene-vinyl acetate copolymer (Elvax 40). All sides were coated with pure polymer except the cavity on the flat surface. Drugs were forced to release from this cavity, shown by the white area of the pellet (left side).

MATERIALS AND METHODS

Materials

Three different proteins, bovine serum albumin (mol wt 69,000), pepsin (mol wt 21,000), and insulin (mol wt 6500) were used in this study. Bovine serum albumin (BSA) and pepsin were obtained from Sigma Chemical Co. (St. Louis, Missouri) and sieved to obtain aggregate sizes ranging from 150 to 180 μm. Sodium insulin, obtained from Elanco Co. (Indianapolis, Indiana), was first agglomerated by adding distilled water in the ratio 4 ml to 1 g of insulin, then lyophilized, and finally sieved to obtain aggregate sizes from 150 to 180 μm. Ethylene-vinyl acetate copolymer (Elvax 40) was obtained from DuPont Chemical Co. (Wilmington, Delaware). A 10% (w/v) polymer solution was made in methylene chloride. Magnets in the shape of hollow cylinders with dimensions of 3 mm OD × 1.5 mm ID × 1.5 mm height were purchased from Permag Northeast Co. (Billerica, Massachusetts).

The molds used for fabricating hemispheric magnetic devices were composed of glass and had a hemispheric bottom (13 mm diameter × 11 mm height). These molds were made from glass test tubes by cutting off the bottoms. To prevent these molds from falling over, an embedding platform was made. This platform was constructed by pouring 15 ml of molten Paraplast into a bacterial petri dish, and then placing empty glass molds into the Paraplast so that they touched bottom. After allowing the Paraplast to harden, the molds were removed and the indentations left behind in the Paraplast could be used subsequently to support the molds (Fig. 2).

Fabrication Procedures

The procedure for preparing the hemispheric magnetic system was adapted from earlier procedures [20,21] and consists of four stages: (1) casting, (2) drying, (3) coating, and (4) opening a cavity. The rationale for the precise procedures used (e.g., the temperatures used in the drying steps) can be found in those earlier papers [17,20,21]. The procedure is shown schematically in Fig. 3 and described in detail below.

Casting A layer of protein-polymer mixture was cast in a glass mold with a hemispheric bottom (13 mm OD × 11 mm ID × 11 mm height) placed on a block of dry ice. The protein loading was one-third of the mixture (w/w). A single hollow-cylinder magnet (3 mm OD × 1.5 mm ID × 1,5 mm height) was then placed in the center after waiting for 1 min. Another layer of protein-polymer mixture identical to the first layer was immediately cast onto it. Controlling the casting time is important to prevent the magnet from settling out and so that the two layers of protein-polymer mixture adhere tightly.

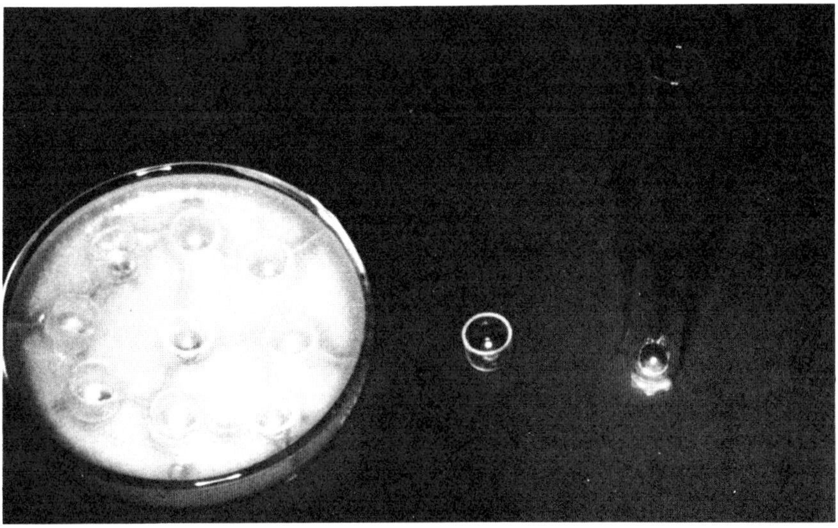

Figure 2 A glass mold (center) having a hemispheric bottom was made from a glass tube (far right) by cutting off the bottom. An embedding platform was constructed with paraffin in a bacterial petri dish (far left). (From Ref. 21.)

Drying The hemispheric magnetic pellet was dried in a freezer (-20°C) for 2 days followed by drying in a desiccator (20°C) under a houseline vacuum (600 mTorr) for 2 days [17]. The finished pellet was approximately 6 mm in height and 8 mm in diameter. Its composition was approximately 51.5 mg of protein, 103. mg of polymer, and 71.6 mg of magnet.

Coating The hemispheric pellets were twice coated with 20% EVA solution (containing no macromolecules) to form an impermeable barrier. (Several coats of concentrated EVA solutions containing *no* macromolecules have been shown to form impermeable barriers [21].) The coating procedure is described as follows:

1. The tip of a cylindrical metal stick (1.8 mm diameter × 30 mm length) was inserted into the center of the flat surface of each hemisphere pellet to a depth of approximately 3 mm.
2. Using the uninserted portion of the stick as a handle, the hemisphere pellets were placed directly on the surface of a block of dry ice for 10 min. (The round bottoms of the pellets were touching the dry ice.)

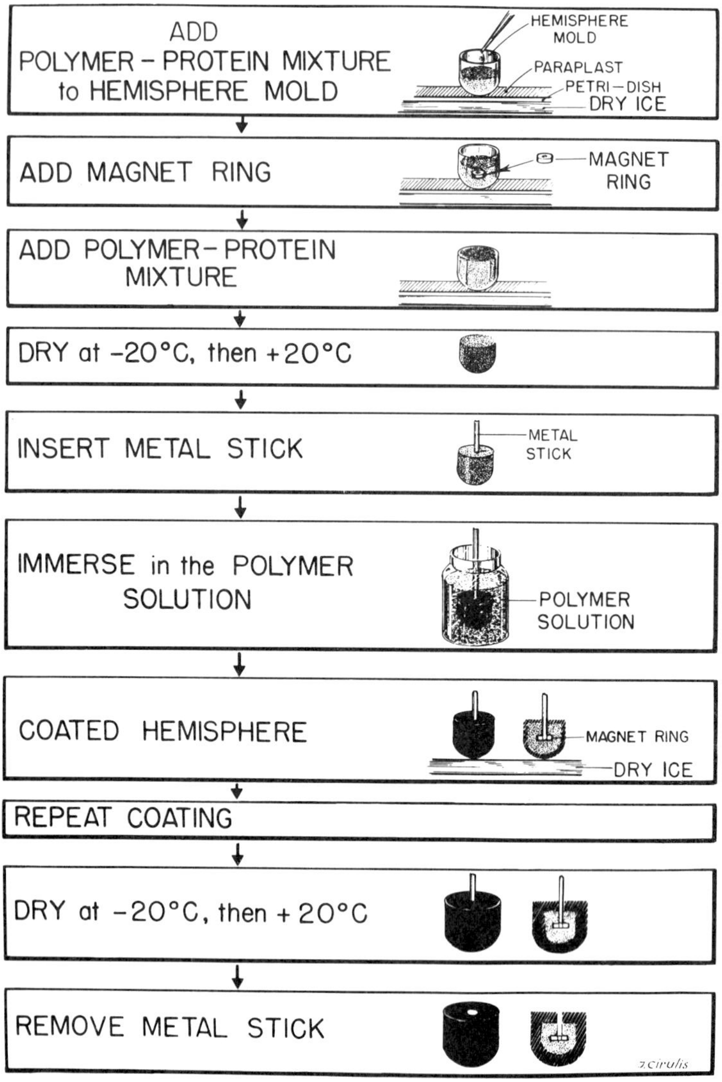

Figure 3 Procedures for making hemispheric magnetic pellets.

3. Again using the metal stick as a handle, the cooled hemisphere was then immersed into 20% EVA solution at 20°C for 10 sec, removed, and then placed immediately on the same dry ice for 10 min.
4. A second layer of coating was done in the same manner as described above.

5. The hemispheres were then put in the freezer (-20°C) for 2 days, followed by further drying at 20°C for 2 days in a desiccator under a houseline vacuum (600 mTorr) to remove residual solvent [17].

Opening a Cavity To create the exposed cavity in the face of the hemisphere pellet, the metal stick was removed by gently encircling the polymer surface immediately surrounding the stick with a scalpel blade. The resulting polymer pellet now appears as shown schematically in Fig. 1.

Kinetic Study

Setup for Release Study To deter motion of the hemispheric magnetic pellets during magnetic triggering, the hemispheric magnetic pellet was fixed and positioned in a plastic tube made of a 10-ml disposable serological pipet (Fig. 4). The flat surface of the hemisphere was toward the outside of the plastic tube and the depth of the insertion of it was about 3 mm. A layer of melted Paraplast (Lancer Co., St. Louis, Missouri) was pipetted onto the pellet inside the tube. The plastic tube was then passed through an opening of a lid of a scintillation vial (Wheaton Scientific Co., Mill ville, New Jersey). Ten milliliters of saline was added as a release medium. The sample was then subjected to alternative triggering and nontriggering for given time intervals.

Triggering Device A triggering device consisting of a motor-driven rotating table with two magnets was employed to create an oscillating magnetic field. Samples were held in slots above the rotating table. The details of the preparation of this table will be discussed in a subsequent report [22].

Triggering The samples were placed in the sample slots on the rotating table prior to triggering. After triggering for a given time (e.g., 5 hr) the sample was transferred into 10 ml of fresh saline solution and placed on a lab bench (not exposed to a magnetic field) for a 19-hr nontriggering period. Before the next triggering, samples were transferred into 10 ml of fresh saline solution and placed onto the triggering device again. The whole experiment was performed at 37°C. The quantity of protein in the released solution was determined by measuring its absorbance with an ultraviolet spectrophotometer at 220 nm [17]. Controls received the same treatment but without exposure to the magnetic field.

RESULTS AND DISCUSSION

In the present study, we have investigated a hemispheric magnetic system which combines a geometric design to achieve a constant baseline level release rate with the magnetically modulated system to obtain

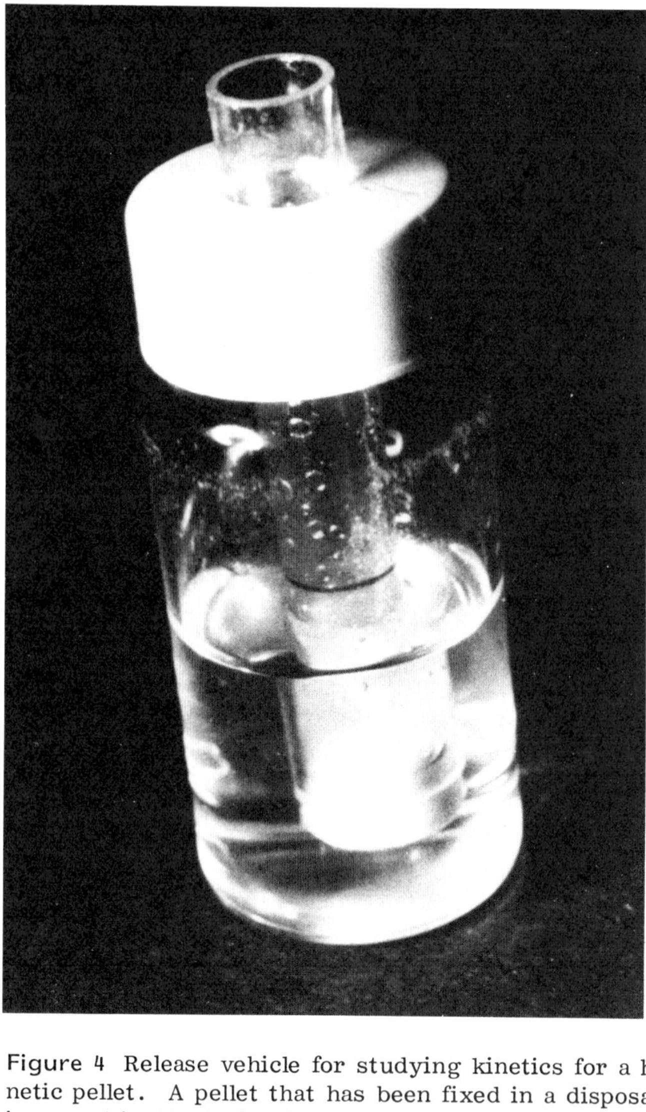

Figure 4 Release vehicle for studying kinetics for a hemispheric magnetic pellet. A pellet that has been fixed in a disposable pellet was immersed in 10 ml of saline solution in a scintillation vial.

a burst of release upon triggering. Three simulated drugs, bovine serum albumin, pepsin, and insulin, were used as model compounds to demonstrate the feasibility of magnetic modulation with this design. The results showed that the average baseline release rates were 14.8, 19.4, and 9.7 μg/hr for BSA, pepsin, and insulin, respectively; and the average burst of modulated release rates were 424.1, 248, and 36.8 μg/hr (Figs. 5-7), respectively. This represents a 29-fold increase (BSA), 13-fold increase (pepsin), and a 4-fold increase (insulin). The systems could delivery drugs for 1 month and the burst of release could be repeatedly modulated when desired. The control pellets which were not exposed to the magnetic field delivered drugs at a constant baseline level release rate without significant fluctuations (Fig. 8).

The major advance of the present study is the use of a hemispheric device impregnated with drug and a single magnetic ring to provide a nearly constant baseline release rate in the absence of a magnetic field and a much higher release rate in the presence of a magnetic field.

The major problem encountered so far in this study is irreproducibilities both with respect to differences in release rates among different pellets within a given triggering period (about 60%) and among the same pellets within different triggering periods (about 54%). The possible causes leading to these irreproducibilities may result from the techniques used to open the cavity on the flat surface of the hemispheric magnetic pellets and from the inconsistencies in manipulations

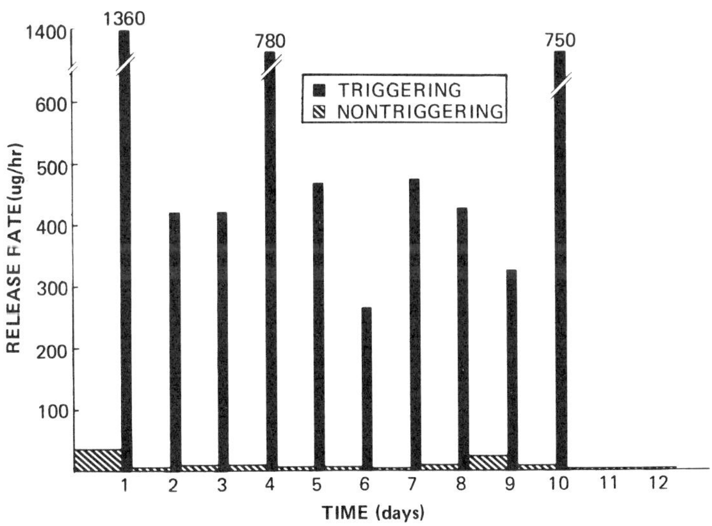

Figure 5 Magnetic modulation of bovine serum albumin release. Prior to triggering, the pellets were prereleased for 1 day. The pellets were triggered for 5 hr, followed by nontriggering for 19 hr. The cycle of triggering and nontriggering was repeated daily. ■, The quantity of BSA release during the magnetic modulation period; ▧, the quantity of BSA released during the nontriggering period.

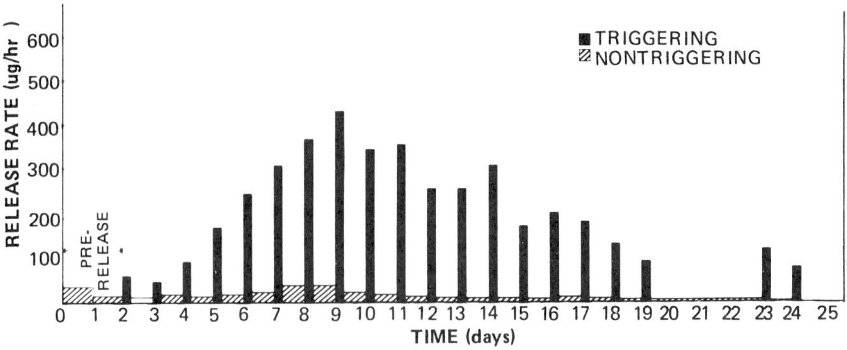

Figure 6 Magnetic modulation of pepsin release. ▨, The quantity of pepsin released during the magnetic modulation period; ■, the quantity of pepsin released during the nontriggering period.

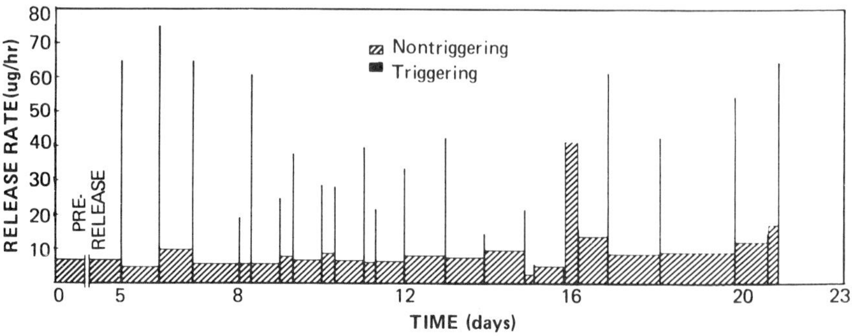

Figure 7 Magnetic modulation of insulin release. ■, The quantity of insulin released during magnetic modulation periods; ▨, the quantity of insulin released during nontriggering periods.

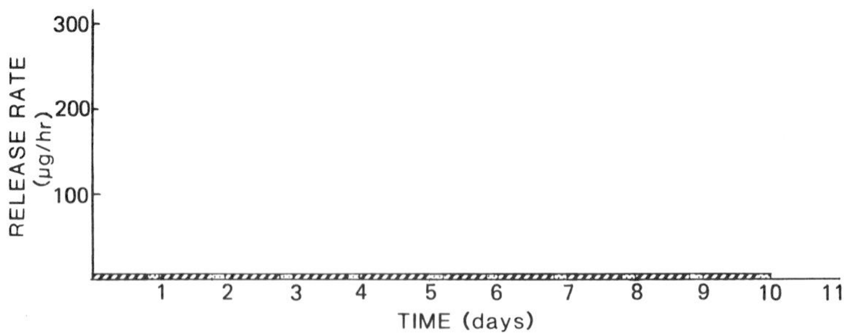

Figure 8 Control experiments for hemispheric magnetic pellets. The pellets containing BSA were prepared in the same manner as shown in Fig. 5. They were not exposed at all to magnetic triggering. The samples were transferred into fresh saline solution in the same intervals as those shown in Fig. 5.

conducted during the magnetic modulation. Improved techniques such as computer-aided drilling may prove useful in opening the cavity; to improve the consistency of magnetic modulation, the use of a degausser may be useful. In addition, future studies will explore the effectiveness of this device as a model system in controlling blood glucose levels in diabetic rats.

ACKNOWLEDGMENTS

Dr. Hsieh is a postdoctoral Fellow at the Juvenile Diabetes Foundation and an awardee of a Starter Grant from the Pharmaceutical Manufacturer's Association. The project was partially supported by National Institutes of Health Grant GM-26698. The authors thank Brian Marasca, Elazer Edelman, and Larry Brown for their assistance.

REFERENCES

1. P. H. Forsham, in *Diabetes Mellitus*, 2nd ed. (M. Ellenberg and H. Rifkin, eds.), McGraw-Hill, New York, 1970, pp. 694-709.
2. M. D. Siperstein, D. W. Foster, H. C. Knowles, Jr., R. Levine, L. L. Madison, and J. Roth, *N. Engl. J. Med.*, *26*:1060 (1979).
3. A. M. Albisser, B. S. Leibel, T. G. Ewart, S. Davidovac, C. K. Botz, and W. Zingg, *Diabetes*, *23*:389 (1974).
4. A. M. Albisser, B. S. Leibel, T. G. Ewart, S. Davidovac, C. K. Botz, W. Zingg, H. Schipper, and R. Gander, *Diabetes*, *23*:397 (1974).
5. G. Slama, M. Hautecouverture, R. Assan, and G. Tchobroutsky, *Diabetes*, *23*:732 (1974).
6. S. Genuth and P. Martin, *Diabetes*, *26*:571 (1971).
7. J. C. Pickup, H. Keen, J. A. Parsons, and K. G. M. Alberti, *Br. Med. J.*, *1*:204 (1978).
8. W. V. Tamborlane, R. S. Sherwin, M. Genel, and P. Felig, *N. Engl. J. Med.*, *300*:573 (1979).
9. K. Irsigler and H. Kritz, *Diabetes*, *28*:196 (1979).
10. P. J. Blackshear, T. Rohde, J. C. Grotting, F. D. Dorman, P. R. Perkins, R. L. Varco, and H. Buchwald, *Diabetes*, *28*:634 (1979).
11. J. Bojsen, T. Deckert, K. Kolendorf, and B. Lorup, *Diabetes*, *28*:974 (1979).
12. P. Raskin, A. Pietri, and R. Unger, *Diabetes*, *28*:1033 (1979).
13. H. Buchwald, R. L. Vario, W. M. Rupp, F. J. Goldenberg, J. Barbosa, R. D. Rohde, R. A. Schwartz, T. G. Rublein, and P. J. Blackshear, *Lancet*, No. 8232, p. 1233 (1981).
14. H. M. Creque, R. Langer, and J. Folkman, *Diabetes*, *29*:37 (1980).

15. D. R. Paul, in *Controlled Release Polymeric Formulations*, ACS Symp. Ser. No. 33 (D. R. Paul and R. W. Harris, eds.), American Chemical Society, Washington, D.C., 1976, p. 1.
16. R. Langer, *Chem. Eng. Commun.*, *6*:1 (1980).
17. W. Rhine, D. S. T. Hsieh, and R. Langer, *J. Pharm. Sci.*, *69*: 265 (1980).
18. W. Rhine, V. Sukhatme, D. S. T. Hsieh, and R. Langer, in *Controlled Release of Bioactive Materials* (R. Baker, ed.), Academic Press, New York, 1980, p. 177.
19. D. S. T. Hsieh and R. Langer, in *Controlled Release of Pesticides and Pharmaceuticals* (D. H. Lewis, ed.), Plenum Press, New York, 1981, pp. 5-15.
20. D. S. T. Hsieh, R. Langer, and J. Folkman, *Proc. Natl. Acad. Sci. USA*, *78*:1863 (1981).
21. D. S. T. Hsieh, W. Rhine, and R. Langer, submitted to *J. Pharm. Sci.*, in press.
22. E. Edelman, D. S. T. Hsieh, and R. Langer, unpublished data.

Chapter 8

A Polymeric Controlled Release Delivery System for Prostaglandins

CHARLES H. SPILMAN and THEODORE J. ROSEMAN The Upjohn Company, Kalamazoo, Michigan

RICHARD W. BAKER,* MARK EDWARD TUTTLE, and HAROLD K. LONSDALE Bend Research, Inc., Bend, Oregon

Prostaglandin vaginal delivery systems are being developed for use as fertility control agents. Most of these systems have been lipid-based vaginal suppositories containing a variety of natural or synthetic prostaglandins [1]. Although clinical efficacy for menses induction, second-trimester abortion, and cervical dilatation has been demonstrated using these suppositories, several problems have been observed with some of these vaginal dosage forms. For example, chemical stability of certain prostaglandins has been difficult to achieve in the suppository vehicles; and the physical stability of suppository bases, and thus the bioavailability of drug, has been reported to be dependent on storage temperature [2]. Thus, some prostaglandin vaginal suppositories have to be stored at refrigerated temperatures, a condition that would limit their use in developing countries. In addition to these stability problems, most prostaglandin vaginal suppositories have to be used in multiple dosing regimens. Furthermore, the release of drug from the suppository is temperature dependent and occurs from a variable surface area as the base changes from a solid to an oil.

Our efforts have been directed toward the design of controlled release vaginal delivery systems that would improve drug administration by (1) controlling the prostaglandin release rate in a predictable and reproducible fashion, (2) allowing the delivery system to be self-administered, (3) providing for termination of drug administration by the facile removal of the delivery module, and (4) requiring only a

*Present affiliation: Membrane Technology and Research, Inc., Palo Alto, California

single administration. The development of a monolithic controlled release delivery system using silicone rubber was reported previously [1,3,4]. Reported here is our experience with the development and preclinical evaluation of a reservoir-type, laminated membrane delivery module containing the p-hydroxybenzaldehyde semicarbazone ester of 16,16-dimethyl prostaglandin E_2 (I, DMPGE). The clinical efficacy of this prostaglandin analog in suppository dosage forms has been documented [5-8].

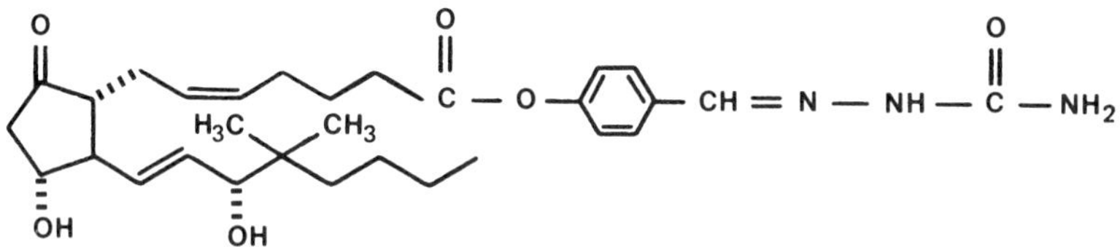

I. 16,16-dimethyl prostaglandin E_2 p-hydroxybenzaldehyde semicarbazone ester.

EXPERIMENTAL

Vaginal Devices

A schematic drawing of the vaginal delivery system is shown in Fig. 1. The delivery module consists of an inner drug reservoir membrane and an outer rate-controlling membrane that are placed around an inert tampon substrate. The laminated sheath was prepared by dip-coating an inverted test tube with drug dissolved in a 10% solution of the

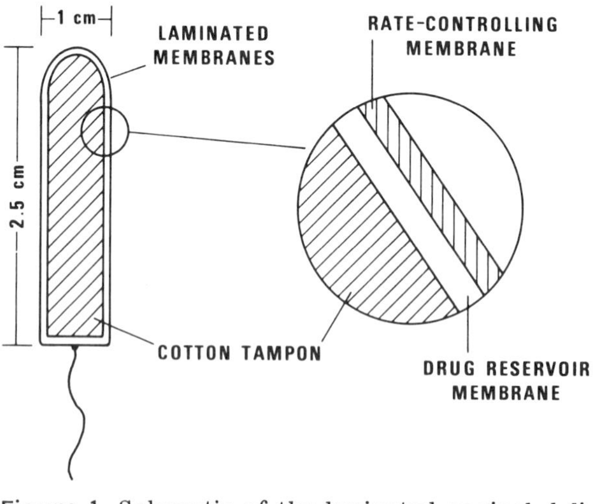

Figure 1 Schematic of the laminated vaginal delivery system.

polymer in tetrahydrofuran. This procedure formed the drug reservoir membrane. The rate-controlling membrane was then applied over the reservoir using a similar dipping process. Membrane wall thicknesses ranged from 1 to 5 mils. The laminated membranes were removed from the test tubes, placed over the tampon substrates, and tied as indicated in Fig. 1. Each device had a surface area of 15 cm^2.

The rate of prostaglandin release was altered by varying the thickness of the rate-controlling membrane. Devices were prepared to release either 20 μg DMPGE/hr or 40 μg DMPGE/hr; the total drug content in these devices was 2.7 and 6.7 mg, respectively. The diffusional properties of the drug-membrane composite were selected so that the major resistance to drug transport resided in the outer membrane, thereby assuring that a zero-order-release profile was achieved. The release rate of the prostaglandin from these devices can be explained by Eq. (1),

$$R = \frac{C_s D_s}{l} \tag{1}$$

where C_s is the solubility of the prostaglandin in the polymer, D_s is the diffusion coefficient of the drug in the polymer, and l is the thickness of the rate-controlling membrane. In vitro release rate curves were determined by agitating the membrane sheaths, while on a test tube, in 1-liter flasks containing distilled water at 37°C and 120 rpm. The volume of the dissolution medium was replaced every 30 to 60 min. The solutions were extracted with ethyl acetate and read on an ultraviolet (UV) spectrophotometer at 290 nm; corrections were made for absorbance readings of blank solutions.

Biological Evaluation

Uterine motility was recorded from four second-trimester pregnant rhesus monkeys (*Macaca mulatta*). A fluid-filled open-ended polyethylene catheter (0.015 in. ID × 0.043 in. OD, Clay Adams) was inserted transabdominally through a 15-g needle into the amniotic cavity. The catheter was attached to a Statham P-23Dc transducer, which was in turn connected to a Grass polygraph. A brief pretreatment recording was obtained before inserting the vaginal delivery system. Thus each animal served as its own control for the uterine motility studies. Although nonmedicated placebo devices were not used in these studies, our previous experience using other placebo vaginal systems demonstrated that the motility recording catheter, anesthesia, and vaginal insertion of a placebo device do not cause abortion. Animals were anesthetized with Sernylan (1.0 mg/kg, Bio-Ceutic Laboratories, Inc.) when recordings were made. The urethras were catheterized in all monkeys to prevent urine from entering the vagina during the uterine motility recording session.

RESULTS AND DISCUSSION

In vitro release curves are shown in Fig. 2 for two different thicknesses of the rate-controlling membrane. The curves are characterized by a biphasic type of behavior; release of drug during the first 3 hr was more rapid than the subsequent steady-state period of zero-order release. The steady-state release rates for the two membrane thicknesses are 20 and 40 μg/hr. As predicted by Eq. (1), the steady-state release rates were inversely proportional to the thickness of the rate-controlling membrane. Scatter in the data is attributed to assay variation of the very dilute solutions that were analyzed. The initially high release rates are due to drug that has diffused into the outer rate-controlling membrane on storage of the devices. The initial release rate, therefore, is more characteristic of non-steady-state release behavior. In contrast, freshly prepared devices would show a time lag before the steady-state portion of the curve is reached [9]. This is graphically illustrated in Fig. 3, where a hypothetical plot of the amount of drug released versus time is presented. Note that after a non-steady-state period, the slopes (i.e., release rates) of the two systems are the same. The time required to reach the steady-state portion of the curve will depend on the diffusion coefficient for the drug and the thickness of the outer membrane.

The biological activities of vaginal devices rated at 20 μg/hr and 40 μg/hr were tested in pregnant rhesus monkeys to provide baseline information on their pharmacological effects. There was a gradual increase in the frequency and amplitude of uterine contractions (Fig. 4)

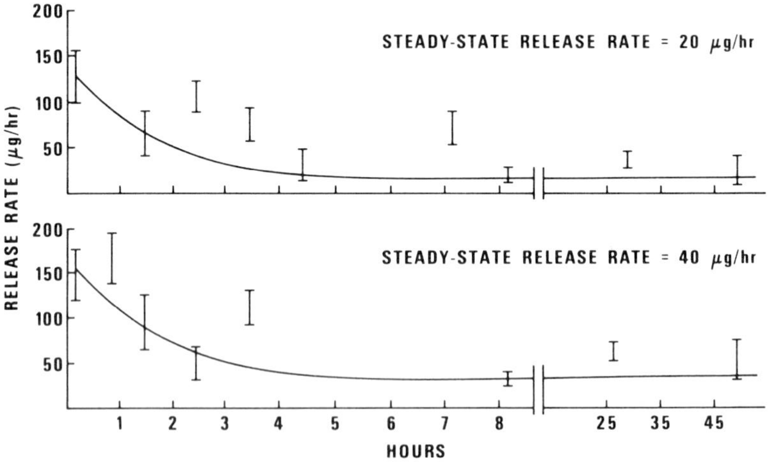

Figure 2 In vitro release rate curves of the p-hydroxybenzaldehyde semicarbazone ester of 16,16-dimethyl prostaglandin E_2 from laminated delivery systems.

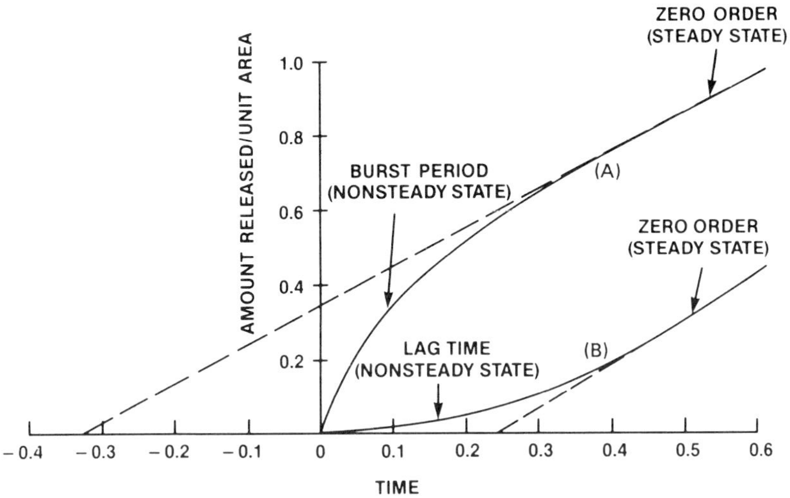

Figure 3 Hypothetical transport patterns for reservoir devices after storage (A) or freshly prepared (B); units are arbitrary. (Adapted from Ref. 9.)

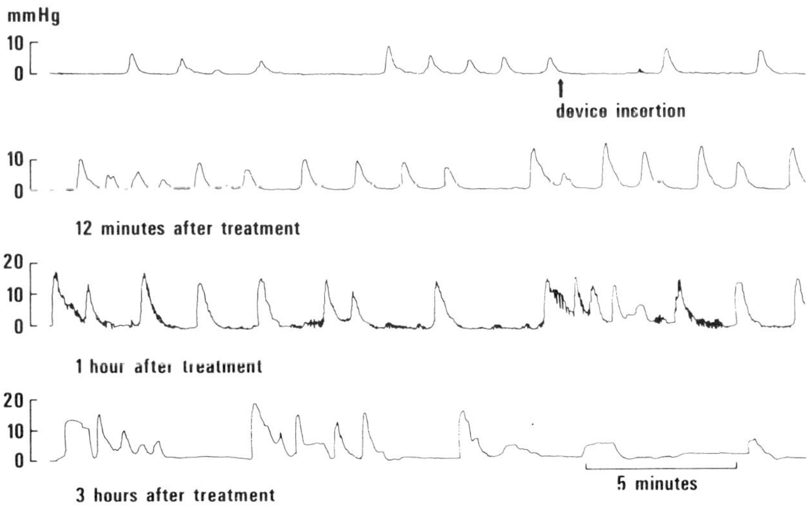

Figure 4 Uterine motility in a pregnant monkey treated with a vaginal device designed to release 20 μg/hr of the p-hydroxybenzaldehyde semicarbazone ester of 16,16-dimethyl prostaglandin E_2.

beginning 15 to 30 min after vaginal insertion of the 20-μg/hr devices. The time of onset of uterine motility corresponded to the non-steady-state portion of the in vitro release curve (Fig. 2). There was no change in basal uterine tone in either of the two monkeys treated with these devices. Therefore, the initial rapid release of drug (Fig. 2) was not reflected in the biological response. This may be explained by the dilution of the prostaglandin in the blood after absorption through the vaginal mucosa. The increase in uterine activity persisted for the duration of the recording session (4.5 hr). A change in the uterine motility patterns was not perceptible toward the end of the recording sessions, when release of drug from the delivery modules would be at a steady state. The vaginal devices were left in place for only 8 hr. Nonetheless, both animals aborted following treatment: one animal aborted within 48 hr, and the second animal aborted 8 days after treatment.

The 40-μg/hr vaginal devices caused a slightly different effect on uterine motility (Fig. 5). Uterine activity began to increase sooner after treatment with the 40-μg/hr devices than in animals treated with the slower-release-rate devices. Beginning approximately 5 min after vaginal treatment with the faster-release-rate devices, there was a significant increase in both the frequency and amplitude of uterine contractions. In one of the two animals treated with these devices the initial response was a slight increase in basal uterine tone, as shown

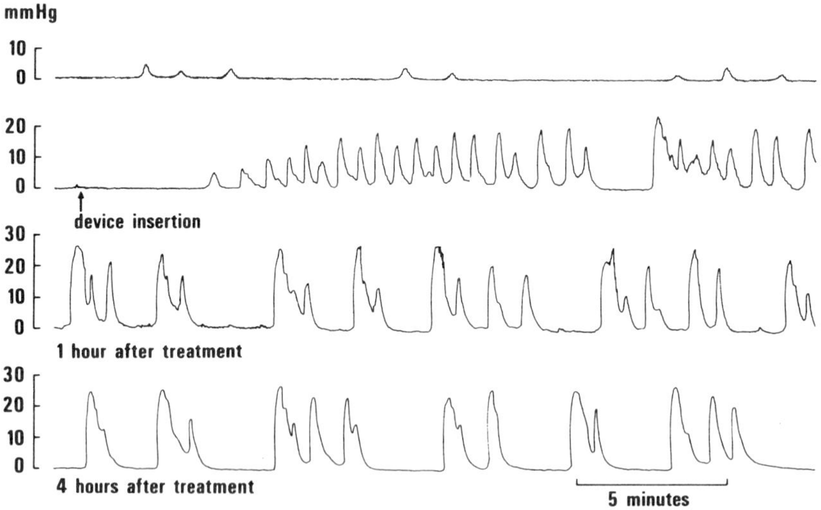

Figure 5 Uterine motility in a pregnant monkey treated with a vaginal device designed to release 40 μg/hr of the p-hydroxybenzaldehyde semicarbazone ester of 16,16-dimethyl prostaglandin E_2.

in Fig. 5. This increase in uterine tone may be a result of higher initial blood levels of drug during the non-steady-state release portion of the curve shown in Fig. 2. However, significant dilution of drug probably occurred since an increase in uterine tone was observed in only one of the animals, and the magnitude of this increase was not representative of the two- to threefold higher release rate of drug during the non-steady state. Uterine activity was characterized by rhythmic, large-amplitude contractions in both animals for the duration of the recording session (4.5 hr). These devices were left in place for approximately 8 hr. Both animals aborted within 7 days after treatment.

SUMMARY AND CONCLUSIONS

The results of this research provide the foundation for the development of novel vaginal delivery systems for prostaglandins. The concepts of diffusion were utilized to control prostaglandin release and to promote a continuous biological response (uterine stimulation) for the duration of vaginal treatment. This biological response was sufficient to terminate pregnancy in all four treated monkeys. This approach offers intriguing possibilities for optimizing drug delivery of the p-hydroxybenzaldehyde semicarbazone ester of 16,16-dimethyl prostaglandin E_2, and for other prostaglandin analogs, for clinical uses.

ACKNOWLEDGMENT

The assistance of A. D. Forbes in performing the monkey experiments is gratefully acknowledged.

REFERENCES

1. T. J. Roseman and C. H. Spilman, in *Controlled Release Systems* (S. K. Chandrasekaran, ed.), AIChE Symp. Ser. No. 206, Vol. 77, New York, 1981.
2. L. J. Coben and N. G. Lordi, *J. Pharm. Sci.*, *69*:955 (1980).
3. C. H. Spilman and T. J. Roseman, *Contraception*, *11*:409 (1975).
4. C. H. Spilman, D. C. Beuving, A. D. Forbes, T. J. Roseman, and L. J. Larion, *Prostaglandins*, *12*(Suppl.):1 (1976).
5. S. M. M. Karim, in *Obstetric and Gynaecological Uses of Prostaglandins* (S. M. M. Karim, ed.), Asian Fed. Obstet. Gynaecol., Proc. First Int. Cong., Eurasia Press, Singapore, 1976.
6. S. M. M. Karim, S. S. Ratnam, W. W. Selvadurai, and R. N. V. Prasad, *Prostaglandins*, *13*:333 (1977).
7. S. M. M. Karim and S. S. Ratnam, *Br. J. Obstet. Gynaecol.*, *84*: 135 (1977).

8. S. M. M. Karim, S. S. Ratnam, R. N. V. Prasad, and Y. M. Wong, *Br. J. Obstet. Gynaecol.*, *84*:269 (1977).
9. A. C. Tanquary and R. E. Lacey, eds., *Controlled Release of Biologically Active Agents*, Plenum Press, New York, 1974.

Chapter 9

Controlled Release of Carcinogens in Heterotopic Tracheal Grafts

BIMAL C. PAL and A. J. P. KLEIN-SZANTO Oak Ridge National Laboratory, Oak Ridge, Tennessee

A major drawback of the conventional approaches to the study of the respiratory tract carcinogenesis by intratracheal injection or instillation is that neither the dose nor the target site can be accurately defined. The tracheal transplant model has been developed in our group to provide a solution to this problem [1]. In this model, rodent tracheas are transplanted under the skin in the scapular region of the isogenic host. The transplants reestablish themselves in the host in 3-4 weeks and survive indefinitely. These tracheas can then be exposed to carcinogens in a controlled and quantitative fashion using monolithic cylindrical pellets. Thus the in vivo progress of carcinogenesis in a preselected site of the respiratory tract can be investigated. The model has a good potential for establishing a more realistic dose-response relationship in respiratory tract carcinogenesis. However, the success of the model depends on the development of devices for the release of carcinogens at a reproducible and predictable rate. This chapter describes various approaches to the solution of this problem. The feasibility of this approach to the study of respiratory tract carcinogenesis has been demonstrated [1-5].

The rat tracheal transplants can easily accommodate cylindrical pellets, 14 mm × 1.4 mm in diameter. Monolithic cylindrical devices are an attractive choice. Any material to be accepted as a vehicle must meet the following requirements: (1) it should not evoke any toxic tissue reaction by itself; (2) it should be easily available and there should be no difficulty in making uniform pellets; and (3) it should not interact with the carcinogen. The selection of the matrix is also determined to a large extent by the physicochemical properties of the carcinogen in question. Unfortunately, the respiratory tract toxicants cover a gamut of chemicals, as evident from the following partial list: CO, NO_x, SO_x, Pb compounds, particulates (asbestos, fly ash, cellulose fibers), benzo[a]pyrene (BP), Mn, N-nitrosodiethylamine, N-nitrosomethylurea, N-nitrosomethylguanidine, nickel subsulfide, As. Water-insoluble carcinogens such as BP and 7,12-dimethylbenz[a]anthracene (DMBA), and tumor promoters such as 12-O-tetradecanoyl-phorbol-13-acetate (TPA), have been incorporated in beeswax, cholesterol/beeswax (9:1), and stearyl alcohol/beeswax (9:1). The polycyclic hydrocarbons (PCHs) have been adsorbed on carbon particles which were subsequently dispersed in beeswax matrix and made into pellets for release studies. Such diffusion-controlled release cannot be resorted to in the case of materials insoluble in any biocompatible medium. In this case, biodegradable materials such as polyglycolic acid (PGA) may provide a solution. Aqueous solutions of water-soluble carcinogens such as As_2O_3 have been filled in plastic tubes and these reservoir-type devices have been used for controlled release. Attempts have been made to lower the release rate further by dip-coating the pellets with polymers, such as cellulose acetate and polystyrene. All these experiments have been designed to provide a release of 20 μg to 30 mg of carcinogen in the tracheal transplant over a period of 1 week to 6 months. The exposure level is determined by the toxicity and severity of the biological effects of different carcinogens. Published data, when available, and trial experiments, in the absence of any information on the exposure level, form the basis of the dose and dose rate. The biological end points in these studies comprise the histopathological examination of the tracheal tissue, including any tumor formation, and will be reported elsewhere. In this chapter we restrict the discussion to the release of PCHs and TPA.

Since the in vivo tests are costly and time consuming, an in vitro test system has also been designed for quick evaluation of the release characteristics of different pellets. In this system, pellets are shaken in fetal calf serum in a shaker water bath at 37°C. Serum is changed daily and the amount of released carcinogen is assayed by radioactivity. We prefer a biological fluid such as serum as a release medium rather than physiological saline or simulated body fluids because serum, with its natural protein and lipid components, provides more realistic release rates which mimic the release rates in vivo.

EXPERIMENTAL

Materials

White (USP grade) beeswax was obtained from Fisher Chemicals, Pittsburgh, Pennsylvania. Molten wax was filtered through a steam-heated funnel with a medium porosity, fritted glass disk under vacuum. BP

(99+%, gold label) was obtained from Aldrich Chemical Co., Milwaukee, Wisconsin, and used without any further purification. DMBA was obtained from Eastman Organic Chemicals, Rochester, New York, and was purified by recrystallization from ethanol as described previously [5]. TPA and [^{3}H]TPA (2 Ci/mmol) were purchased from P. Borchert, University of Minnesota, Minneapolis, Minnesota. NCS, [^{14}C]BP (specific activity, 25 mCi/mmol), and [^{14}C]DMBA (21.2 mCi/mmol) were obtained from Amersham/Searle Corp., Arlington Heights, Illinois. The last two chemicals were purified on silica gel plates using benzene: n-hexane (1:15; solvent A). Heat-inactivated fetal calf serum, human serum, and rat serum were obtained from Grand Island Biological Co., Grand Island, New York. PPD (scintillation grade) was received from Packard Instrument Co., Downers Grove, Illinois. Carbon particles (Barnaby Cheney Catalog No. JF) were passed through sieve No. 200 and sieve No. 325 and the particles retained on the latter were used. Cholesterol was obtained from three sources (Aldrich Chemical Co., Milwaukee, Wisconsin; Fisher Chemicals, Pittsburgh, Pennsylvania; and Eastman Organic Chemicals, Rochester, New York). Stearyl alcohol was obtained from Sigma Chemical Co., St. Louis, Missouri. Polystyrene and polyglycolic acid were obtained from Aldrich Chemical Co., Milwaukee, Wisconsin, and Davison and Geck (Division of American Cyanamide), Danbury, Connecticut, respectively. Silastic materials were obtained from Dow Corning Corp., Midland, Michigan. All other chemicals were reagent grade.

Animals

Ten-week-old isogenic Fischer 344 rats were bred and reared in an animal isolation facility. These animals were demonstrated to be free of the common infectious diseases of rats, including pneumonia.

Assay of BP, DMBA, and TPA

Spectrophotometry Beeswax, beeswax/cholesterol (1:9), and beeswax/stearyl alcohol (1:9) pellets containing BP or DMBA were dissolved in benzene. Pellets containing carbon particles coated with BP or DMBA were extracted with benzene for 2 hr in a Soxhlet apparatus with double-thickness cellulose thimbles. The following molar extinction coefficients were used for determining the concentrations of different carcinogens in benzene: for BP, λ_{max} (benzene), 388 nm (ε = 30,960); for DMBA, λ_{max} (benzene), 301 nm (ε = 79,000). Beeswax, cholesterol, stearyl alcohol, and benzene do not interfere with the spectrophotometric assay at these wavelengths.

Radioassay Concentrations of [^{3}H]TPA, [^{14}C]BP, and [^{14}C]DMBA in fetal calf serum were assayed by dissolving 0.2-ml aliquots in 1 ml NCS followed by the addition of 10 ml of scintillation cocktail (0.5% PPD in toluene) and counting in a Beckman LS-233 liquid scintillation counter. All three compounds had a specific activity of approximately 200 dpm/μg.

Preparation of Pellets

Beeswax, beeswax/cholesterol (1:9), and beeswax/stearyl alcohol (1:9) pellets containing BP, DMBA, or TPA were made by using a pellet maker (Fig. 1) as described previously [1], with some modifications. Weighed amounts of carcinogen and the matrix media were heated in a glass scintillation vial placed in a cavity in an aluminum block placed on a thermostatically controlled hot plate. The aluminum block had a thermometer placed in a central hole to monitor the temperature. A clear homogenous melt was obtained at 80°C in the case of beeswax and beeswax/stearyl alcohol. In the case of cholesterol pellets it was necessary to heat up to 150°C. An appropriate aliquot of the melt was transferred to the recess in the bottom half of the preheated pellet maker. The top half was placed on the bottom half when the melt rose to fill the cylindrical cavities in the top half. The mold was then rapidly cooled by placing it on a cylindrical copper block (3 in. × 3 in. diameter) cooled in ice. When the melt solidified, the two halves were separated and the pellets were pushed out with the push pin. The uniformity of the pellets was determined by assaying three pellets selected at random. Pellets made in the pellet maker were fairly uniform [e.g., the average weight of beeswax pellets was 24.48 mg ± 0.62 SD (95% confidence range, 23.24 to 25.72)]. Pellets containing PCH were individually weighed, and those that did not fall within ±2.0% of the mean pellet weight were rejected. Thus, a pellet labeled as 100 μg BP beeswax actually contained 98 to 102 μg BP. We had about 30% rejections for every batch of pellets processed with the pellet maker.

The cholesterol/beeswax (9:1) pellets are rather fragile. For ease of handling, these pellets may be encased in thin-walled silastic tubing (medical grade; catalog No. 602-234; ID 1.47 mm, OD 1.96 mm) and sealed at the ends with silastic type A medical adhesive silicone (catalog No. 891). Results of in vitro experiments (not reported herein) with both bare and silastic-enclosed PCH/beeswax pellets indicated that silastic did not significantly influence the release rates. The carbon pellets cannot be made in the pellet maker because these particles have a tendency to settle and agglomerate. In this case, the weighed matrix was melted in a hot mortar and the carbon particles loaded with PCH were mixed up thoroughly using the mortar and pestle and allowed to cool until the mix congealed. It was then scraped out from the mortar and packed in the cell of a Greenerd Arbor Press (Fisher Scientific Co.) fitted with a disk with a 1.5-mm-diameter hole in the middle. The cell was warmed up to a suitable temperature (below the melting point of the mix) and extruded quickly. The extruded material was cut into proper lengths by using a channeled Teflon block, very much like a carpenter's miter box.

BP and DMBA Coating of Carbon Particle Carbon particles have been internally coated by heating and stirring with PCH in acetone solution

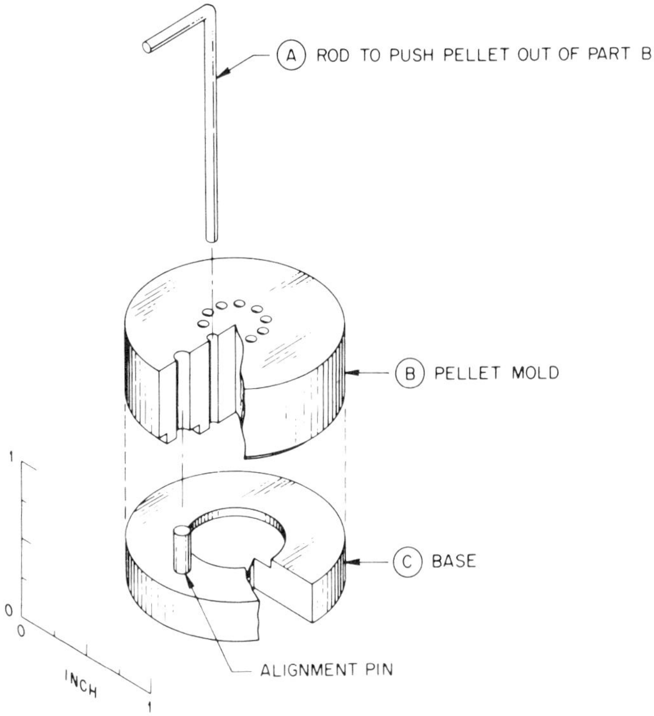

PELLETIZER

Figure 1 Schematic diagram of a pellet maker used to make uniform carcinogen pellets. (From Ref. 1.)

as described in Report II TRI-C6184 of June 1970 under Contract NIH-60-0275.

Carbon particles (2.0 g) were added with stirring to a hot solution of PCH (2.2 g) in acetone in a beaker. Acetone was allowed to evaporate in the hood at room temperature. All of the dried, caked mixture from the walls of the beaker was scraped down, and the side of the beaker was rinsed with 1 ml of acetone. The mixture was heated gently with constant stirring and scraping. After all the acetone was evaporated, the mixture was heated at 40°C above the melting point of the PCHs for about 1 min. The final product was cooled in a desiccator. The PCH content was assayed by extracting a weighed portion of the sample for 2 hr with benzene in a Soxhlet extractor with a double-thickness cellulose thimble. The recovery and the ultraviolet (UV) absorption spectra indicated negligible degradation of the PCH during this process.

Dip Coating of the Pellets A circular Teflon block (4 in. diameter × 0.5 in. thickness) is fitted with 20 stainless steel pins (1 in. length × 1/10 in. diameter). The pellets to be dip-coated are attached to the pins by means of short lengths of silastic tubing. The other side of the Teflon block carries a shaft (0.25 in diameter × 5/8 in. length) at the center. A 5% solution of cellulose acetate (acetyl 40.0%, ASTM viscosity 25) in acetone is placed in a petri dish. Using a Payne dip coater, the Teflon block containing the pellets is lowered into the dish so that slightly more than half of the pellet is immersed in the solution. The block is raised and rotated vertically by using a stirring motor and warming the pellets at the same time with an infrared lamp. The process is repeated several times. The pellets are removed and reinserted in the Teflon block to dip-coat the other end in a similar fashion. A slight overlap is formed in the middle. The thickness of the coating is expressed in the weight of the coating (milligrams) per pellet. All traces of solvents are removed from the pellets by keeping them in a desiccator under high vacuum. Polystyrene coating of the pellets was achieved in a similar manner using a 5% solution of the resin in ethyl acetate.

Procedure for Release Experiments

In Vitro Carcinogen pellets were shaken in 25-ml Erlenmeyer flasks with 6 ml of fetal calf serum at 37°C in a shaker water bath at 100 rpm (Model G86; New Brunswick Scientific Co., New Brunswick, New Jersey). Serum was changed every 24 hr and the amount of released carcinogen was determined by radioassay. Sterile conditions were observed as far as practicable.

In Vivo Pellets containing a known amount of carcinogen were inserted into established tracheal grafts as described by Kendrick et al. [6] and as shown in Fig. 2 [5]. The pellets were recovered at 1-, 2-, 4-, 6-, 8-, 12-, and 16-week intervals and the remaining carcinogen was assayed by spectrophotometry or radioactivity.

Solubility of BP

In Serum Four milliliters of serum was shaken in a stoppered 10-ml Erlenmeyer flask in a shaker water bath at 37°C and 100 rpm with about 20 mg [^{14}C]BP (specific activity, 2500 dpm/μg). Aliquots, 0.4 ml, were withdrawn at 8-, 24-, 32-, and 48-hr intervals and filtered under pressure through a fine-fritted glass disk (pore diameter 4-5.5 μm). A 0.2-ml aliquot of the filtrate was counted for radioactivity. The filtrate was also counted for radioactivity after centrifugation at 250 × g for 30 min to rule out the presence of fine BP particles. Practically no difference was observed in the radioactivity of the filtrate before and after centrifugation. Samples were withdrawn and counted

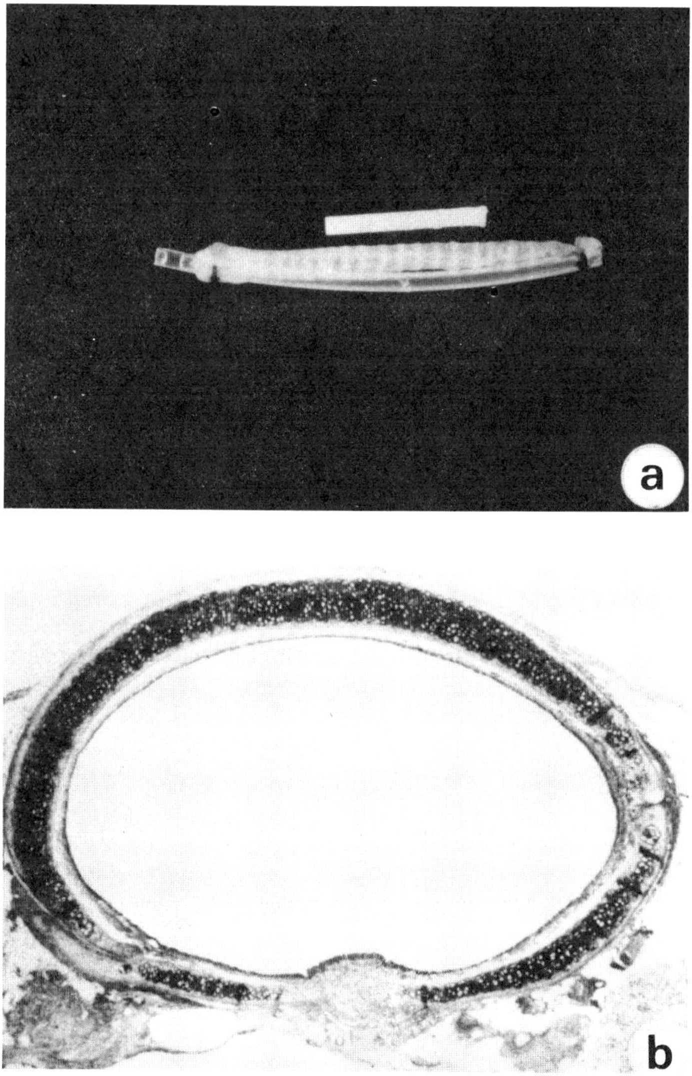

Figure 2 (a) Rat trachea sutured to polyethylene tubing. These were implanted subcutaneously for tracheal transplant studies. Next to it is a beeswax pellet of the type placed in the lumen of established transplants for determining in vivo release characteristics. 1.5 X. (b) Cross section of an established tracheal transplant showing normal epithelial morphology. Hematoxylin and eosin, 32 X. (From Ref. 5.)

until the concentration of BP in the serum leveled off. These experiments were repeated with a Millipore syringe filter (catalog No. XX-3001200) and a filter with an average porosity of 0.22 μm (catalog No. GSWP-01300), with essentially similar results.

In Beeswax Weighed amounts of BP and beeswax were heated together until the mixture formed a clear homogenous melt; it was then transferred into the mold, and 5-μm-thick sections were prepared from the BP-beeswax mixture and contained 0.4, 0.5, 0.6, 0.7, 0.8, 0.9, and 4% (w/w) BP. The sections were observed and photographed at 37°C under a Zeiss UV epifluorescence microscope (UV source, halogen bulb; excitation filter, KP 490-500, barrier filter, LP 528). The maximum concentration at which BP crystals were not discernible under the microscope was taken as the solubility of BP in beeswax at 37°C.

RESULTS AND DISCUSSION

Solubility of BP in Different Sera and Beeswax

Since the in vitro release of BP was carried out in fetal calf serum, it was necessary to determine the solubility of BP in serum. Solubility was found to be lowest in fetal calf serum (35 μg/ml) and highest in human serum (214 μg/ml), as shown in Table 1. Solubility of BP in human serum was reported to be 50 μg/ml by Obrikat and Wettig [7]. Since these authors did not mention the temperature at which the solubility was determined, presumably it was done at room temperature and this may partly explain the difference from our data recorded at 37°C. Unfasted rat serum showed slightly higher solubility, 147 μg/ml,

Table 1 Solubilities of BP in Various Sera at 37°C

Serum[a]	Equilibrium solubility (μg/ml)
Fetal calf	35.6 ± 6.9[b] (3)[c]
Fasted rat	131.6 ± 3.2 (3)
Unfasted rat	147.4 ± 9.4 (4)
Human	214.6 ± 3.6[d]

[a]Fetal calf serum (Batch C-962918) and human serum (Batch C-467124) were obtained from Grand Island Biological. Unfasted and fasted rat sera were obtained from Fischer 344 rats in the laboratory.
[b]Mean ± SD.
[c]Numbers in parentheses indicate numbers of measurements.
[d]Reported 50 μg/ml at room temperature [7].
Source: Ref. 5.

compared with fasted rat serum, 131 μg/ml, probably because of the higher lipid content of the former. We have found that most of BP is bound to serum albumin, the major carrier protein present in the serum (unpublished observation).

The solubility of BP in beeswax was carried out at 37°C by putting the microscope and the sections from BP-beeswax mixture in a thermostatically controlled hot room. At a concentration of 0.5% (w/w) or below, no crystals of BP could be observed at a magnification of 400 whereas at higher concentrations BP crystals of various sizes could be discerned. We took this to indicate that the solubility of BP in beeswax was about 0.5% at 37°C. The 100-μg BP-beeswax pellets containing 0.41% (w/w) BP did not show BP crystals (Fig. 3a), whereas the 1000-μg BP-beeswax pellets containing 4.1% (w/w) BP showed many large and small crystals (Fig. 3b).

In Vitro and In Vivo Release of BP and DMBA from Beeswax Pellets

We anticipated that the in vivo release of carcinogens such as BP and DMBA would be complicated by the changes in the surrounding tissue brought about by these agents. Both in vitro and in vivo release experiments were carried out in parallel to evaluate this situation. Physiological saline or pseudoextracellular fluid containing physiological concentrations of Na^+, K^+, Cl^-, HCO_3^-, and phosphate has been used as a release medium by previous investigators [8-10]. Since PCHs are practically insoluble in aqueous medium, we decided to use fetal calf serum, which with its protein and lipid components, more closely resembles the extracellular fluids surrounding the pellets in vivo. The concentration of BP was kept sufficiently below the saturation level of 35 μg/ml by changing the serum daily (6 ml of serum was used in the in vitro tests, which means that saturation would occur at 6 × 35 μg BP). This schedule of serum changes created a situation resembling an infinite sink not much different from the continuous flow system used by Roseman and Higuchi [11].

Release rates of BP and DMBA from beeswax pellets at two different concentrations, 0.41 and 4.10% (i.e., 100 and 1000 μg PCH per pellet, respectively), are reported in Figs. 4 and 5. The findings can be summarized as follows.

The rate of in vitro release of BP from 100-μg BP-beeswax pellets is faster (100% released in 2 weeks) than that from 1000-μg BP-beeswax pellets (80% released in 2 weeks). Although the percentage of BP released in the former case is higher, the amounts released are lower than those in the latter case at different time points (Fig. 4A and B). The Higuchi model [12] for release of dissolved and dispersed drug from monolithic devices provides an explanation for this finding. In the former case, BP is completely in solution in beeswax and the release

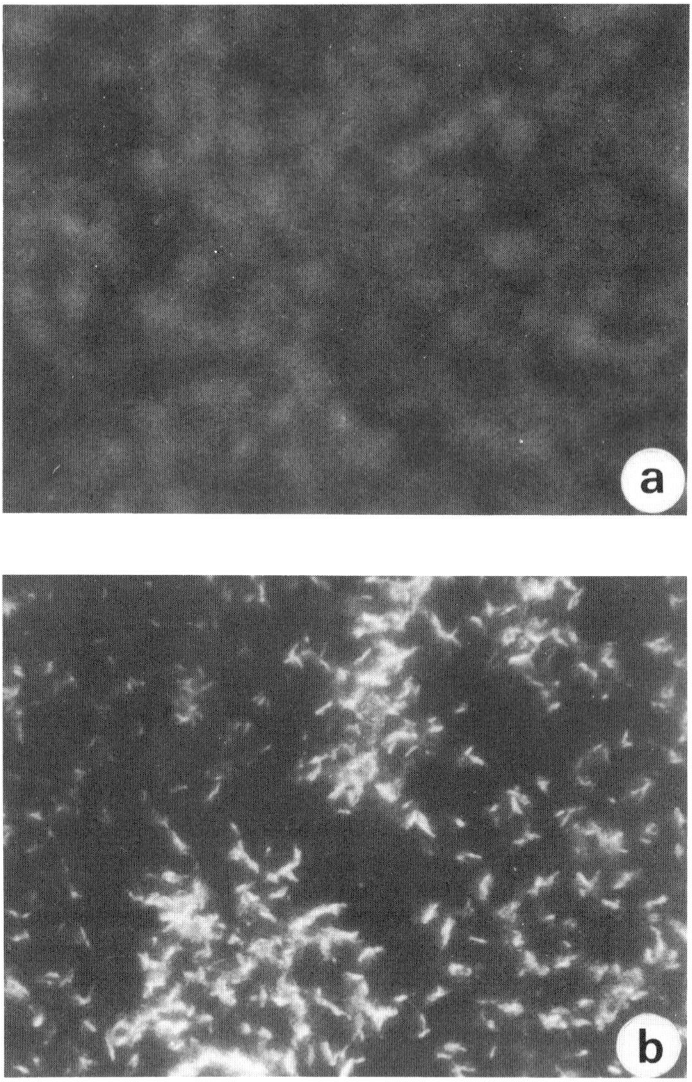

Figure 3 (a) Photomicrograph of a 5-μm-thick section of BP/beeswax matrix [0.40% (w/w) BP] taken with a reflecting microscope and UV and showing absence of any crystalline undissolved BP. 400 X. (b) Photomicrograph of a 5-μm-thick section of BP/beeswax matrix [4.0% (w/w) BP] showing the presence of undissolved BP crystals. 400 X. (From Ref. 5.)

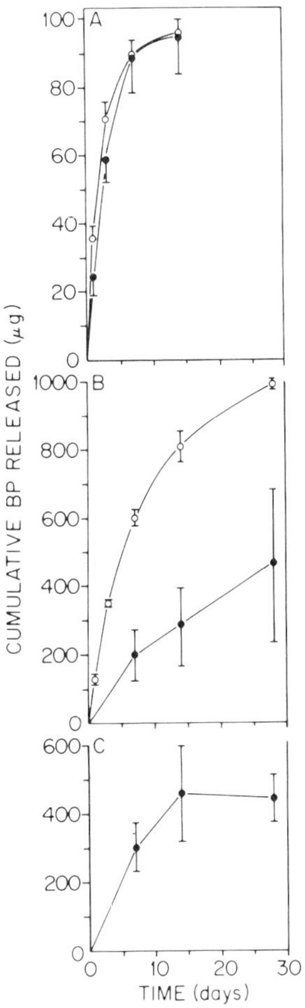

Figure 4 Cumulative release of BP from beeswax pellets. (A) Pellets containing 100 μg BP. O, in vitro release; ●, in vivo release in tracheal grafts. Each point represents the mean observation from four pellets in vitro ± SD and six pellets in vivo ± SD. (B) Pellets containing 1000 μg BP. O, in vitro release; ●, in vivo release in tracheal grafts. Each point represents the mean observation from three pellets in vitro ± SD and 12 pellets in vivo ± SD. (C) Pellets containing 1000 μg BP implanted subcutaneously. Each point represents the mean observation from six pellets ± SD. (From Ref. 5.)

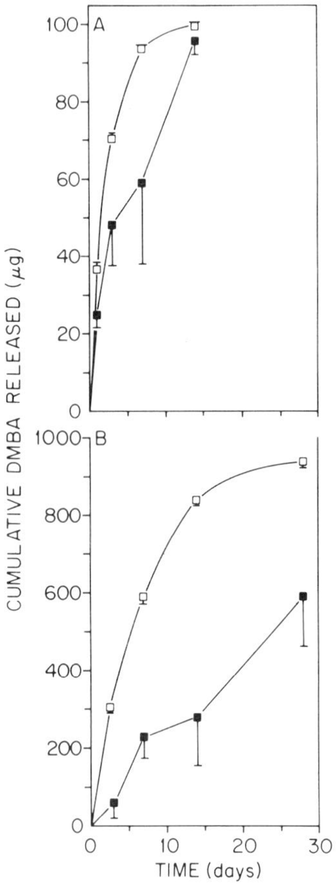

Figure 5 Cumulative release of DMBA from beeswax pellets. (A) Pellets containing 100 μg DMBA. □, in vitro release; ■, in vivo release in tracheal grafts. Each point represents the mean observation from four pellets in vitro ± SD and six pellets in vivo ± SD. (B) Pellets containing 1000 μg DMBA. □, in vitro release; ■, in vivo release in tracheal grafts. Each point represents the mean observation from three pellets in vitro ± SD and six pellets in vivo ± SD. (From Ref. 5.)

involves a two-phase system; whereas in the latter case, most of the BP is in crystalline dispersed form and the release involves a three-phase system (Fig. 3a and b). In addition, these pellets also demonstrate the phenomenon of the burst effect. At low concentrations of PCH, the in vitro and in vivo rates are very similar. In vitro release rates of BP show only a minor degree of variability at both low and high concentrations; the maximum percentages of standard deviation (SD) are 18 and 23, respectively. In contrast, in vivo variability is high, maximum percentages of SD are 45 and 91 at low and high concentrations, respectively.

In general, the release rates of BP and DMBA are very similar except that, at low concentration, the in vivo DMBA release shows pronounced variability. Pellets containing a high concentration of BP implanted subcutaneously show a slow release rate with high variability, similar to that of BP pellets inserted into tracheal grafts (Fig. 4B and C). These in vitro and in vivo studies indicate the deficiency of beeswax pellets as vehicles for protracted delivery of the two PCHs, BP and DMBA. Release rates are too rapid at low concentration and at high concentration the release shows great pellet-to-pellet variability, which must be due to the changing environment in the transplant since it does not occur in vitro.

Retardation of PCH Release Rate by Dip-Coating the Pellets with Polymers

We have attempted to slow down the release rate of BP from beeswax pellets by dip-coating them with cellulose acetate or polystyrene. The results are shown in Figs. 6 and 7. The in vitro tests were very promising; as the coating thickness was increased, the release rate consistently went down further and further and the percentage standard deviation was also consistently low; but the in vivo tests were rather disappointing, particularly in the case of cellulose acetate coating. The pellets quit releasing BP at a certain stage due to encapsulation. Encasing the pellets in silastic tubing did not help very much. Polystyrene coating, on the other hand, is not as bad as cellulose acetate. The pellets did continue releasing BP in vivo (Fig. 7).

BP Release from Carbon Particles Incorporated into Beeswax Pellets

BP was adsorbed on carbon particles in BP/carbon ratios of 1:1, 1:3, and 1:9. The BP/carbon was then incorporated into beeswax pellets, and the release of BP from the pellets was studied in vitro. As shown in Fig. 8A, at the BP/carbon ratios of 1:3 and 1:9, the release rates are markedly reduced, compared to the release of BP from beeswax pellets. At the highest carbon concentration, <40% of the BP was released within 4 weeks.

Release of TPA from Beeswax Pellets

The tracheal transplant model was eminently suitable for demonstration of tumor promotion and this prompted us to study the release of the classical tumor promoter TPA from beeswax pellets. The in vitro and

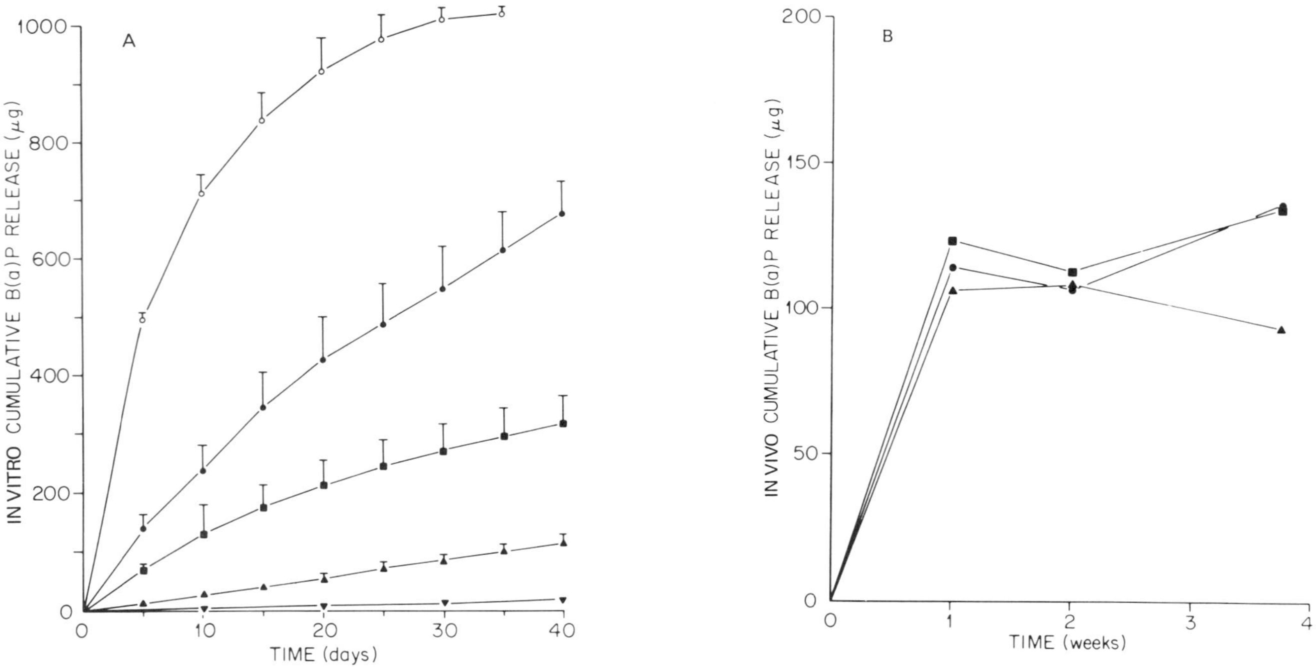

Figure 6 Cumulative release of BP from 1000-μg BP/beeswax pellets dip-coated with different thicknesses of cellulose acetate expressed in milligrams of coating weight per pellet. (A) In vitro release, beeswax pellet without any coating, ○, with different weights of cellulose acetate coating per pellet; ●, 0.55 mg, ■, 0.80-0.90 mg, ▲, 2.30-2.40 mg, ▼, 5.10 mg. Each point represents the mean observation from three pellets ± SD. (B) In vivo release, beeswax pellet without any coating, ○, with different weights of cellulose acetate coating per pellet; ●, 0.5 mg, ■, 2.5 mg, ▲, 3.6 mg. Each point represents the mean observation from six pellets.

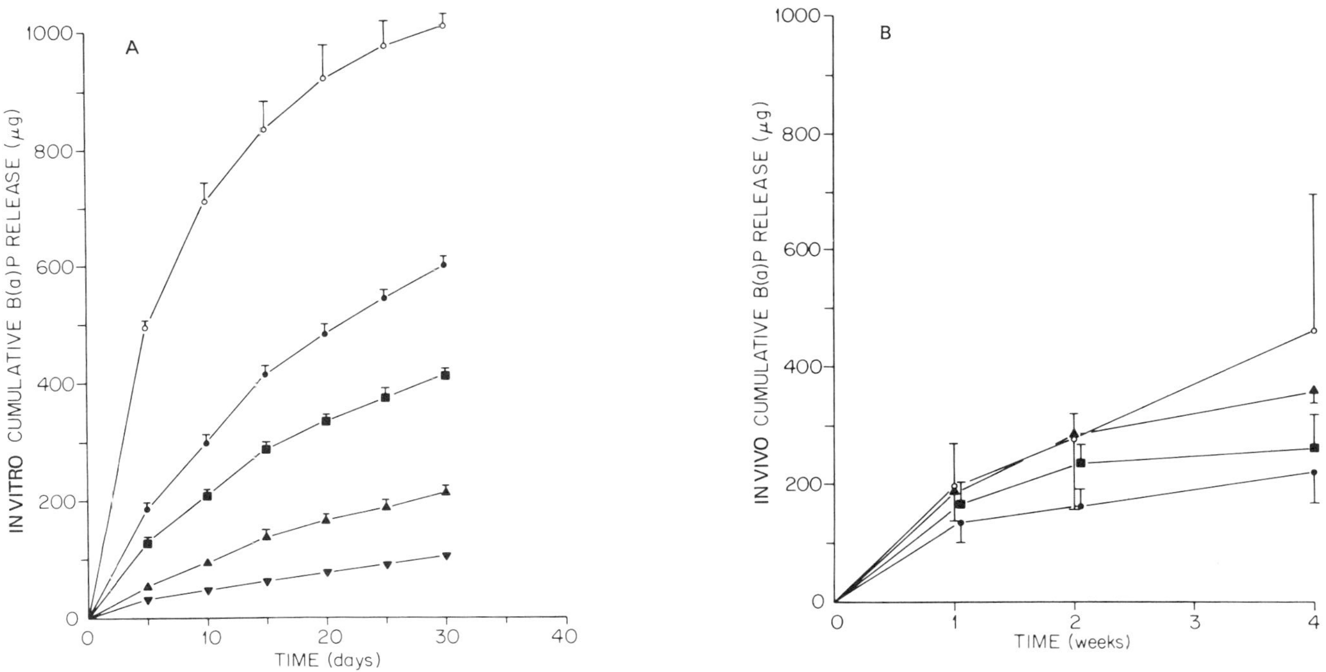

Figure 7 Cumulative release of BP from 1000-μg BP/beeswax pellets dip-coated with different thicknesses of polystyrene expressed in milligrams of coating weight per pellet. (A) In vitro release, beeswax pellet without any coating, O, with different weights of polystyrene coating per pellet: ●, 1.75 mg, ■, 3.15-3.30 mg, ▲, 5.30-5.50 mg, ▼, 10.10-10.35 mg. Each point represents the mean observation from four pellets ± SD. (B) In vivo release, beeswax pellet without any coating, O, with different weights of polystyrene coating per pellet: ▲, 2.30-2.55 mg, ■, 5.20-5.40 mg, ●, 10.20-10.50 mg. Each point represents the mean observation from six pellets ± SD.

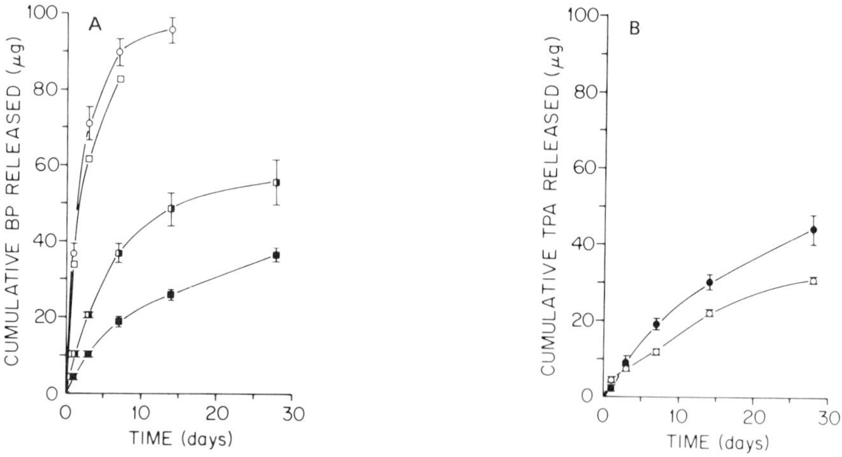

Figure 8 (A) In vitro release of BP from carbon/beeswax matrix. BP was absorbed to carbon particles in varying ratios, at 100 μg BP per pellet. ○, BP in beeswax; □, BP/carbon at a ratio of 1:1 in beeswax; ◧, BP/carbon at a ratio of 1:3 in beeswax; ■, BP/carbon at a ratio of 1:9 in beeswax. Each point represents the mean observation from two to four pellets ± SD. (B) Cumulative release of TPA from beeswax pellets, at 100 μg TPA per pellet. ○, in vitro release; ●, in vivo release in tracheal grafts. Each point represents the mean observation from four pellets in vitro ± SD and six pellets in vivo ± SD. (From Ref. 5.)

in vivo release of TPA from 100-μg TPA-beeswax pellets are shown in Fig. 8B. The amount of TPA released in 4 weeks was 31% in vitro and 45% in vivo. The percentages of SD ranged from 3 to 11 in vitro and 7 to 25 in vivo for different time points. Thus the release of TPA from beeswax is much slower than that of two PCHs, BP and DMBA, and the in vivo variability is also much less. It appears that, with a starting concentration of 0.4% TPA, the transplants can be exposed to this promoter for at least 2-3 months.

Retardation of PCH Release by Modification of Pellet Matrix

Cholesterol has been previously used as a matrix for controlled release of steroids [13] and luteinizing hormone-releasing hormone [14]. We preferred to retain at least 10% beeswax in the cholesterol matrix for ease of pellet fabrication. Cholesteryl laurate has also been used in place of cholesterol, but it was not very effective in slowing down the release rate (Fig. 9). Cholesterol effectively reduced the release rate

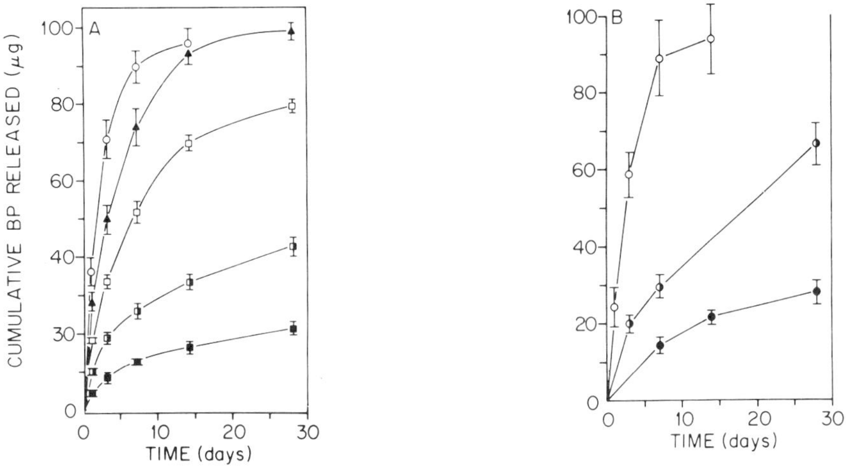

Figure 9 Cumulative release of BP from pellets with modified matrix, at 100 µg BP per pellet. (A) In vitro studies. ○, beeswax pellets; ▲, beeswax/cholesteryl laurate pellets at a ratio of 1:9; □, beeswax/cholesterol pellets at a ratio of 1:1; ◧, beeswax/cholesterol pellets at a ratio of 1:3; ■, beeswax/cholesterol pellets at a ratio of 1:9. Each point represents the mean of two to five observations ± SD. (B) In vivo studies in tracheal grafts. ○, beeswax pellets; ◑, beeswax/cholesterol pellets at a ratio of 1:3; ●, beeswax/cholesterol pellets at a ratio of 1:9. Each point represents the mean of four to six observations ± SD. (From Ref. 5.)

of DMBA, about 30 µg being released over a period of 4 weeks from 100-µg DMBA-cholesterol/beeswax (9:1) pellets. This is remarkable when one considers that in 1 week, ∿90% DMBA is released from beeswax pellets, whereas only about 13% is released from cholesterol matrix (Fig. 9). The rate of release can be reduced further by heating the cholesterol/beeswax (9:1) matrix for 6 hr at 150°C in a nitrogen atmosphere (data not reported). Presumably, cholesterol undergoes some type of polymerization under these conditions. Transesterification may also take place with the components of beeswax, but this cannot be responsible for slower release. Unfortunately, cholesterol has been found to have some drawbacks. It readily undergoes autoxidation and these products have been shown to be mutagenic in an Ames test [15], although the particular components in the mixture responsible for mutagenic activity have not been identified. These autoxidation products have also been found to be angiotoxic [16]. Terzaghi et al. have observed in our laboratory that cholesterol causes an undesirably high background in the epithelial foci assay of the preneoplastic lesions in tracheal transplants [17] (unpublished observations). For these reasons, we made a detailed investigation of cholesterol from three different commercial sources: Aldrich, Fisher, and Eastman Kodak. The GC analysis of cholesterol on a Supelcoport 3% SP-2250 column (3 ft × 2 mm) revealed that Aldrich product has some impurities, while Fisher and Eastman Kodak product showed a homogeneous peak. Nonetheless, Eastman Kodak cholesterol (assay 99.5% minimum by differential scanning calorimetry) was further purified by the dibromide method of Fieser [18] and stored in the deep freeze in a nitrogen atmosphere. The findings of Terzaghi et al. cited above were confirmed by using the highest-purity cholesterol. The cholesterol-beeswax matrix, when heated during the preparation of the pellets in a nitrogen atmosphere, did not show the formation of autoxidation products, whereas when the matrix was heated in air, formation of several autoxidation products was detected by TLC [silica gel, ether, R_f's 0.23, 0.37, 0.49, 0.55, 0.65, 0.74, 0.85 (cholesterol); spots were visualized by exposure to iodine vapor]. These results led us to find an alternative for cholesterol in controlling the release of PCHs. Stearyl alcohol has been found to be a suitable substitute, although the release rates are not as low as one can obtain with cholesterol [75% PCH is released in 4 weeks from stearyl alcohol/beeswax (9:1) compared with 30% from cholesterol/beeswax (9:1) in 4 weeks].

SUMMARY AND CONCLUSIONS

The attractiveness of the tracheal transplant model as a tool in experimental lung cancer research is apparent since several other laboratories have adopted it with minor modifications [19,20]. However, serious shortcomings of the model were realized and most of these were related to the carcinogen delivery system used to bring the test substance in direct contact with the tracheal epithelium. Beeswax was used initially as a matrix for release of PCHs, BP, and DMBA and it was found that low-dose exposure cannot be realized with 100-μg PCH-beeswax pellets. Practically 100% of the PCHs was released in 2 weeks, whereas protracted release over >4 weeks was realized with 1000-μg PCH-beeswax pellets. The anomaly was resolved when it was found that the release characteristics of the pellet rather than the in vivo environment were responsible for this difference in release. The solubility of BP in beeswax at 37°C was found to be about 0.5%; at a lower dose level (0.41%), most of the BP was in solution in beeswax, whereas at higher dose levels (4.1%), most of the BP was in crystalline form. The release of PCHs from these pellets follows the course predicted by the Higuchi model [12]. The solubility of BP in fetal calf serum, rat serum, and human serum has been found to be 35, 147, and 214 μg/ml, respectively, at 37°C. It was found that at high release rates of highly potent carcinogens such as BP and DMBA, the severity of the tissue reaction and changes in the circulating fluid caused high variability in the release rates in vivo. Apparently, the solution lies in the slower protracted release of the carcinogens in vivo. Three different approaches to achieve this goal were tried:

1. *Dip-coating the PCH-beeswax pellets with cellulose acetate or polystyrene.* The in vitro results were very promising but the in vivo results were disappointing, particularly with cellulose acetate. The pellets stopped releasing due to encapsulation.
2. *Changing the matrix composition.* Cholesterol has been incorporated in beeswax up to the extent of 90%, and this matrix dramatically slows down the release of the PCHs, from 7 μg/day to 1 μg/day in vivo. Since cholesterol itself was found to cause undesirably high background in the epithelial foci assay of the preneoplastic lesions of the tracheal epithelium, an acceptable alternative to cholesterol was found in stearyl alcohol. The release rate with stearyl alcohol/beeswax (9:1) is two and a half times higher than that obtainable with cholesterol/beeswax (9:1). Stearyl alcohol does not cause any high background in the above-mentioned assay.
3. *Adsorbing PCHs on the carbon particles followed by dispersion of these particles in beeswax.* The problem of uniform dispersion of these particles in beeswax has been solved simply by triturating the mix in a hot mortar and pestle until it congeals. Release rates from these pellets were comparable to those obtained with cholesterol/beeswax (9:1) matrices. Beeswax alone was found to be a suitable matrix for release of TPA, releasing about 1 μg/day in vivo, although the severity of the tissue reaction indicates that slower rates are desirable. In carrying out in vitro experiments on the release of PCHs, it was found that fetal calf serum was a more suitable medium for release than was physiological saline or simulated extracellular fluid, and the in vitro rates were more realistic and mimicked the rates in vivo.

We conclude that a satisfactory solution to the problem of exposing tracheal transplants at a controlled rate to carcinogens, BP and DMBA, and promoter, TPA, has been found. Controlled release of gases such as SO_2 and NO_x, fly ash, asbestos, cellulose fibers, coal liquids, and water-soluble carcinogens such as dimethylnitrosamine in the tracheal transplant are challenging problems for the future. The tracheal transplant model may also serve as a useful method for evaluating various controlled release devices in vivo.

ACKNOWLEDGMENTS

Thanks are due to R. A. Griesemer, P. Nettesheim, and Ann Marchok for advice and encouragement and to F. R. Nelson, R. H. Martin, and C. Howard for their expert technical assistance. This research was supported in part by the Environmental Protection Agency (81D-X0533) and by the Department of Energy under contract with the Union Carbide Corporation.

REFERENCES

1. R. A. Griesemer, J. Kendrick, and P. Nettesheim, Tracheal grafts, in *Experimental Lung Cancer: Carcinogenesis and Bioassays* (E. Karbe and J. F. Park, eds.), Springer-Verlag, New York, 1974, pp. 539-547.
2. P. Nettesheim, R. A. Griesemer, D. H. Martin, and J. E. Caton, Jr., *Cancer Res.*, *37*:1272 (1977).
3. R. A. Griesemer, P. Nettesheim, D. H. Martin, and J. E. Caton, Jr., *Cancer Res.*, *37*:1266 (1977).
4. D. C. Topping, B. C. Pal, D. H. Martin, F. R. Nelson, and P. Nettesheim, *Am. J. Pathol.*, *93*:311 (1978).
5. B. C. Pal, D. C. Topping, R. A. Griesemer, F. R. Nelson, and P. Nettesheim, *Cancer Res.*, *38*:1376 (1978).
6. J. Kendrick, P. Nettesheim, and A. S. Hammons, *J. Natl. Cancer Inst.*, *52*:1317 (1974).
7. H. Obrikat and K. Wettig, *Arch. Geschwulstforsch.*, *35*:326 (1974).
8. C. A. Homsy, *J. Biomed. Mater. Res.*, *4*:341 (1970).
9. I. B. Rubin and M. R. Guerin, *J. Natl. Cancer Inst.*, *58*:641 (1977).
10. J. T. Veal and G. E. Dagle, *Toxicol. Appl. Pharmacol.*, *35*:157 (1976).
11. T. J. Roseman and W. I. Higuchi, *J. Pharm. Sci.*, *59*:353 (1970).
12. T. Higuchi, *J. Pharm. Sci.*, *52*:1145 (1963).
13. F. A. Kincl, K. Sunderam, C. C. Chang, and H. W. Rudel, *Acta Endocrinol.*, *64*:253 (1970).
14. J. S. Kent, B. H. Vickery, and G. I. McRae, *Abstr. 7th Int. Symp. Controlled Release Bioact. Mater.*, July 28-30, 1980, p. 67.
15. L. L. Smith, V. B. Smart, and G. A. Ansoni, *Mutat. Res.*, *68*: 23 (1979).
16. H. Imai, N. T. Werthessen, V. Subramaniyam, P. W. LeGuerre, A. M. Solway, and M. Kanisawa, *Science*, *207*:651 (1980).
17. M. Terzaghi and P. Nettesheim, *Cancer Res.*, *39*:4003 (1979).
18. L. F. Fieser, in *Organic Synthesis*, Collected Vol. 4 (N. Rabjohn, ed.), Wiley, 1963, p. 195.

19. B. P. Lane and M. J. Mass, *Cancer Res.*, *37*:1476 (1977).
20. B. T. Mossman and J. E. Craighead, *Proc. Am. Assoc. Cancer Res.*, *18*:222 (1977).

Chapter 10

Development of a Controlled Absorption Quinidine Drug Delivery System

O. I. CORRIGAN Trinity College School of Pharmacy, Dublin, Ireland

ADRIAN DUNNE and HUGH McLAUGHLIN University College, Dublin, Ireland

EDWARD J. GEOGHEGAN, CHRISSIE A. KILLIAN, and DONALD E. PANOZ Elan Corporation, Ltd., Monksland, Athlone, Ireland

The anti-arrhythmic drug quinidine has been in use for some 50 years. Conventionally, quinidine is administered in a regimen of 200 mg, three or four times daily. A narrow margin exists between the serum levels required to elicit the desired effect and those producing drug toxicity. The ratio of the median lethal dose to the median effective dose has been reported to be less than 2. A similar difference exists between the maximum desired concentration ($C^*_{max} \sim 8^\dagger$ μg/ml) and minimum effective concentration ($C^*_{min} \sim 4^\dagger$ μg/ml) [1]. The therapeutic index of quinidine is therefore of the order of 2: that is,

$$TI = \frac{C^*_{max}}{C^*_{min}} \sim 2$$

When the therapeutic index of a drug is known, the proper dosage interval (τ) is dictated by [2]

$$\tau \le t_{1/2} \frac{\ln TI}{\ln 2}$$

This approach suggests that for quinidine (the half-life of which is $\sim$ 6 hr) a dosing interval of about 6 hr is appropriate—a finding consistent with conventional therapy.

---

†Values based on double-extraction technique.

The objective of the current work was therefore to design an oral delivery system which could lengthen the dosage interval to a more convenient span, while minimizing fluctuations in the maximum-to-minimum plasma concentrations (C_{max}/C_{min} ratio) and without significantly reducing the bioavailability. The C_{max}/C_{min} ratio during repetitive drug administration has been called the dosage form index DI_{τ} and is a function of the dosage form, the pharmacokinetics of the drug, and the dosing interval. The ideal C_{max}/C_{min} ratio to use is that pertaining at the steady state. In product development work this is impractical and therefore the corresponding values following a single dose (DI_s) are used in the current work: the ratio of the peak serum concentration to the serum concentration after 12 or 24 hr (DI_{s12} or DI_{s24}, respectively). If linear pharmacokinetics are operative, this apparent dosage form index (DI_s) should reflect the steady-state situation. A properly designed dosage form should have a dosage form index equal to or smaller than the therapeutic index. It also follows , when comparing dosage forms, that the system with the lowest dosage form index should be therapeutically superior, provided that C_{min} during treatment is larger than or equal to the minimum effective concentration (C^*_{min}).

Possible factors limiting the development of an optimal quinidine product include the reported incomplete bioavailability of the drug, about 70% reaching the systemic circulation [1,3], as a consequence of either first-pass metabolism in the liver or slow dissolution in the gastrointestinal tract.

EXPERIMENTAL

The dosage forms investigated were Quinora Tablets (Key) 300 mg, Lot 900821; Quinidex Extentabs (A. H. Robins) 300 mg, Lot 802486; and four dosage forms developed by Elan, which have been designated A, B, C, and D. The release characteristics of the latter products were controlled by the nature of the drug excipient mixture, the multiparticulate nature of the drug delivery system, and the properties of the rate-controlling membranes employed. All dosage forms administered contained 300 mg of quinidine sulfate except product D, which contained 400 mg. The data reported for the latter product have therefore been dose-corrected throughout the report.

Each product was tested in six healthy male volunteers, Quinora, Quinidex, and product A being compared initially in a crossover study. During the development work on products B, C, and D, volunteers were replaced on the volunteer panel such that three subjects were common to trials on all products. The data from these three volunteers formed the basis of comparisons involving these products.

Dosage forms were administered 30 min before a light breakfast. Plasma quinidine concentrations were determined by high-pressure liquid chromatography on a C-18 reverse phase column using 5:45:50, 0.13% ammonium phosphate solution/acetonitrile/methanol as mobile phase and ultraviolet (UV) detection at 236 nm. The plasma samples were extracted using a modification of the method of Kessler et al [4]. Dihydroquinidine and the 3-hydroxy metabolite of quinidine did not interfere with the chromatographic peaks of quinidine. Differences in bioavailability (AUC_∞) and DI_s were assessed using analysis of variance. Terminal loss rate constants were obtained using NONLIN from the terminal Quinora data.

Quinidine sulfate dissolution profiles were obtained using a modified United States Pharmacopeia (U.S.P.) XIX procedure having a basket rotating rate of 75 rpm and dissolution media of pH 1.5, 3.0, 6.0, and 7.5. Dissolved quinidine was assayed at 250 nm by UV spectroscopy. Reproducibility (products A, C, and D) of replicate determinations was generally within 8%, when more than 10% of the drug had dissolved. The coefficients of variation of product B (n = 4) were approximately 11%.

RESULTS AND DISCUSSION

Figure 1 shows the plasma level versus time profiles obtained from a preliminary bioavailability crossover trial (n = 6) comparing a currently available solid oral dosage form with immediate release characteristics (Quinora Tablets, 300 mg) and a conventional sustained release form (Quinidex Extentabs, 300 mg). Both products had equivalent bioavailability but differed significantly in C_{max}/C_{min} 12-hr ratio, reflecting differences in rate of absorption.

While the pharmacokinetics of intravenous Quinidine show a short alpha phase ($t_{1/2\alpha} \approx 3$ min) [5,6], the pharmacokinetics of quinidine following oral administration have been represented by the one-compartment open model [7] and comparisons of the relative rate of quinidine absorption have, in the absence of intravenous data, been made [7] using the Wagner-Nelson function, A_T/V [8]:

$$\frac{A_T}{V} = C_P(T) + K \int_O^T C_P(t)\, dt$$

where A_T is the amount absorbed at time T, V is the volume of distribution, $C_P(T)$ is the plasma level at time T, and K is the terminal rate constant. From the plots obtained, the average rate of absorption at each sampling interval was estimated. Quinora was most rapidly absorbed in the first hour following drug administration, absorption being virtually complete after 4 hr. The maximum absorption rate of Quinora was three to four times more rapid than that of Quinidex. Peak rate of

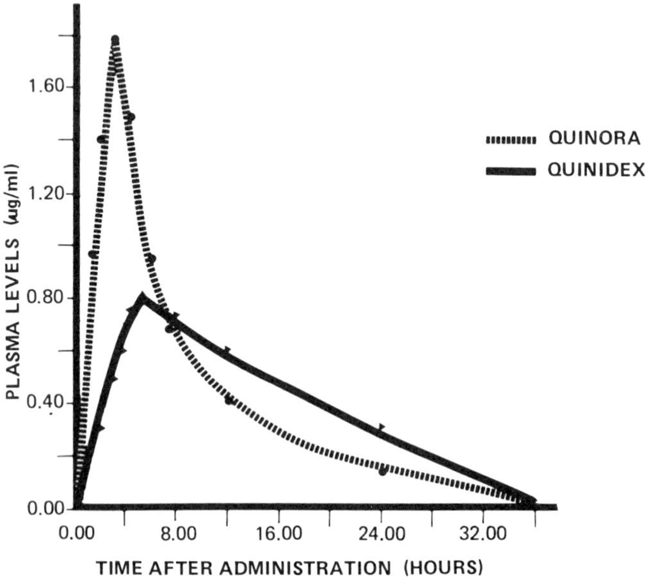

Figure 1 Plasma level versus time profiles of immediate release (Quinora) and sustained release (Quinidex) quinidine sulfate products.

absorption from Quinidex occurred between the first and second hour following drug administration.

In outlining requirements for quinidine bioequivalence the FDA points to rapid metabolism of the drug in the intestinal wall or liver during the process of absorption [1]. They state that about 70% of drug reaches the systemic circulation after oral administration, and imply that poor bioavailability may be due to saturable first-pass metabolism. If this reasoning is correct, one would have expected a significantly higher bioavailability from the more rapidly absorbed product, Quinora, than from Quinidex.

The dissolution profiles obtained for these two products at pH 1.5, 3.0, 6.0, and 7.5 are shown in Fig. 2. Over 90% of quinidine was dissolved from Quinora in 10 min, the percentages ranging from 100 to 94% in the pH range cited. By contrast, the percentage of drug released from Quinidex after 6 hr ranged from 73% at pH 1.5 to only 35% at pH 7.5. Even after 12 hr, when complete dissolution had occurred at pH 1.5, less than 50% dissolution had taken place at the higher pH values.

The Elan Corporation has been involved in a research project with the aim of developing a quinidine dosage form that would overcome this apparently limited dissolution at higher pH values. This has entailed

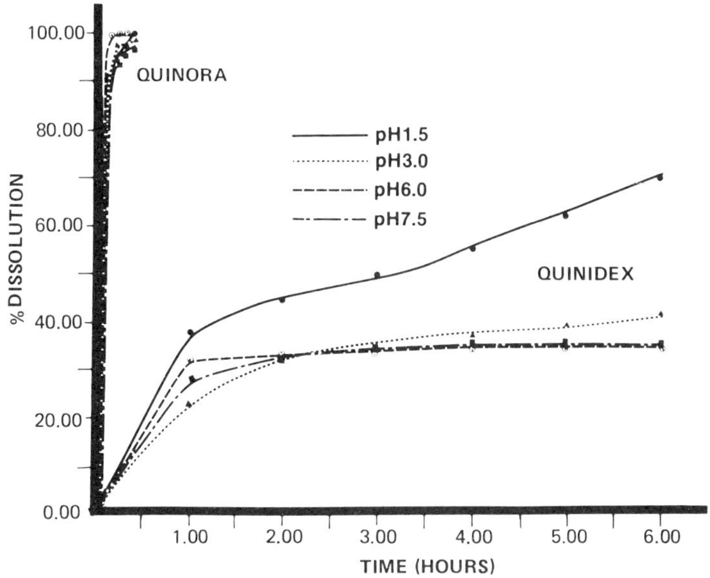

Figure 2 Effect of pH on the dissolution profiles of Quinora and Quinidex.

developing and testing a sequence of formulations, including those which we have designated products A to D. Each product was tested in vitro and in vivo, and on the basis of the results obtained by these screening procedures, the next product in the series was designed.

The basic dosage form chosen was multiparticulate, the active principle being dispersed in a large number of microgranules, contained in a hard gelatin capsule. The size and density of the granules are designed to ensure a consistent rate of travel through the stomach and into the upper intestine.

The core of each granule consists of active principle, physically complexed with excipients to enhance and control its dispersion and solubility. A membrane is then applied, to control further the rate of dissolution, and the sequential development process leading from product A to product D involved modifications in the composition and thickness of the membrane.

The excipients incorporated in the formulation are specific to the drug involved, and in the present case they were selected to cater for the relevant properties of quinidine, including its pH-related solubility and dissolution. The dissolution profiles under varying conditions for products A to D are shown in Fig. 3.

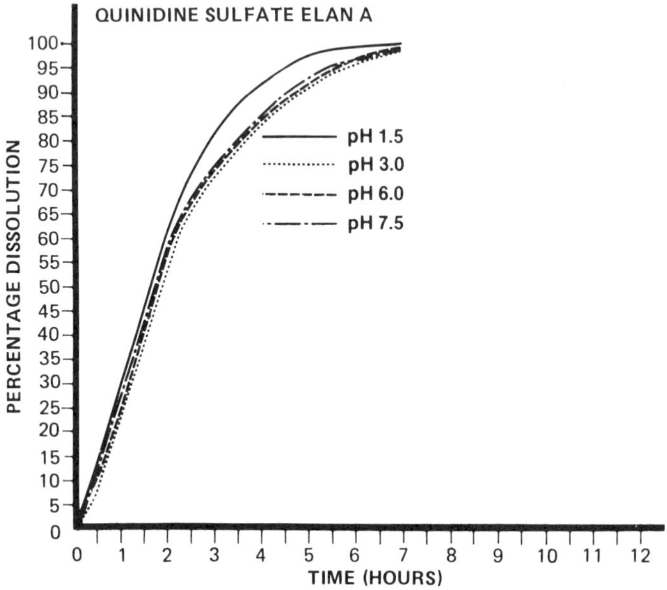

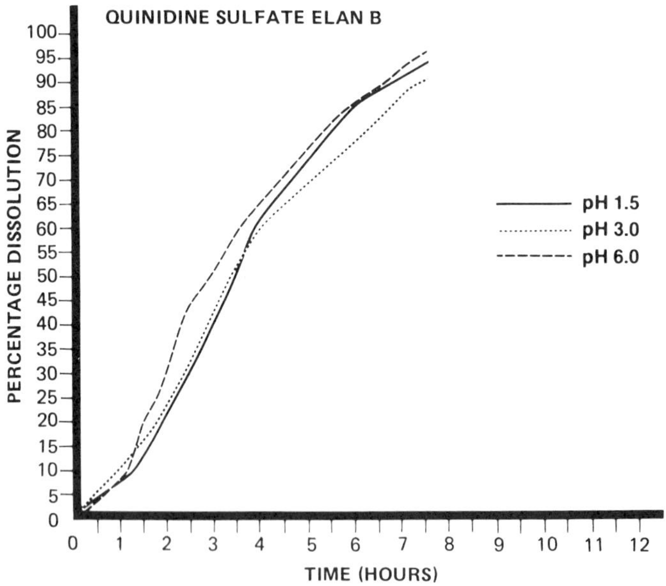

Figure 3 Influence of pH on the dissolution properties of four Elan quinidine sulfate products, A, B, C, D.

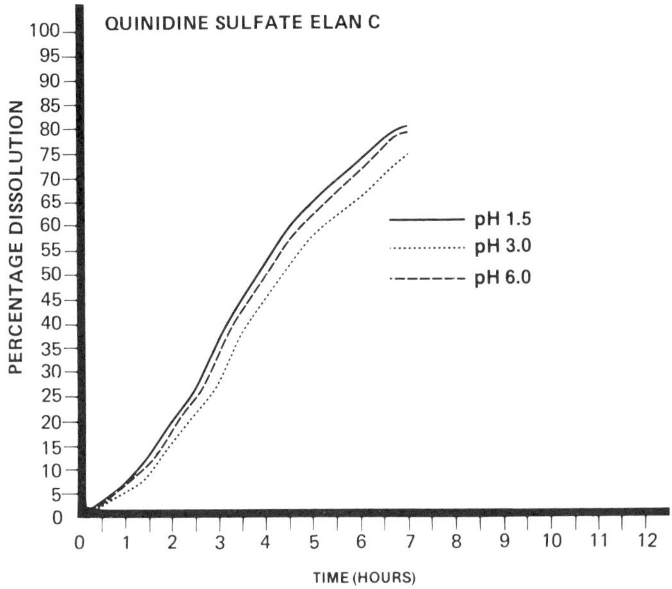

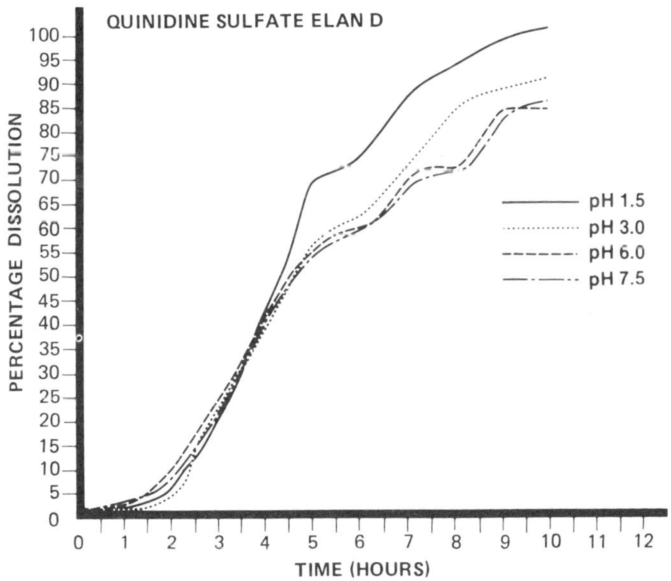

Figure 3 Continued.

Product A gave linear drug release up to about 70% dissolved, the average time for 50% quinidine drug release ($T_{50\%}$) being 108 min. Because of the less favorable environment for dissolution and absorption in the lower gastrointestinal tract, the products were designed to give slightly more rapid drug release at higher pH. Products B, C, and D were formulated to give slower overall drug delivery rates and have $T_{50\%}$ values of 195, 243, and 270 min, respectively.

Decreasing the drug delivery rate has tended to introduce an initial lag in release rate, with slower rather than faster release at high pH relative to low pH. The average plasma level versus time curves obtained in the same subjects (n = 3) using these four formulations are shown in Fig. 4. The bioavailability of all products was compared by calculating the area under the plasma level versus time curve ($AUC_{0 \rightarrow \infty}$). Relative bioavailabilities are tabulated in Table 1. None of the Elan products had a significantly lower bioavailability than either Quinora or Quinidex. Indeed, Elan A had a significantly greater ($P < 0.05$) bioavailability than Quinora and Quinidex.

Products B, C, and D, with progressively decreasing drug dissolution rates, show reduction in peak height, with prolonged time to peak. A trend toward decreasing bioavailability was also apparent.

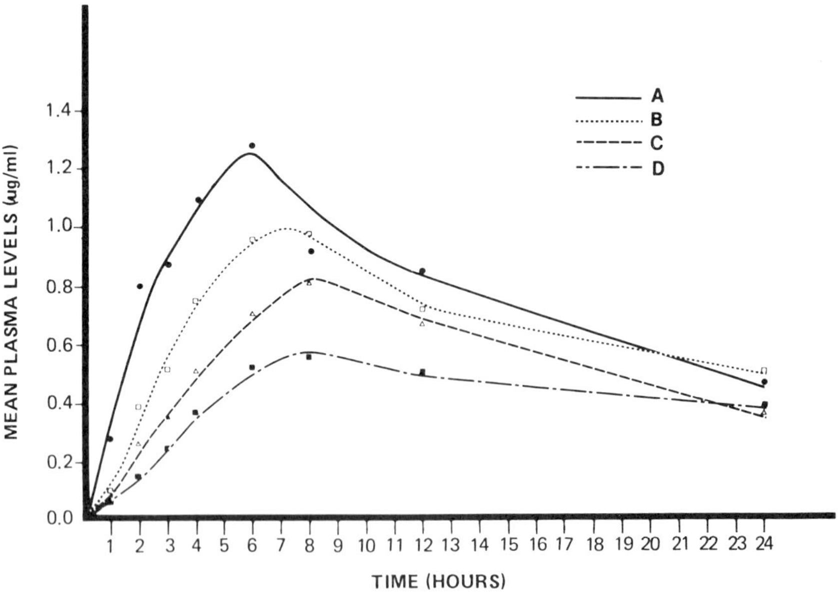

Figure 4 Average plasma level versus time profiles for formulations A, B, C, and D.

Table 1 Comparison of Relative Bioavailability of Six Quinidine Sulfate Preparations Using Quinora as Standard

Formulation	Relative bioavailability (%)
Quinora	100.0
Quinidex	92.0
Elan A	129.9
Elan B	107.2
Elan C	87.1
Elan D	73.3

Wagner-Nelson plots for six formulations are shown in Fig. 5. Absorption for products A to D are in rank-order agreement with the dissolution rates (Fig. 3). These profiles were not first order; initial absorption was reasonably linear, and absorption continued beyond 12 hr, while in the more slowly dissolving products it continued beyond 24 hr.

The change in relative rate of absorption with time for these products is shown in Fig. 6. As with Quinidex, the maximum absorption rate for products A and B occurred between the first and second hours following administration. Peak absorption rates for products C and D, however, occurred between the third and fourth hours following dosing.

Reducing the drug dissolution rate can be seen to result in a more even rate of drug absorption, whereas maintaining drug dissolution at higher pH tended to result in a higher absorption rate at later times after drug administration. The early 1- to 2-hr absorption peak present in products A to C may represent gastric dissolution of the drug, since the absorption rates in this period are in rank-order agreement with the dissolution rates in acid media during the same time period.

In vitro dissolution testing is important not only in drug dosage form development, but also because in many cases such tests are required by regulatory agencies, particularly the U.S. Food and Drug Administration (FDA) [9]. With reference specifically to quinidine, the FDA recently proposed to establish dissolution testing criteria for certain immediate release solid oral dosage forms, as part of a Quinidine Bioequivalence Requirement [1]. The proposed test, to be carried out in 0.1 N HCl, requires not less than 85% drug dissolution in 30 min. The controlled release products examined in this chapter, having acceptable bioavailability, do not comply with these limits, and this underscores the problems inherent in defining dissolution test conditions.

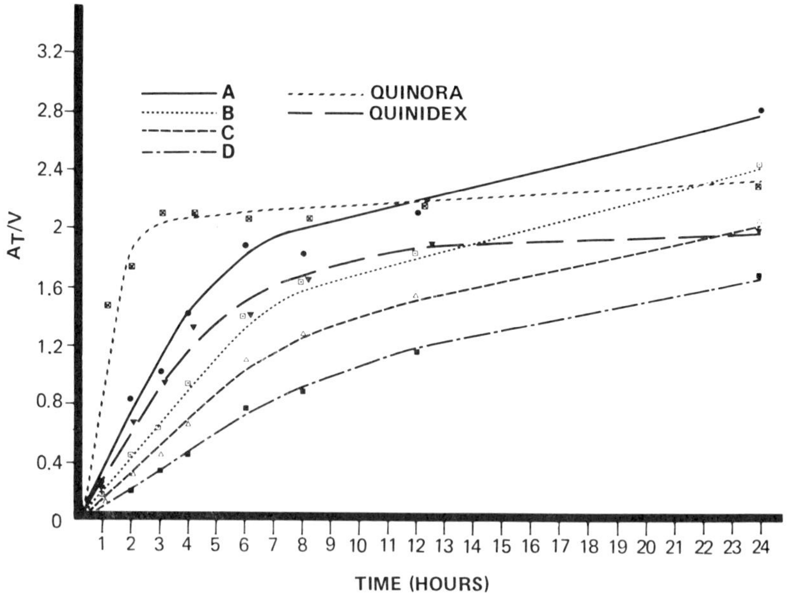

Figure 5 Absorption versus time profiles for Quinora, Quinidex, and formulations A, B, C, and D obtained using the Wagner-Nelson function.

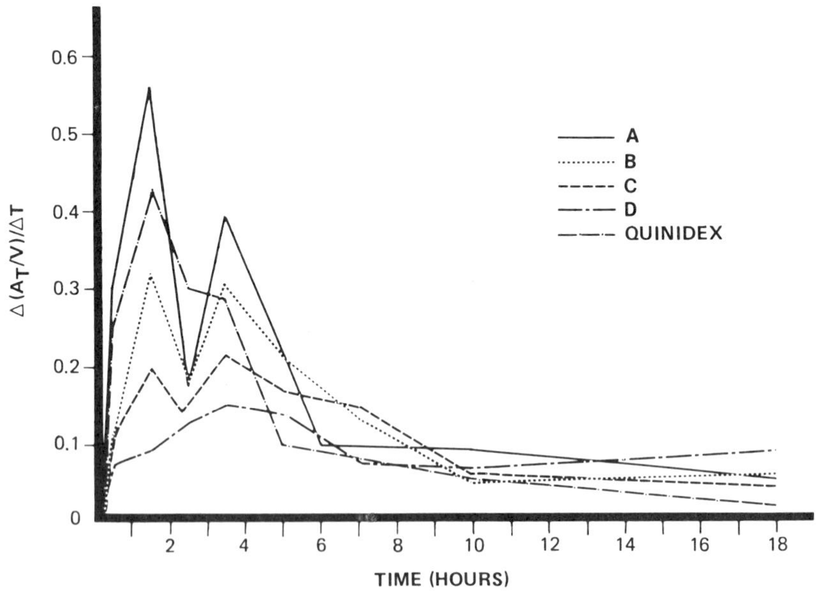

Figure 6 Changes in relative rate of absorption with time for formulations A, B, C, D, and Quinidex.

The dissolution test employed in the current work is basically similar to the USP procedure but employs a lower basket rotation rate of 75 rpm.

In Fig. 7 the relationship between quinidine absorbed (A_T/V) at a given time after drug administration and the amount dissolved in vitro is plotted for the Elan products. The good linearity of the plot ($r = 0.923$, $n = 20$) strongly indicates that in vitro dissolution rates directly dictate in vivo absorption for these products. The Quinidex data are also included in Fig. 7, but here there is no comparable relationship. These results show clearly that dissolution profiles for the Elan products are good indicators of absorption. They also illustrate the sequential development process by which Elan arrived at a final formulation.

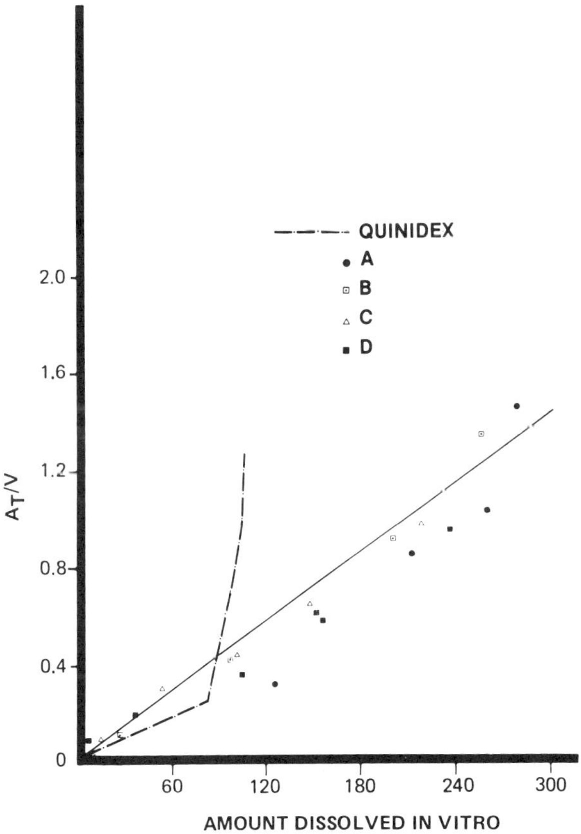

Figure 7 Relationship between Quinidine absorbed (A_T/V) at a given time after drug administration and the amount dissolved in vitro at the same time.

The influence of dosage form modification on DI_{s12} is shown in Fig. 8. As expected, the rapidly absorbed product Quinora has an unsatisfactory DI_{s12} of 4, twice the therapeutic index, while Quinidex has a value below 2. In the case of the Elan formulations, the systematic reduction in drug dissolution rate and hence in absorption rate brought about a corresponding reduction in DI_{s12}. All these controlled release products had DI_{s12} values significantly ($P < 0.05$) lower than Quinora, while the value for product D was significantly ($P < 0.05$) lower than that of Quinidex.

We have also calculated the DI_{s24} values for all these formulations. They are shown in Fig. 9. The ratios for products B, C, and D were significantly ($P < 0.05$) lower than that of Quinidex. The value for product D is not only less than 2 (the therapeutic index) but is also lower than the DI_{s12} of Quinidex (Fig. 8).

These observations suggest that product D has potential as a once-a-day product, given in a single dose every 24 hr. However quinidine pharmacokinetics may require fitting with different models in different

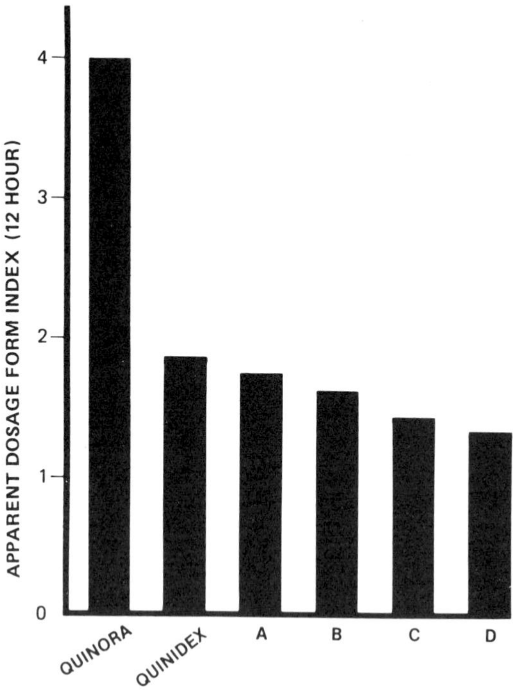

Figure 8 Influence of formulation on the apparent 12-hr dosage form index (DI_{s12}) of the six quinidine sulfate dosage forms.

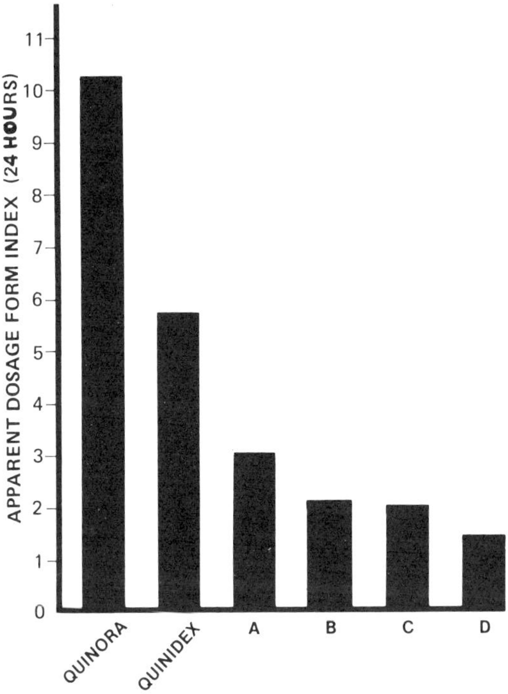

Figure 9 Influence of formulation on the apparent 24-hr dosage form index (DI_{S24}) of the six quinidine sulfate dosage forms.

subjects and often give poor prediction of steady-state levels. None of the plasma levels (Figs. 1 and 4) reached the reported C^*_{min} value of 4 μg/ml because this value is based on the non-specific double-extraction assay technique and because of the single-dose (non-steady-state) nature of the present study [10]. Thus confirmatory steady-state studies with product D are desirable.

REFERENCES

1. J. A. Halperin, *Fed. Reg.*, *45*:72200 (1980).
2. F. Theeuwes and W. Bayne, *J. Pharm. Sci.*, *66*:1388 (1977).
3. C. T. Ueda, B. J. Williamson, and B. S. Dzindzio, *Clin. Pharmacol. Ther.*, *20*:260 (1978).
4. K. M. Kessler, D. T. Lowenthal, H. Warner, T. Gibson, W. Briggs, and M. M. Reidenberg, *N. Engl. J. Med.*, *290*:706 (1974).

5. D. J. Greenblatt, H. J. Pfeifer, H. R. Ochs, K. Franke, D. S. McLaughlin, T. W. Smith, J. Koch-Weser, *J. Pharmacol. Exp. Ther.*, *202*:365 (1977).
6. T. W. Guentert, W. H. G. Halford, P. E. Coates, R. A. Upton, and S. Riegelman, *J. Pharmacokinet. Biopharm.*, *7*:315 (1979).
7. I. J. McGilveray, K. K. Midha, M. Rowe, M. Beaudoin, and C. Charette, *J. Pharm. Sci.*, *70*:524 (1981).
8. J. G. Wagner and E. Nelson, *J. Pharm. Sci.*, *52*:610 (1963).
9. B. E. Cabana and Y. W. Chien, Regulatory Considerations in controlled release medications, in press (1981).
10. M. E. Winter, in *Basic Clinical Pharmacokinetics*, Applied Therapeutics, San Francisco, 1980.

Chapter 11

Stability of Controlled Release Pharmaceutical Microcapsules

JOSEPH A. BAKAN and THOMAS C. POWELL Eurand America, Inc., Dayton, Ohio

Microencapsulation of pharmaceutical materials by coacervation/phase separation has been used academically and industrially for many years. As a process, it is a means of applying relatively thin film forming polymeric coatings to small particles of solid, droplets of liquids, or dispersions. Microencapsulation is arbitrarily differentiated from macroencapsulation in that the former involves the coating of particles ranging dimensionally from several tenths of a micrometer to about 5000 μm. Microcapsules provide a means to convert liquids to solids, separate reactive components, and control the release of materials.

The uniqueness of microcapsules lies in the smallness of the coated particles and their subsequent use and adaptation to a wide variety of dosage forms. Table 1 shows the large number of particles per gram of various diameter microcapsules. Because of the number and smallness of the microcapsules, drug moieties can be widely distributed throughout the gastrointestinal tract, thus potentially improving drug absorption.

The recent radiological studies of microencapsulated barium sulfate by Galeone et al. [1] graphically demonstrate this fact. Figure 1 shows microencapsulated barium sulfate being released from a dissolving hard gelatin macrocapsule shortly after ingestion. Figure 2 shows the microcapsules of barium sulfate having been released from the dissolved hard gelatin capsule and distributed as small-particle entitics (microcapsules) throughout the intestines.

Table 1 Microcapsule Diameter versus Number of Microcapsules per Gram

Microcapsule diameter (μm)	Approximate number of microcapsules per gram of material[a]
5	15,279,000,000
25	122,230,000
50	15,279,000
100	1,909,800
200	238,730
300	70,736
400	29,841
500	15,277
600	8,842
700	5,568
800	3,730
900	2,620
1000	1,910

[a]Assumes that the density = 1.
Source: Reprinted with permission from A. F. Kydonieus, *Controlled Release Technologies: Methods, Theory, and Applications*, vol. 2, CRC Press, Boca Raton, Florida, 1980. Copyright, The Chemical Rubber Company, CRC Press, Inc.

EXPERIMENTAL

The microencapsulation process to be discussed here is a phase separation technique from organic solvent using ethylcellulose, cyclohexane, and polyethylene [2-4]. This method of preparing microcapsules uses the demixing phenomenon of incompatible polymer pairs and temperature change as depicted in Fig. 3. The ethylcellulose and polyethylene are insoluble in cyclohexane at low temperatures. By raising the temperature to about the boiling point of the solvent, the polymers dissolve. By slowly cooling the mixture, the ethylcellulose comes out of solution as a liquid phase, which in turn coats a dispersed solid core particle. A schematic of this microencapsulation process can be found in Fig. 4. This batch microencapsulation process is carried out under controlled conditions of temperature and agitation. The ethylcellulose is added to the cyclohexane at

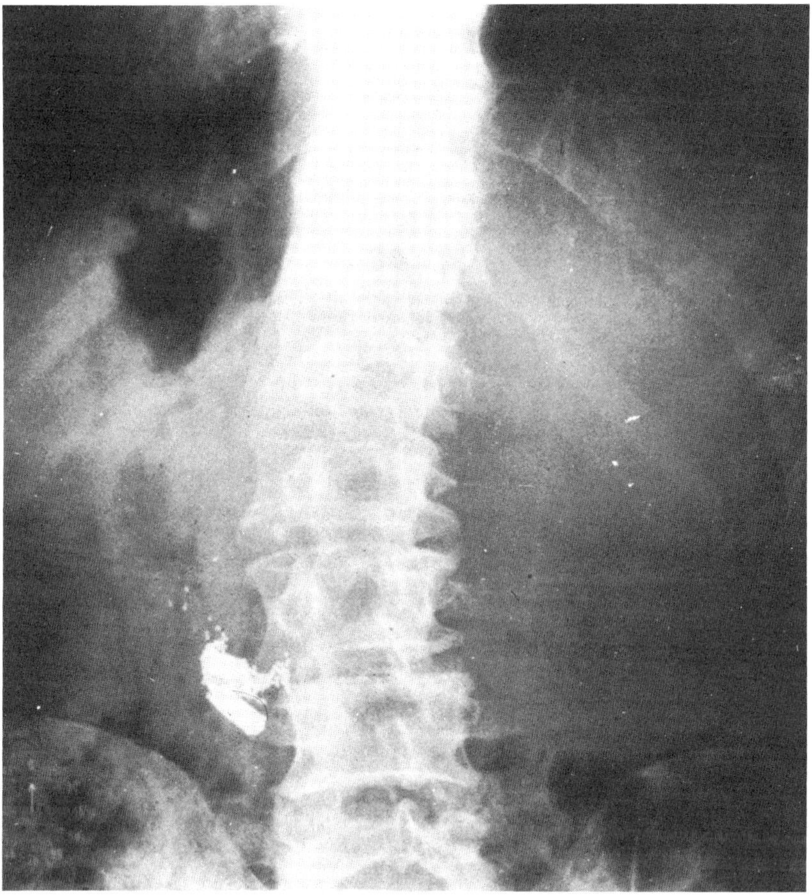

Figure 1 Barium sulfate particles in stomach. (From Ref. 1.)

room temperature in concentration ranges from about 0.3 to 4%. Polyethylene is then added to this mixture in the same concentrations. A quantity of solid drug core material is dispersed in this mixture to achieve the desired percent activity and release rate properties. The mixture is agitated while heating it to approximately 80°C to dissolve the polymers and maintain a good dispersion of core material and polymer solution. The heat is then removed and with continued agitation the dispersion is cooled slowly at a controlled rate to achieve microencapsulation. During the cooling stage, the ethylcellulose comes out of solution as a liquid phase. The mechanical stirring brings the liquidous concentrated ethylcellulose solution to the near

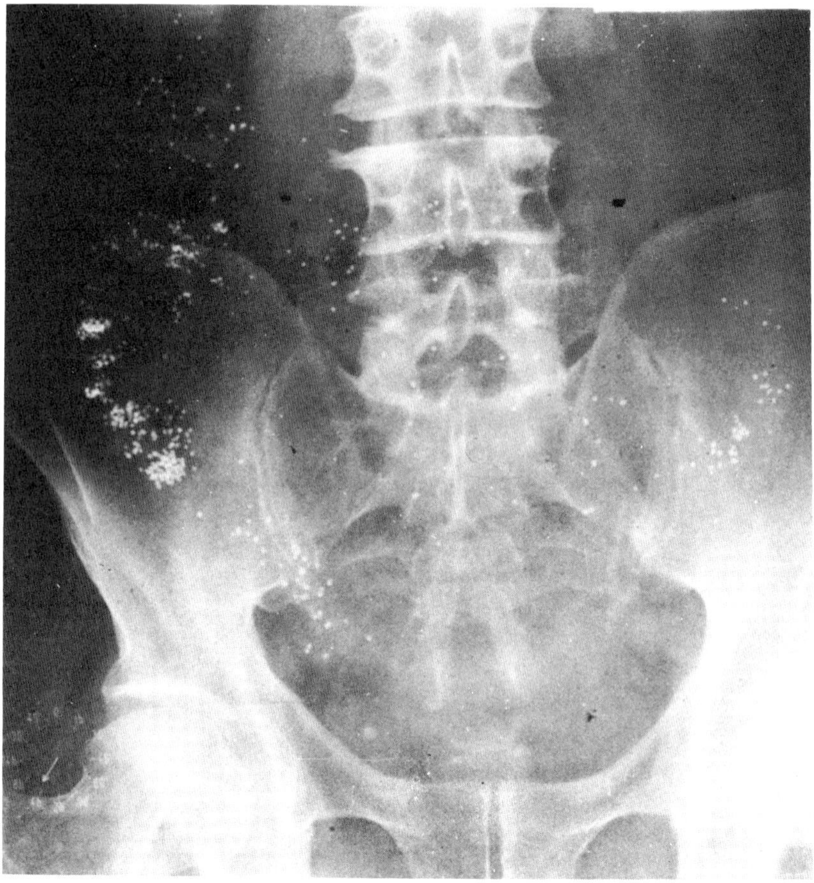

Figure 2 Barium sulfate particles in intestines. (From Ref. 1.)

proximity of the interface, where the polymer comes in contact with the core material and is sorbed at the solid-liquid interface, thus forming microcapsules. The driving force for microencapsulation at this point is a total reduction in the total free interfacial energy of the system. In the latter stages of the cooling cycle, the ethylcellulose solidifies to form solid microcapsules. The microcapsules are separated from the polyethylene-cyclohexane mixture. They may be washed with pure solvent if desired prior to drying to remove free polyethylene particles.

The release from microcapsules of water-soluble or partially water soluble drugs in water or gastrointestinal (GI) fluids is believed to

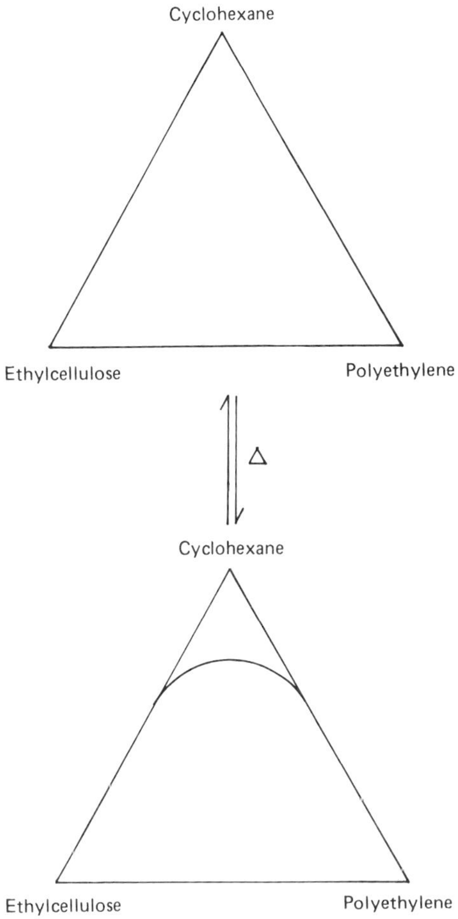

Figure 3 Phase diagram.

be primarily diffusion controlled. A simplified release mechanism is shown in Fig. 5. In the initial stages of the process, water permeates the coating, an aqueous solution of the water-soluble solid is formed within the microcapsule, and this solution permeates into the continuous water phase due to the concentration gradient existing across the membrane. The desired *in vitro* release rate is controlled primarily by the ethylcellulose film thickness around the core material. Other factors influencing the release rate include the solubility of the drug in water or GI fluid, microcapsule size, shape and structure of the core materials, the rate of solution of the drug in the aqueous media

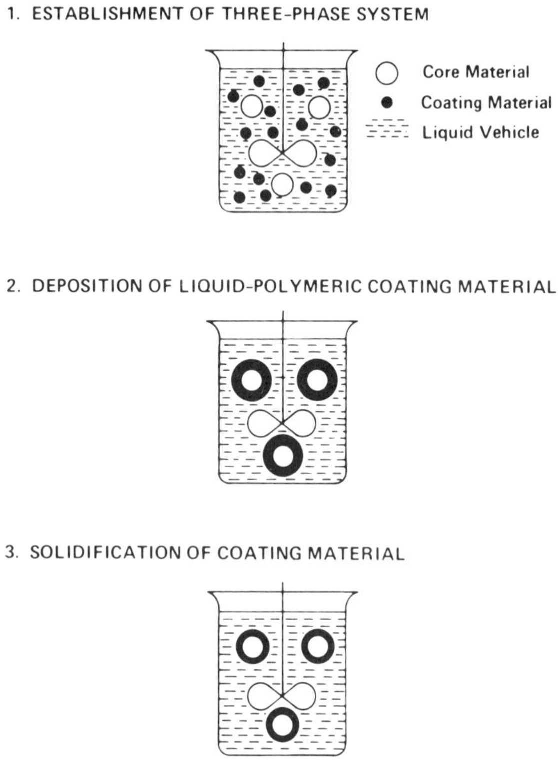

Figure 4 Process schematic. (From R. Kronenthal, Z. Oser, and E. Martin, *Polymers in Medicine and Surgery*, Plenum Press, New York, 1975.)

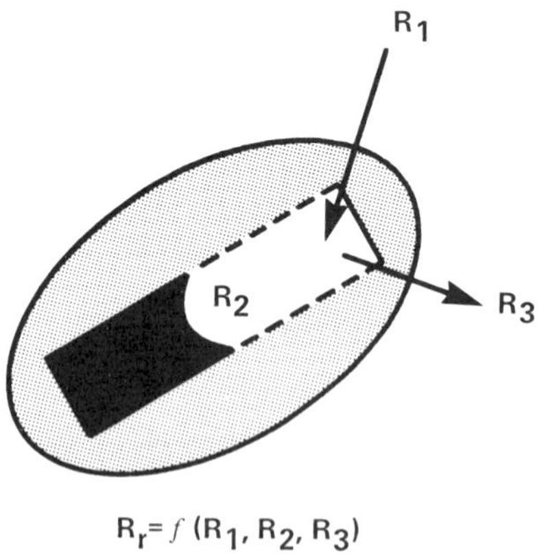

Figure 5 Release mechanism. (From R. Kronenthal, Z. Oser, and E. Martin, *Polymers in Medicine and Surgery*, Plenum Press, New York, 1975.)

inside the microcapsule, polymer concentrations and thermal rates used in the microcapsules process, and lot-to-lot variations in the ethylcellulose.

The concentration gradient across the microcapsular membrane (driving force) and in vitro test method are yet other important considerations. The kinetics of the release rate is essentially pseudo-first order throughout the majority of the release curve provided that dilute microcapsule dispersions are used.

Numerous drugs have been microencapsulated by the technique described above. The long-term stability of microcapsules of the analgesic-antipyretic acetaminophen and aspirin, the potassium supplement potassium chloride, and the smooth muscle relaxant anhydrous theophylline are discussed in this chapter. The storage conditions for the bulk microencapsulated materials were screw-capped polyethylene bottles stored in the laboratory at ambient conditions. All samples tested were lots from production picked at random. In vitro test methods used for the pharmaceutical materials included a modified United States Pharmacopeia (U.S.P.) disintegration method, a rotating bottle method, and a modified National Formulary (N.F.) paddle method.

RESULTS AND DISCUSSIONS

Various samples of microencapsulated acetaminophen (APAP) were stored for various periods up to slightly over 3.8 years. The microcapsule samples were analyzed for APAP activity and were found to be essentially the same as when manufactured. Infrared analysis of the microencapsulated APAP was identical to raw APAP for the periods tested. As can be readily ascertained from Table 2, the 1/2-hr release rate remained essentially unchanged over the storage time. The p-aminophenol content of none of the samples during the period of storage exceeded 50 ppm.

Two types of microencapsulated aspirin (crystalline and granular) were evaluated for periods up to 4.75 years. The activities of both types of microencapsules were checked and found to be unchanged by chemical analysis. Infrared analysis of aspirin microcapsules showed spectra identical to unencapsulated aspirin standards. Table 3 demonstrates that the first-hour release point of the microencapsulated crystalline aspirin was unaltered with time. The aspirin granules used to prepare these microcapsules were 100% aspirin. The data presented in Table 4 again show excellent 1-hr release rate stability.

The average salicylic acid (SA) buildup rate of all the microencapsulated aspirin crystal samples is depicted in Fig. 6. The average SA buildup rate of all the microencapsulated aspirin granule samples is illustrated graphically in Fig. 7. Upon close examination of the set of SA curves it is interesting to note that the slopes of both types of aspirin microcapsules are essentially linear and almost identical. This

Table 2 Microencapsulated Acetaminophen

Elapsed time (days)	Percent release in 1/2 hr
Initial	47.3
646	47.1
988	45.0
1400	48.7
Initial	48.6
329	52.9
671	48.6
1083	48.8
Initial	47.1
252	49.9
594	47.2
1006	47.9
Initial	47.9
22	50.2
435	50.2

Table 3 Microencapsulated Aspirin Crystals

Elapsed time (days)	Percent release in 1 hr
Initial	75.1
947	76.8
1304	75.4
1709	77.2
Initial	77.1
441	74.1
798	77.2
1203	72.2
Initial	75.6
224	73.4
584	73.3
986	76.8
Initial	79.3
188	80.2
591	75.6

Table 4 Microencapsulated Aspirin Granules

Elapsed time (days)	Percent release in 1 hr
Initial	50.2
975	51.8
1328	51.4
1735	51.9
Initial	52.4
518	50.4
874	50.0
1278	53.6
Initial	47.9
204	43.3
560	46.3
965	48.8
Initial	54.0
165	52.2
570	52.2

is a little surprising in that the surface area of the crystalline material is somewhat larger than the granular material. In any case, the SA values are considerably below those permitted by the U.S.P. for formulated aspirin products.

A series of samples of microencapsulated potassium chloride were stored for numerous periods of time up to and exceeding 3.2 years. The samples were analyzed for KCl activity and found to be identical before and after the storage periods. The multipoint release rate data presented in Table 5 demonstrate essentially unaltered rate patterns for the time periods tested.

The microencapsulated process used for theophylline was essentially the ethylcellulose system with one minor modification: that a paraffinic wax was incorporated into the cellulosic coating after the microencapsules were formed. Samples of microencapsulated theophylline were tested for periods up to and exceeding 3 years. The theophylline activity was checked before and after the storage periods and found to be identical within experimental error. Infrared analysis of the microencapsulated theophylline was identical to reference standards. The rate data in Table 6 once again show in vitro pattern stability. It should be noted that the assay method for theophylline is not quite as accurate as the other materials referenced in this chapter.

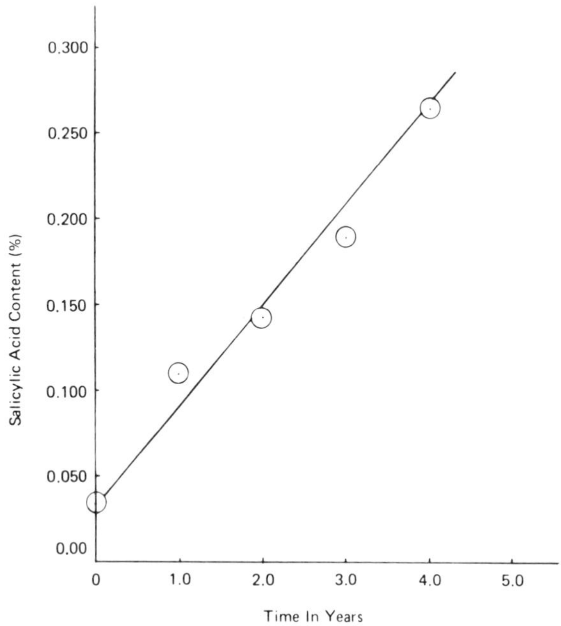

Figure 6 SA curve for microencapsulated aspirin crystals.

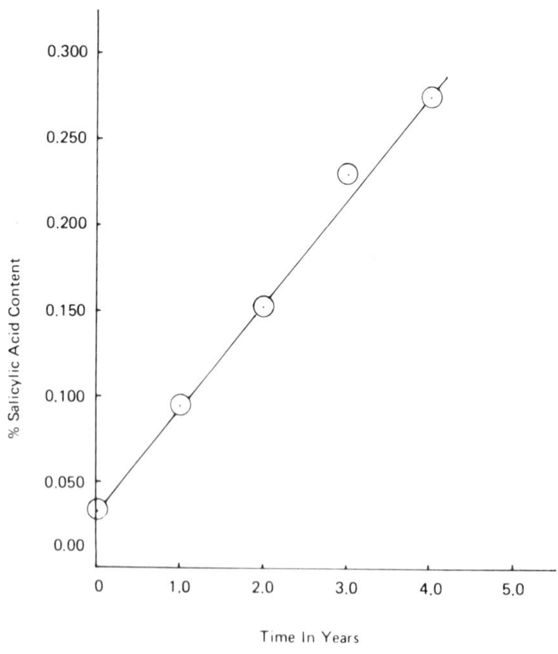

Figure 7 SA curve for microencapsulated aspirin granules.

Table 5 Microencapsulated Potassium Chloride

Elapsed time (days)	Percent release in:		
	1 hr	4 hr	8 hr
Initial	20.1	75.9	93.1
178	19.9	75.3	93.3
Initial	23.1	80.5	95.6
165	21.6	76.9	96.2
Initial	25.4	71.7	94.4
161	25.9	70.5	94.5
Initial	23.0	84.3	98.1
194	21.3	78.0	95.2
Initial	27.8	69.2	93.1
991	28.8	70.1	93.1
1184	27.8	69.8	94.4
Initial	26.3	68.8	92.8
990	26.7	65.3	91.6
1183	24.7	66.3	92.0
Initial	29.0	73.8	97.5
185	33.8	76.0	95.0
278	33.4	76.0	95.0

Table 6 Microencapsulated Theophylline

Elapsed time (days)	Percent release in:	
	1 hr	2 hr
Initial	64.4	89.8
352	68.3	87.5
701	64.9	84.6
1113	62.8	81.9
Initial		83.8
233		86.0
582		80.7
994		76.3
Initial	62.4	84.2
89	59.3	79.9

CONCLUSIONS

The data graphically demonstrate that microcapsules produced by the ethylcellulose-cyclohexane-polyethylene phase separation technique are indeed stable in bulk storage containers for long periods of time. The contributions microcapsules make to the drug materials include taste masking, controlled release, reduced gastric irritation, and separation of incompatibles. These microencapsulated drug materials are ultimately formulated into rapidly disintegrating tablets, chewable tablets, powders, and hard gelatin macrocapsule dosage forms.

REFERENCES

1. M. Galeone, L. Nizzola, D. Caciola, and G. Moise, *Curr. Ther. Res.*, *29*(1): (1981).
2. J. L. Anderson, G. L. Gardner, and N. H. Yoshida, U.S. Patent No. 3,341,416 (1967).
3. T. C. Powell, M. E. Steinle, and R. A. Yoncoskie, U.S. Patent No. 3,415,758 (1968).
4. J. A. Bakan and J. L. Anderson, Microencapsulation, in *The Theory and Practice of Industrial Pharmacy*, 2nd ed. (L. Lachman, H. A. Lieberman, and J. L. Kanig; eds.), Lea & Febiger, Philadelphia, 1976.

Chapter 12

Antiviral Activity of an Interferon Inducer in a Biosoluble Ophthalmic System

RICHARD J. HARWOOD, HELEN CAROL B. PERRY, and A. KIRK FIELD
Merck Sharp & Dohme Research Laboratories, West Point, Pennsylvania

The double-stranded complex of polyriboinosinic acid and polyribocytidylic acid (poly I:C) has been successfully used to induce resistance to systemic as well as localized viral infections through production of endogenous interferons [1]. Of particular interest, poly I:C has successfully been applied topically for clinical treatment of herpetic infections of the cornea and conjunctiva of the eye [2]. However, a disadvantage associated with topical ophthalmic application of poly I:C has been the apparent need for frequently repeated applications to ensure adequate exposure of the infected tissue. Major improvements in ophthalmic medication systems can be realized either by providing for the controlled release of drug subsequent to instillation of the medication in the eye [3-9] or by increasing the contact time for the drug with the eye tissues [10,11].

This report describes the preliminary studies that were initiated to evaluate poly I:C incorporated in a solid, biosoluble ophthalmic dosage form designed to provide for prolonged contact of poly I:C with ophthalmic tissues.

EXPERIMENTAL

Chemicals

Lyophilized polyriboinosinic acid, potassium salt (poly I), and lyophilized polyribocytidylic acid potassium salt (poly C) were obtained from P-L Biochemicals (Milwaukee, Wisconsin). Hydroxypropylcellulose was pharmaceutical grade (Klucel HF, Hercules, Inc., Wilmington, Delaware). Dibasic sodium phosphate (J. Baker Chemical Co., Phillipsburg, New Jersey), monobasic sodium phosphate (Merck and Co., Rahway, New Jersey), and sodium chloride (Merck and Co., Rahway, New Jersey) were reagent grade.

Preparation of Poly I:C/Hydroxypropylcellulose Units

In separate beakers, poly C (225 mg) and poly I (216 mg) were each added to 10 ml of distilled water. Both mixtures were placed in a cold vault (2-8°C) for 18 hr so that each polymer could hydrate completely to form thick gels.

The hydroxypropylcellulose (3970 mg) was slowly added to 100 g of boiling distilled water. The slurry of hydroxypropylcellulose was stirred while it cooled, until a gel formed. Poly I gel and the poly C gel were combined with the hydroxypropylcellulose gel by stirring at room temperature.

The mixture was dried to a cake by freeze drying in a portable lyophilization cabinet (Model 650L1, Hull Corporation, Hatboro, Pennsylvania). The dried cake was compressed into a 1-mm-thick flat sheet using a hydraulic press (Model C, Fred S. Carver, Menomenee Falls, Wisconsin). Rectangular pieces were cut from the film using a special punch (Hoggson and Pettis Co., Wallingford, Connecticut). Each piece weighed approximately 11.5 mg and was stored in a cold vault (2-8°C) until used.

Assay of Poly I:C Released from Poly I:C/ Hydroxypropylcellulose Units

A poly I:C/hydroxypropylcellulose unit was dissolved in phosphate buffered saline (PBS) (0.15 M, pH 7.0). The concentration per unit was determined by ultraviolet absorption spectrum (Beckman DB-G Spectrophotometer, Beckman Instruments, Irvine, California). Poly I:C in PBS has a characteristic absorption spectrum with maxima at 248 and 265 nm, an absorption minimum at 228 nm [12], and an $E_{1\%}$ of 140 at 265 nm.

In addition, antiviral activity was determined by incubation of monolayers of primary rabbit kidney cell cultures for 18 hr at 36°C with medium [Minimal Essential Medium (Eagle's) with Earle's salts (Gibco, Grand Island, New York), containing 2% fetal calf serum and 100,000 units of neomycin per milliliter] containing serial dilutions of the poly I:C sample under test. After removal of the medium, cultures were challenged with 10 infectious doses of vesicular stomatitis virus (10 $TCID_{50}$) in fresh medium. Following a 3-day incubation period at 36°C, cell cultures were observed for inhibition of viral-induced cytopathology. Antiviral activity was expressed as the minimum protective concentration of poly I:C (μg/ml) to elicit complete inhibition of viral cytopathology development.

Release of Poly I:C from Hydroxypropylcellulose Units

Units containing poly I:C were placed in 10 ml PBS at 37°C in 20-ml vials, and stirred sufficiently with a magnetic stirrer to maintain constant mixing. One-milliliter aliquots were sampled at 30-min intervals for determination of poly I:C concentration using ultraviolet absorption at 265 nm. At each sampling time the sampling aliquot was replaced with an equivalent volume of PBS (prewarmed at 37°C).

Infection of Rabbit Eyes by Herpes Simplex Virus

Herpes simplex virus type 1, strain Schooler (HSV-1), was used to infect 4- to 5-lb New Zealand white rabbits by dropping approximately 10 infectious doses into the cul-de-sac of each unscarified eye, followed by gently massaging the closed eyelids against the globe for about 10 sec [13].

Monitoring of Herpes Simplex Virus Infection

The infection was monitored by observing the development of eye disease. Infected eyes developed heavy exudate formation and conjunctival inflammation. No slit-lamp biomicroscopic evaluations of the eyes were carried out. In addition, virus infection was monitored by assay of viral infectivity in isolates obtained daily. The cul-de-sac of each eye was swabbed daily prior to drug treatment. Swabs were eluted into 5 ml of cell culture medium, and stored frozen at -70°C until assay. Assay for infectious virus was conducted by incubating guinea pig embryo cell monolayers with serial 10-fold dilutions of the eye swab eluates in similar culture medium at 36°C for 5 days. Virus titers were expressed as $\log_{10}$ of the infectious virus concentration, $TCID_{50}$, determined by development of viral cytopathology.

RESULTS AND DISCUSSION

The hydroxypropylcellulose units containing poly I and poly C were prepared using homopolynucleotides not previously complexed. Since complex formation of the double-stranded poly I:C is essential for induction of antiviral activity [1], it was important to determine whether complex formation occurred upon dissolution of the poly I:C-containing hydroxypropylcellulose units. As shown in Fig. 1, the absorption spectrum of polynucleotides eluted from the units was that expected for complexed poly I:C, as previously reported by Field et al. [12]. Absorption maxima were at 248 and 265 nm; absorption minimum was at 228 nm. The average content of poly I:C recovered from dissolved units was about 78% of theoretical yield and was fully active in protecting monolayers of primary rabbit kidney cells against vesicular stomatitis virus infection (minimum protective concentration - 0.06 μg/ml).

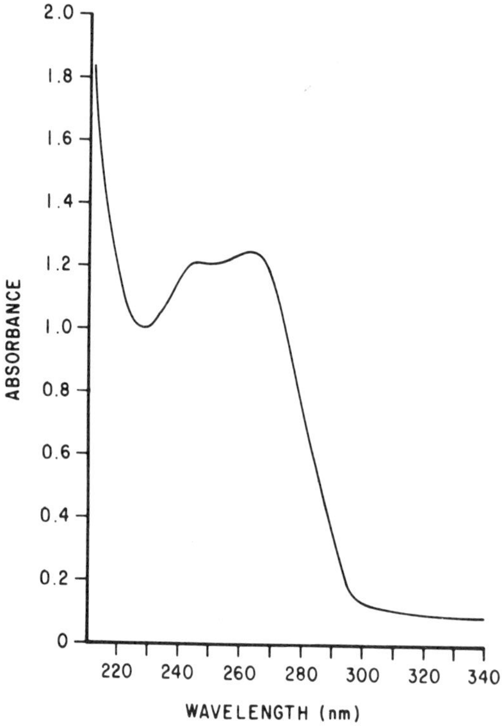

Figure 1 Absorption spectrum of a dissolved unit containing poly I, poly C, and hydroxypropylcellulose.

The dissolution profile (determined spectrophotometrically), as shown in Fig. 2, indicated that the poly I:C was released from the matrix into PBS over a 2-hr period. To further demonstrate that the poly I:C-containing hydroxypropylcellulose units were an effective means to deliver poly I:C, units containing approximately 400 μg of poly I:C (as determined by mass of the unit and confirmed by spectrophotometric analysis of the released poly I:C) were inserted into the cul-de-sac of each eye of two unanesthetized animals at 6 hr prior to HSV-1 infection and daily for 4 days. Two animals were similarly treated with placebo hydroxypropylcellulose units. The course of infection was monitored by observing development of symptoms of eye disease and by monitoring the shedding of infectious HSV-1 as described in the experimental section. Typically, placebo-treated infected eyes developed inflammation initially at 3-4 days following infection and resulted in heavy exudation and inflammation of the conjunctiva by 8 days (Fig. 3A). By contrast, the eyes treated with units containing

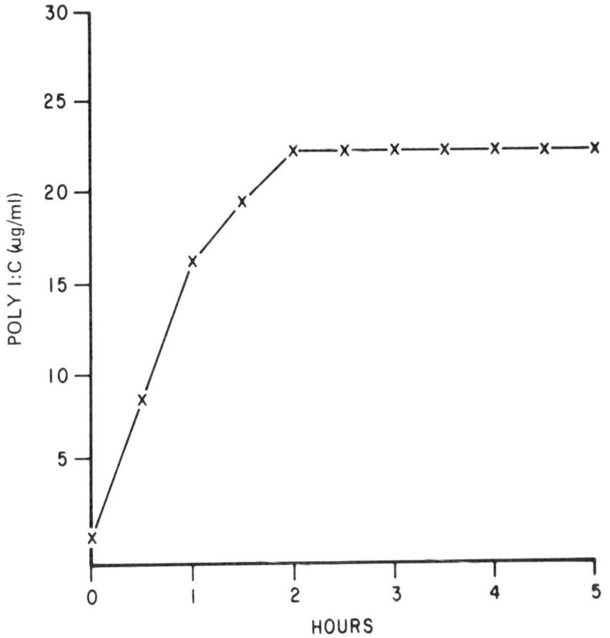

Figure 2 Poly I:C release from hydroxypropylcellulose unit into phosphate buffered saline (0.15 M, pH 7.0).

poly I:C remained normal (Fig. 3B). The protective activity of the units containing poly I:C was further demonstrated by inhibition of virus shedding during the first 4 days of infection (Fig. 4). Compared to treatment with placebo units, treatment of eyes with units containing poly I:C reduced recovered virus by as much as 10,000-fold (Table 1).

The present studies have demonstrated that the antiviral substance, poly I:C, can be effectively incorporated as uncomplexed homopolynucleotides into a matrix of hydroxypropylcellulose and recovered as the biologically active double-stranded RNA. In addition, in vitro data suggest that the poly I:C-containing unit provided sustained delivery of poly I:C to the eye tissues. This is a potentially important advantage over the frequent treatment schedule usually used for eye drop delivery of medication [14].

In rabbit studies treatment of keratitis four times per day with drops of concentrated poly I:C were only poorly effective in promoting healing [14]. However, poly I:C was effective in treating herpes keratitis in patients using eye drops for treatment at 10-min intervals for the first hour and hourly thereafter [2]. The potential of a

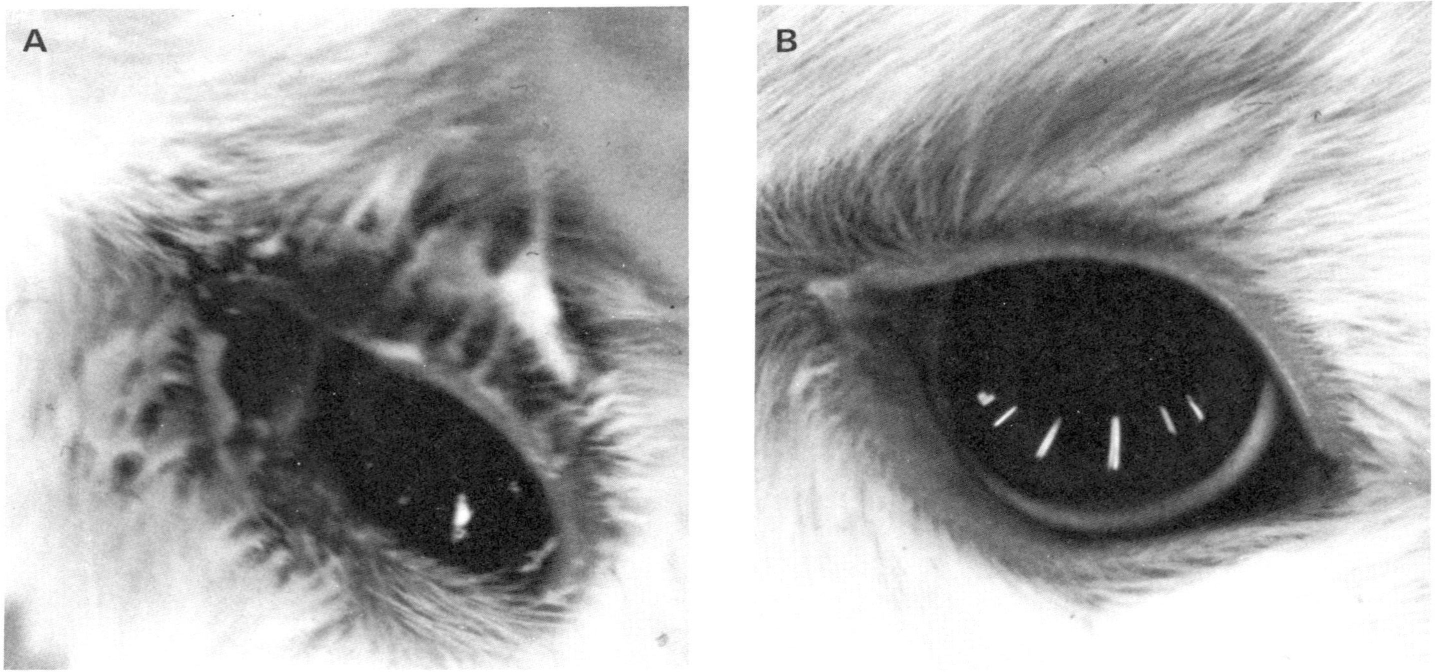

Figure 3 Photographs of rabbit eyes 8 days following infection with herpes simplex virus type 1. (A) Placebo-treated eye. (B) Poly I:C unit-treated eye.

Table 1 Protective Effect of Poly I:C/Hydroxypropylcellulose Ophthalmic Unit Against Herpes Simplex Virus Rabbit Eye Infection

Rabbit eye[a] treatment	Rabbit eye identification		Herpes simplex virus titer[b]			
	Rabbit	Eye	Day 1	Day 2	Day 3	Day 4
Poly I:C ophthalmic unit	1	L	-0.3	0.9	0.9	1.9
		R	-0.3	0.7	-0.3	-0.3
	2	L	0.4	0.0	0.7	-0.3
		R	-0.3	0.7	1.0	1.7
GMT[c]			-0.1 ± 0.2	0.6 ± 0.2	0.6 ± 0.3	0.8 ± 0.6
Placebo units	3	L	-0.3	2.0	4.0	3.9
		R	-0.3	1.4	3.9	4.0
	4	L	-0.3	2.7	3.0	3.7
		R	0.0	1.0	0.9	3.0
GMT[c]			-0.2 ± 0.1	1.8 ± 0.4	3.0 ± 0.7	3.7 ± 0.2

[a]New Zealand white rabbits were treated (two animals/group, four eyes total) with eye inserts each containing approximately 400 μg of poly I:C or placebo eye inserts. The first treatment occurred 6 hr prior to infection and continued once daily for 4 days. Infection was initiated with herpes simplex virus type 1 (HSV-1) by dropping 0.05 ml containing approximately 10 infectious doses onto the unscarified cornea of each eye. Prior to treatment each day, each eye was swabbed to recover infectious virus.

[b]Titers are expressed as $\log_{10}$ of the infectious virus concentration ($TCID_{50}$) determined following exposure of cultures of guinea pig embryo cells to serial 10-fold dilutions of virus samples and incubation at 36°C for 5 days. -0.3 was assigned to those samples containing no infectious virus.

[c]GMT, geometeric mean titer ± standard error of the mean.

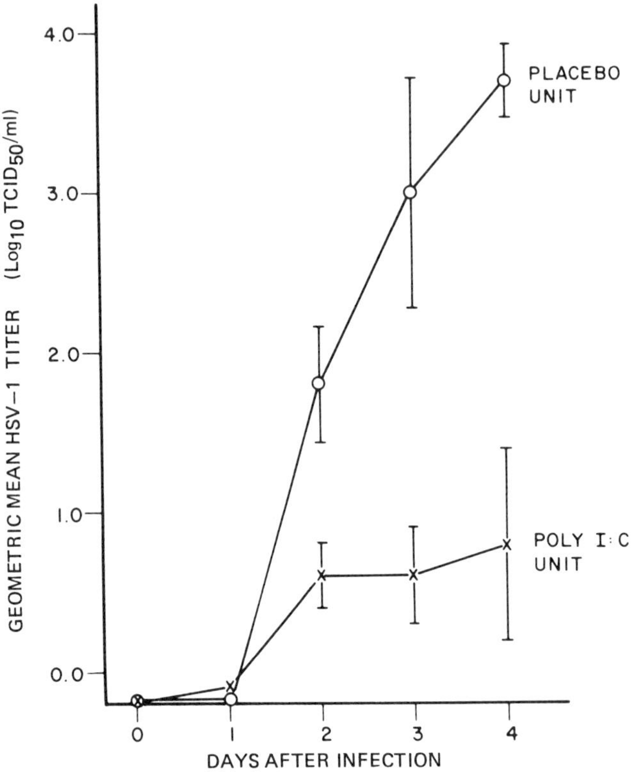

Figure 4 Protective effect of poly I:C containing unit against herpes simplex virus type 1 eye infection. Mean ± standard error of mean. ○, placebo unit; X, poly I:C ophthalmic unit.

sustained release of medication provided by the system described in this chapter could provide a more convenient and more effective therapy for human herpetic keratitis.

CONCLUSION

These studies indicate that a water-soluble matrix such as hydroxypropylcellulose is an effective vehicle to provide an antiviral substance such as poly I:C to the eye. In vitro data suggest that such a matrix provided sustained release of the interferon inducer to the eye tissues. The system described in this report effectively protected cell cultures and the eyes of rabbits against virus infection.

ACKNOWLEDGMENT

The authors wish to thank G. P. Lampson for technical assistance and advice during these studies.

REFERENCES

1. A. K. Field, *Selective Inhibitors of Viral Functions* (W. A. Carter, ed.), CRC Press, Cleveland, Ohio, 1973, pp. 149-176.
2. M. A. Galin, E. Chowchuvech, and B. Kronenberg, *Ann. Ophthalmol.*, *8*:72 (1976).
3. C. H. Dohlman, D. Pavan-Langston, and J. Rose, *Ann. Ophthalmol.*, *4*:823 (1972).
4. M. F. Armaly and K. R. Rao, *Invest. Ophthalmol.*, *12*:491 (1973).
5. R. L. Friederich, *Ann. Ophthalmol.*, *6*:1279 (1974).
6. H. A. Quigley, I. P. Pollack, and T. S. Harbin, *Arch. Ophthalmol.*, *93*:771 (1975).
7. V. A. Place, M. Fisher, S. Herbst, L. Gordon, and C. Merrill, *Am. J. Ophthalmol.*, *80*:706 (1975).
8. T. Higuchi, A. Hussain, and J. W. Shell, U.S. Published Patent Application B 520, 277, February 17, 1976.
9. D. Pavan-Langston, R. H. S. Langston, and P. A. Geary, *Arch. Ophthalmol.*, *93*:1349 (1975).
10. I. M. Katz, personal communication.
11. Y. T. Maichuk, *Antibiotiki, 12*(5):432 (1967).
12. A. K. Field, A. A. Tytell, G. P. Lampson, and M. R. Hilleman, *Proc. Natl. Acad. Sci. USA*, *58*:1004 (1967).
13. A. B. Nesburn and P. J. Ziniti, *Am. J. Ophthalmol.*, *72*:821 (1971).
14. H. E. Kaufman, E. D. Ellison, and S. R. Waltman, *Am. J. Ophthalmol.*, *68*:486 (1969).

Chapter 13

Controlled Release of Dapsone by Intramuscular Injection

E. S. M. MODDERMAN, F. W. H. M. MERKUS, and J. ZUIDEMA
University of Amsterdam, Amsterdam, The Netherlands

H. HUIKESHOVEN and D. L. LEIKER Royal Tropical Institute, Amsterdam, The Netherlands

Controlled release of dapsone [diaminodiphenylsulfone (DDS)] by intramuscular administration has been studied extensively by Huikeshoven [1] and by Modderman [2,3] and their coworkers. This chapter presents some of the recent studies of these research groups on the release of dapsone after intramuscular administration of aqueous dapsone suspensions in volunteers and patients, and discusses the reason for developing an intramuscular depot injection in leprosy treatment. Since 1949 dapsone has been the drug of first choice in the treatment of leprosy. It is a very effective and inexpensive drug, administored predominantly as tablets, usually in a dose of 25-100 mg/day. Leprosy is still a serious problem in the world, especially in developing countries. The World Health Organization estimates that more than 10 million people are suffering from this chronic infectious disease: estimated cases in Africa, 3.5 million; the Americas, 0.4 million; Southeast Asia, 4.5 million; and Western Pacific area, 2 million.

Leprosy is caused by *Mycobacterium leprae*, a microorganism that multiplies very slowly. After infection, the first symptoms of leprosy may take 3-5 years to develop. The pattern of symptoms depends on the immune response in the patient. When cell-mediated immunity is strong, the pattern is called *tuberculoid*: the disease is localized to one or a few sites in the body and bacteria are difficult to find (paucibacillary). When there is no cell-mediated immunity, the pattern is called *lepromatous*. In this case many organs are affected, especially the skin, peripheral nerves, eyes, upper respiratory mucosa, lymph nodes, and testes, and it often involves superficial muscles of the face, hands, and feet. Bacteria are numerous in all these organs (multibacillary). Between these two types there are a number of intermediate forms called *borderline* types. The lepromatous, and to a lesser extent the borderline types, are the main reservoirs of new infections.

PATIENT COMPLIANCE

In spite of the fact that the effective drug dapsone has been available for more than 30 years, leprosy has not yet been eradicated. This can be attributed to problems which have become evident in the past 10-15 years: patient noncompliance, dapsone resistance, and persistence of viable bacteria. The first investigations of patient compliance yielded such alarming results that attention was immediately attracted to this aspect of dapsone therapy. The conclusions of subsequent investigations were no less disappointing; the percentage of doses not taken amounted in Malawi, for example, to 40-50%; Ethiopia, 58%; Tanzania, 50%; and Burma, 24-74%. These investigations were carried out with registered patients who attended their clinic regularly. This picture would get worse if patients who seldom or never come to their clinic were included. Irregular dapsone intake is not confined to single areas but occurs generally [1]. *Noncompliance* results in an impaired therapeutic effect; additionally, when a patient is grossly noncompliant, he or she may continue to be a focus of infection.

Also, the development of *resistance* is probably favored by low and irregular blood levels resulting from irregular dapsone intake. Another point of concern is the *persistence* of viable bacteria in the body of leprosy patients in spite of treatment with chemotherapeutic agents. This is especially a problem for multibacillary, lepromatous, and borderline lepromatous patients. The tuberculoid patients are usually cured after a few years of chemotherapy. In lepromatous patients, however, a number of viable bacteria persist in nerve and muscle tissue despite the use of drugs. This is why dapsone has to be given for life to lepromatous and borderline lepromatous patients, as a kind of maintenance therapy.

PHARMACOKINETICS OF DAPSONE

In 1966, with the aid of the mouse-footpad test, the minimum inhibitory concentration (MIC) of dapsone for *M. leprae* was determined to be very low, about 10 ng/ml. Following this finding a prodrug of dapsone was introduced: acedapsone (diacetyldiaminodiphenylsulfone). Injection of 225 mg of this drug resulted in an average dapsone release of 2 mg/day and blood levels higher than 15 ng/ml for 11 weeks. But although these concentrations lay well above the MIC, such low levels are no longer desirable because of the risk of development of resistance.

At the moment dapsone is administered predominantly in oral form, usually in a dose of 25-100 mg/day. The resulting blood levels vary between 0.5 and 2 μg/ml. Dapsone is slowly but almost completely absorbed from the gastrointestinal tract and peak levels are reached 1-4 hr after administration. In the liver, acetylation takes place to give monoacetyldapsone (MADDS). The rate of acetylation may vary widely between different people and rapid and slow acetylators can be classified. Also N-hydroxylation takes place, the extent and importance of which have yet to be established. Dapsone is bound to protein for 50-80% and MADDS for 97-100%.

Dapsone is bacteriostatic or weakly bactericidal and its mechanism of action is probably similar to that of the sulfonamides. Dapsone and metabolites are excreted predominantly in urine, partly as sulfates and glucuronides. The half-life may vary widely, between 10 and 50 hr, but is not related to acetylation capacity. Few adverse reactions are seen with the dosage presently used. Anorexia, nausea, and vomiting may occur, and sometimes headache, nervousness, and insomnia are reported. A slight rise in the percentage of methemoglobin is common but not serious.

INTRAMUSCULAR DAPSONE DEPOT INJECTION

The need for a more reliable route of administration led us to investigate the possibility of an intramuscular dapsone depot injection. Dapsone is almost insoluble in water and in oil. Therefore, only suspensions can be made. Also in the 1950s dapsone injections were given intramuscualrly.

Various oils were used, sometimes gelled with aluminum stearate to prolong the action. Because oily injections are often painful or difficult to inject, some leprosy workers prepared aqueous suspensions. They used large dapsone particles in an aqueous medium. Nevertheless, these injections finally disappeared from leprosy therapy in favor of dapsone tablets. Our investigations were focused on the preparation of an aqueous suspension of dapsone with different particle sizes for intramuscular injection and control of the resulting blood levels of DDS and MADDS for about 1 month by high-pressure liquid chromatography (HPLC).

After a pilot study in volunteers, we performed a trial in 20 leprosy patients at the Leprosy Control and Training Centre at Zaria, Kaduna State, Nigeria. All patients involved in this study were in a quiet stage of their disease and they all had been treated with oral dapsone before the start of this trial. The injections consisted of a sterile suspension of dapsone in an aqueous medium. Sodium chloride was present to obtain isotonicity and methylcellulose to enhance the viscosity. Dapsone bulk powder was sieved (wet) to obtain fractions of different particle sizes. An injection of 900 mg of dapsone, particle size 90-125 μm (80%) + <90 μm (20%), was administered to 10 patients; following the results of these injections 5 patients received an injection of 1200 mg, particle size 90-125 μm (80%) + <90 μm (20%), and 5 patients received an injection of 1200 mg, particle size <90 μm.

Blood samples were drawn at day 0, 1, 2, 3, 4, 5, 6, 7, 9, 12, 14, 16, 19, 23, 25, and 28, after an injection of 900 mg of dapsone or at day 0, 1, 2, 3, 4, 5, 6, 8, 11, 15, 18, 22, 25, and 28, after an injection of 1200 mg of dapsone. The samples were determined instantly in Nigeria by a semiquantitative ELISA method for sulfones, developed by Huikeshoven et al. [4,5]. In Amsterdam the concentrations of DDS and of MADDS in the samples were measured using a nonextractive HPLC method, as described by Zuidema et al. [6]. The dapsone injections were not painful and were well tolerated by all 20 participants. Only a few patients reported a slight local tenderness during the first days after injection. The results of the HPLC analysis are summarized in Table 1. A representative serum level curve resulting from injection B is shown in Fig. 1. As a criterion for the effectivity of our injection we have taken the period during which the dapsone level above 0.5 μg/ml was maintained, which corresponds with the levels yielded after oral therapy. As a maximum we have chosen arbitrarily 5 μg/ml, which is generally thought to be the maximum level tolerated without serious side effects. As can be seen from Table 1, injection B resulted in effective levels for 3-4 weeks. With injection C (relatively small particles), once a peak level of 5.0 was reached and once one of 5.1 μg/ml. This indicates the necessity of using large particles when doses of 1200 mg of dapsone are injected.

After these encouraging results, we studied the use of crystals of dapsone of different particle sizes. The dissolution rate in vitro of the crystals, prepared by recrystallization, is considerably slower than that of the bulk powder (Roussell) and also slower than that of the particle size mixture used in the Nigeria injections, which was prepared by sieving bulk powder. Injections of the crystals were prepared with particle size ranges of 38-63 and 63-90 μm, and administered to volunteers in dosages of 300, 600, 900, and 1200 mg. These injections gave an excellent sustained release of dapsone, without high peak levels in the first week.

In these experiments also methemoglobin formation was studied, which appeared to be absent or moderate. No difference in the results with the particle sizes 38-63 and 63-90 μm was observed. This was not very surprising because the difference in dissolution rate in vitro was only very small. A representative curve is given in Fig. 2.

At the therapeutic dosage level of 1200 mg, however, with an injection volume of 4 ml, injectability gave some problems, caused by obstruction of the injection needle. These problems had to be solved before the injections would be suitable for application in leprosy therapy.

Table 1 Dapsone Peak Concentrations in the Serum of 20 Leprosy Patients and the Number of Days the Dapsone Serum Level, Measured by HPLC, Was Above 0.5 μg/ml

	Patient number	Peak concentration (μg/ml)	Number of days the dapsone level was above 0.5 μg/ml
900 mg dapsone	1	2.7	19
[90-125 μm (80%) +	2	4.1	13
<90 μm (20%)]	3	3.9	18
injection A	4	2.2	12
	5	2.4	27
	6	2.1	20
	7	4.2	15
	8	0.9[a]	23
	9	3.6	14
	10	2.3	22
	Mean ± SD	3.1 (±0.9)	18 (±5)
1200 mg dapsone	11	1.9	28
[90-125 μm (80%) +	12	4.2	22
<90 μm (20%)]	13	1.7	28
injection B	14	2.5	25
	15	3.2	22
	Mean ± SD	2.7 (±1.0)	25 (±3)
1200 mg dapsone	16	2.5	28
(<90 μm)	17	5.0	15
injection C	18	2.9	24
	19	5.1	18
	20	4.2	21
	Mean ± SD	3.9 (±1.2)	21 (±5)

[a]This patient received only 800 mg.
Source: Ref. 3.

The dapsone crystals, as obtained from the recrystallization process, had a somewhat oblong shape, as can be seen in Fig. 3A, which is unfavorable for the rheological properties of the injection. Therefore, the solution of this injectability problem was searched for in the modification of the shape of the particles.

For this purpose a milling step was introduced in the preparation procedure. The crystals, obtained from recrystallization of bulk powder, were milled in a porcelain ball mill for 1 hr. Subsequently, the fraction with particle size 38-63 μm was separated by wet sieving

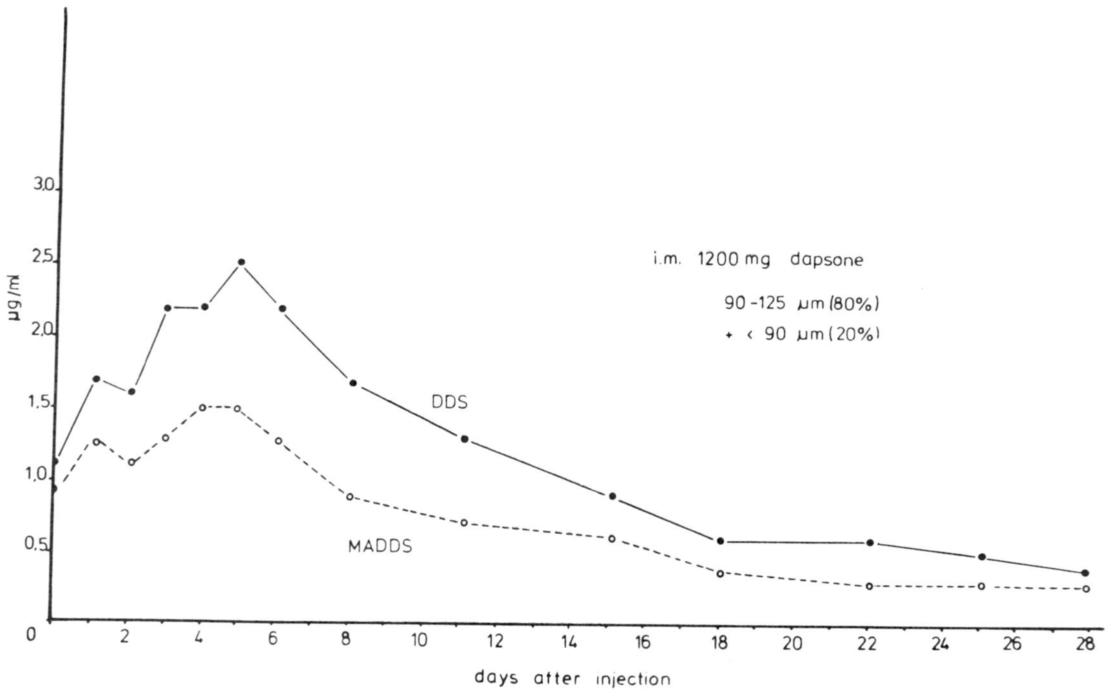

Figure 1 Representative serum level curve of dapsone (DDS) and monoacetyldapsone (MADDS) during 28 days after intramuscular injection of 1200 mg of dapsone, 90-125 µm (80%) + <90 µm (20%) (leprosy patient). (From Ref. 3.)

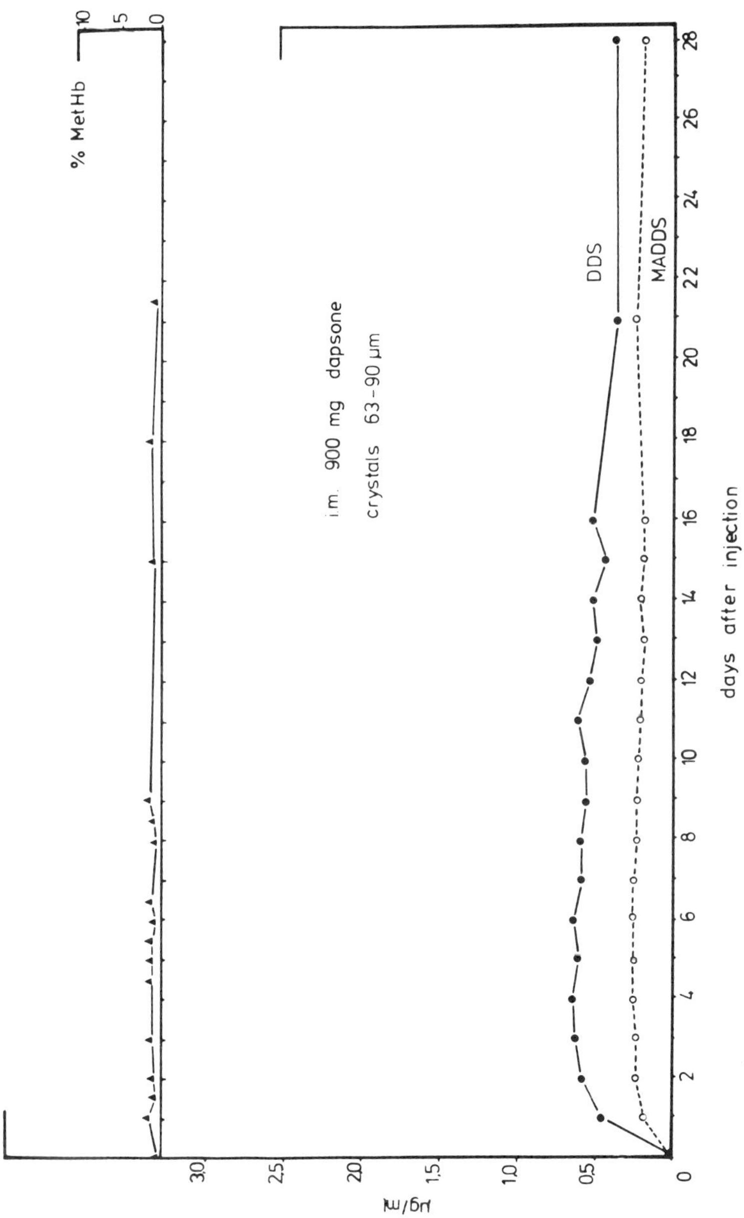

Figure 2 Representative serum level curve of dapsone (DDS) and monoacetyldapsone (MADDS), with corresponding methemoglobin percentages, during 28 days after intramuscular injection of 900 mg of dapsone crystals, 63-90 μm (healthy volunteer).

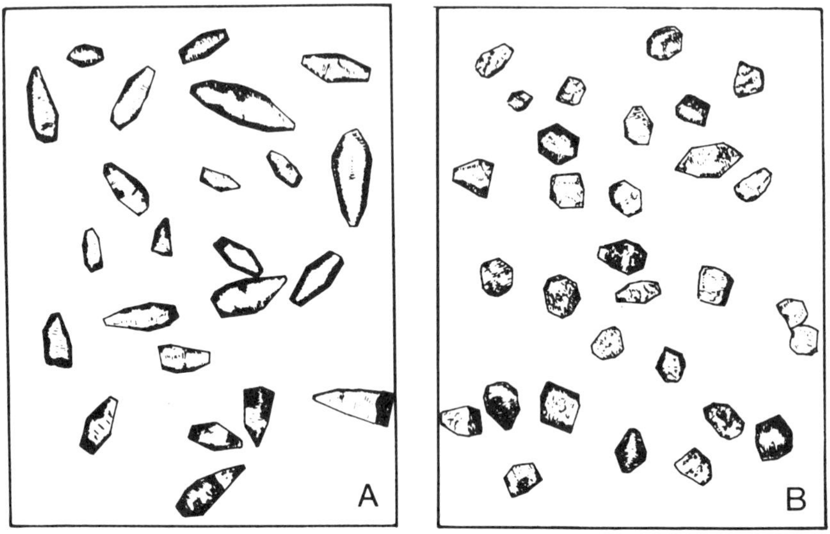

Figure 3 (A) Dapsone crystals 38-63 μm, magnification 119. (B) milled dapsone crystals 38-63 μm, magnification 119. (Copies from microscopic photographs.)

in an electromagnetic sieve. This way, particles of a more rounded form were obtained, as can be seen in Fig. 3B.

New injections were prepared with these particles. Two groups of three volunteers received 600 and 900 mg, respectively, and nine volunteers received 1200 mg. With these new injections the blood level curves showed no pronounced change, as can be seen from a comparison of Figs. 2 and 4. At the moment a trial with these injections in leprosy patients in Ethiopia is being prepared.

ACKNOWLEDGMENT

This investigation received financial support from the Chemotherapy of Leprosy (Thelep) component of the UNDP/World Bank/WHO Special Programme for Research and Training in Tropical Diseases.

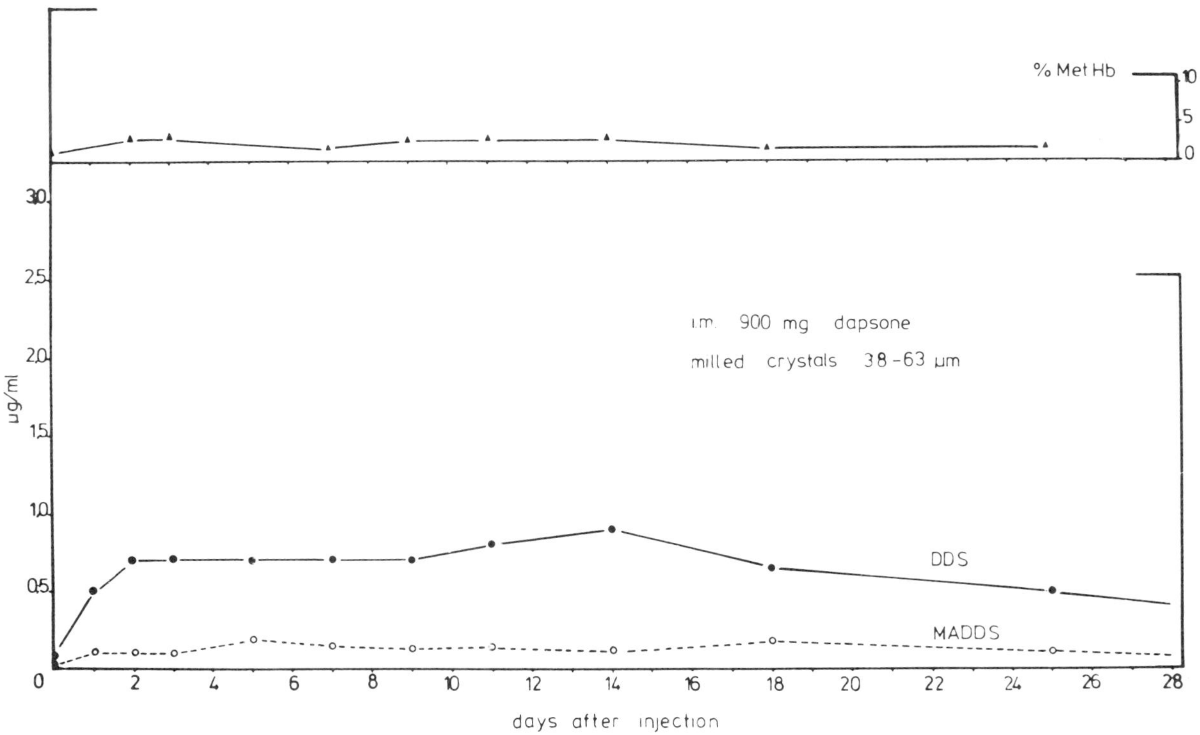

Figure 4 Representative serum level curve of dapsone (DDS) and monoacetyldapsone (MADDS), with corresponding methemoglobin percentages during 28 days after intramuscular injection of 900 mg of milled dapsone crystals, 38-63 µm (healthy volunteer).

REFERENCES

1. H. Huikeshoven, Ph.D. thesis, University of Amsterdam, 1980.
2. E. S. M. Modderman, *Pharm. Int.*, *1*:198 (1980).
3. E. S. M. Modderman, H. Huikeshoven, J. Zuidema, D. L. Leiker, and F. W. H. M. Merkus, *Int. J. Clin. Pharmacol. Ther. Toxicol.*, *20*:51 (1982).
4. H. Huikeshoven, M. de Wit, A. Soeters, T. A. Eggelte, J. E. Landheer, and D. L. Leiker, *Leprosy Rev.*, *50*:275 (1979).
5. H. Huikeshoven, M. de Wit, A. Soeters, J. E. Landheer, and D. L. Leiker, *Leprosy Rev.*, *52*:11 (1981).
6. J. Zuidema, E. S. M. Modderman, H. W. Hilbers, and F. W. H. M. Merkus, *J. Chromatogr. (Biomed. Appl.)*, *182*:130 (1980).

Chapter 14

Radioisotope Labeling: A Unique Technique for Polymer Characterization

ALBERT DORSKY,* RON L. HALE, and STEVEN A. de KECZER†
Dynapol, Palo Alto, California

Over the past several years there has been a rapidly growing interest in the functionalization of polymers through chemical reactions. Increasingly, these chemical modifications are directed toward preparation of materials tailored for specific uses in the pharmaceutical, biomedical, and other health and environmental-related areas. Our specific interest at Dynapol is the development of polymeric food additives. An important phase of our research involves determining the absorption, metabolism, and excretion of our direct food additives in radiolabeled form. Radioisotopes provide the only sufficiently sensitive, accurate, and convenient means of doing this. In addition, radioisotopes can be used to study the stability, distribution, and nonvolatility of polymeric additives in complex food systems under the conditions of production and usage. We are indeed fortunate at Dynapol to have the capability of synthesis from very basic sources, ($Ba^{14}CO_3$, $^3H_2$). Thus our involvement in the preparation of radiolabeled polymers has been largely oriented toward the goal of providing suitably labeled materials for these studies. At the same time these syntheses have provided many interesting examples of the ways in which radioisotopes can be applied to the study of these complex polymeric systems.

Present affiliations
*Cooper-Lipotech, Inc., South San Francisco, California
†Syntex (U.S.A.), Inc., Palo Alto, California

EXPERIMENTAL

Liquid scintillation counting was performed with a Packard Tri-Carb Model 2420 instrument. Analytical thin-layer chromatography (TLC) was carried out on prelayered silica gel LQ6DF plates (Quantum Industries). The plates were developed and examined with a Packard Model 7201 radiochromatogram scanner or zones were scraped into scintillation vials containing Instagel (Packard Instrument Company) and counted in the Tri-Carb 2420. Purification of synthetic polymers was by ultrafiltration in an Amicon (Amicon Corp.) apparatus using PM-10 membranes. High-pressure liquid chromatography (HPLC) was performed with a Waters Associates instrument constructed from a U6K universal injector, a Model 660 solvent flow programmer, and two Model 6000 pumps using a Waters Associates 30 cm × 4 mm ID reverse-phase μBondapak C-18 column. Gel permeation chromatography (GPC) was done on a CGP-10 porous glass column (Electro-Nucleonics) with 0.05 M phosphate as the mobile phase which was delivered by a high-pressure mini-Pump (Milton-Roy). In both HPLC and GPC the column effluent was monitored by differential refractometry (Waters Associates Model R401) and fractionated into scintillation vials for radioassay. The results were processed with a Tektronix Model 31 calculator and plotted on a Tektronix Model 4661 X-Y plotter.

[^{14}C]Poly Y-607 (I, Fig. 1) was synthesized from [^{14}C-ring]acetanilide according to the scheme shown in Fig. 1. The [^{14}C-ring]acetanilide was prepared from barium [^{14}C]carbonate (General Electric Co.) in six steps via the labeled intermediates barium carbide, acetylene, benzene, nitrobenzene, and aniline. The synthesis of [^{14}C]Poly AO-79 (II, Fig. 6) has been reported elsewhere [8]. [^{14}C-sulfanilamide ring] Poly ASA-171 (VII, Fig. 9) was synthesized from [^{14}C-ring]N-acetylsulfanilyl chloride according to the scheme shown in Fig. 9, the sulfonyl chloride being derived from barium [^{14}C]carbonate as described above (see Fig. 1). [^{14}C-salicylic acid ring]Poly ASA-171 (VIII, Fig. 10) was prepared by coupling [^{14}C-ring]salicylic acid (ICN Chemical and Radioisotope Division) to the intermediate polymeric diazonium salt [2].

RESULTS AND DISCUSSION

Figure 1 shows the radiosynthesis of one of our polydyes where the label is in the pendant chromophore. By the simple technique of scintillation counting, it was possible to establish easily and accurately the efficiency of the ultrafiltration purification procedure [1] as well as the efficiency of chromophore use (Table 1), a task that could be exceedingly difficult without the use of a label. The extent of chromophore attachment to the backbone (mer %* chromophore) was also

---

*In reporting polymer composition, the term *mer* % is used. This term may be defined as follows: The polymer is considered to be a series of

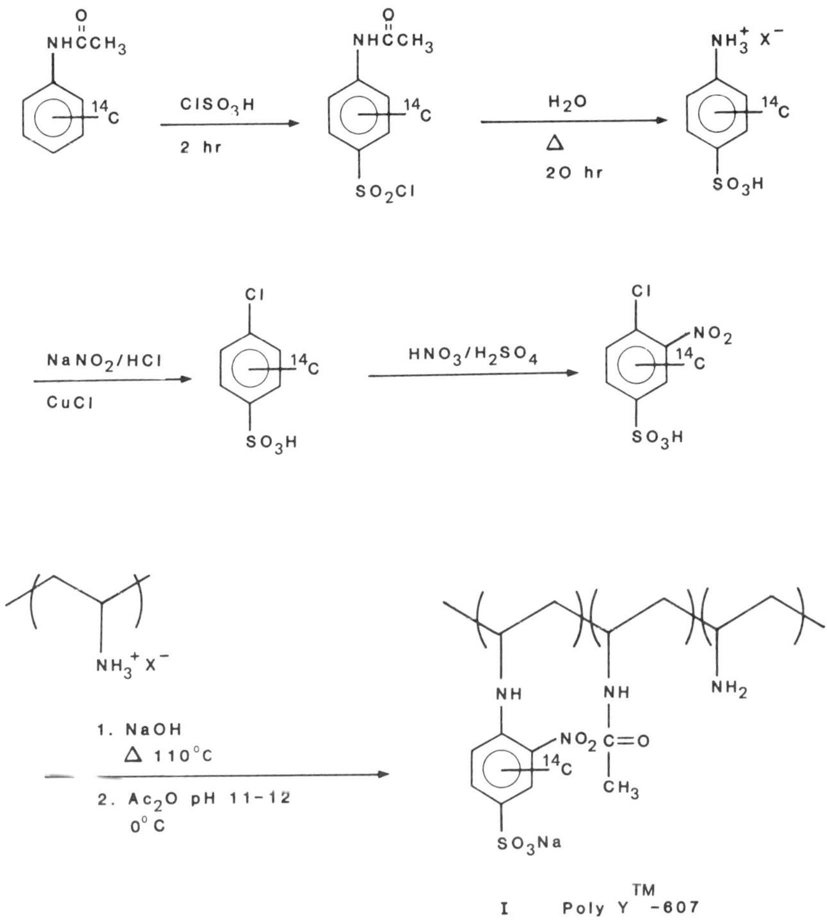

Figure 1 Synthesis of [^{14}C]Poly Y-607 (I).

---

units, each of which is based on a two-carbon segment of the polymer backbone. Each unit is called a *mer unit*. In a given polymer there may be several different types of mer units, corresponding to the different chemical functional groups based on the two-carbon backbone units. The composition of any polymer of this type may be conveniently expressed in terms of mer % of each functional group, where for a functional group A, mer % A = mer units of A per 100 mer units of polymer.

Table 1 [^{14}C]Poly Y-607 Synthesis Yield Data

Start: 3.0 mCi chromophore		
Recovery from ultrafiltration, 40 diavolumes		
Ultrafiltrate	1.08 mCi	36.0%
Retentate	1.89 mCi	63.0%
	2.97 mCi	99.0%
Yield freeze-dried material	1.10 g	1.83 mCi
(12% H_2O)	(61 % if 58 mer % dye)	(61% radiochemical yield)
Mer % chromophore (calc.) 58%		

readily determined by scintillation counting techniques, as shown in Table 2. The analysis required three simple determinations: the specific activity of the chromophore, the specific activity of the polydye, and the water content of the polydye. Figure 2 represents the gel permeation chromatography molecular weight determination of the polydye and Fig. 3 shows a low molecular weight impurity analysis, both of which were carried out by fractionation of the column effluent and scintillation counting analysis of the fractions. Using this technique it is a simple matter to quantitate the amount of polymer in any given molecular weight range.

Figure 4 illustrates a stability study of a model anthrapyridone polydye [2] in pH 7 water which was simply and effectively carried out by applying aliquots of the test solutions to TLC plates, eluting the plates, scraping sections of the plate into scintillation vials, and counting the solutions. This procedure not only provided the stability data, but enabled us to identify the major decomposition product as well (4-amino-3'-carbethoxy-2-methylanthrapyridone).

Figure 5 serves to illustrate the quality of data that can be obtained even in complex food systems under usage conditions. In this case, a polymeric dye was prepared by a sequence of synthetic steps carried out on a copolymer of aminoethylene (AE) and sodium ethylene sulfonate (SES). The final product contained a variety of units, including AE units with the attached chromophore (group A, 30 mer %), the comonomer SES units (group B, 35 mer %), unreacted AE units (group C, 5 mer %), and units made up of AE with an intermediate linking group attached (group D, 5 mer %). As a final step in the synthesis of this polymeric dye, unreacted AE units are acetylated leading to a fifth unit (group X). The use of [^{14}C]acetic anhydride for the acetylation provided a means of determining the number of units acetylated (25 mer %). In addition, this provided a tracer for studying the stability of the acetate group toward hydrolytic cleavage in food systems, an important factor affecting the solubility of the dye. The polymeric dye containing labeled pendant groups was dissolved in the uncolored soft

Table 2 Calculations

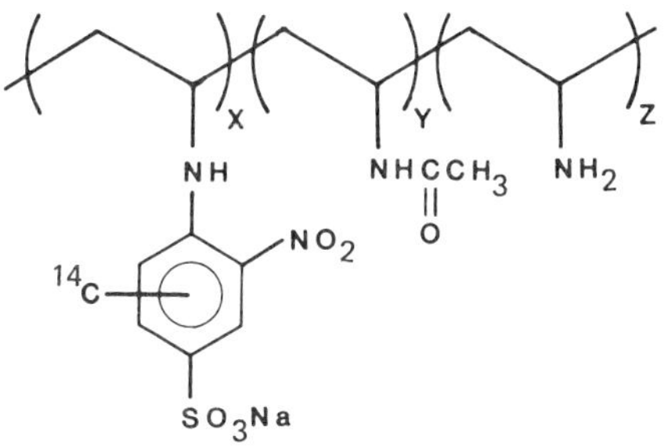

(I)

X	Y	Z
$C_8H_7N_2O_5SNa$	C_4H_7NO	C_2H_5N
266.209	85.106	43.069

For no free amine

X = mer % chromophore

$$\text{Equivalent weight (EW)} = \frac{(266.209)(X) + 85.106(1 - X)}{X}$$

Solving,

$$X = \frac{85.106}{EW - 181.503}$$

Specific activity chromophore = 618 μCi/mmol

Specific activity of polydye (dry) = 1.89 μCi/mg

$$\frac{1.892\ \mu Ci/mg}{618\ \mu Ci/mmol} = 3.061 \text{ mEq chromophore/g polydye}$$

Therefore, equivalent weight = 326.64

X - 58.64 mer %

Assuming 5% free amine

$$EW = \frac{(266.209)(X) + 85.106(0.95 - X) + 43.069(0.05)}{X}$$

$$X = \frac{83.004}{EW - 181.503}$$

= 57.19 mer %

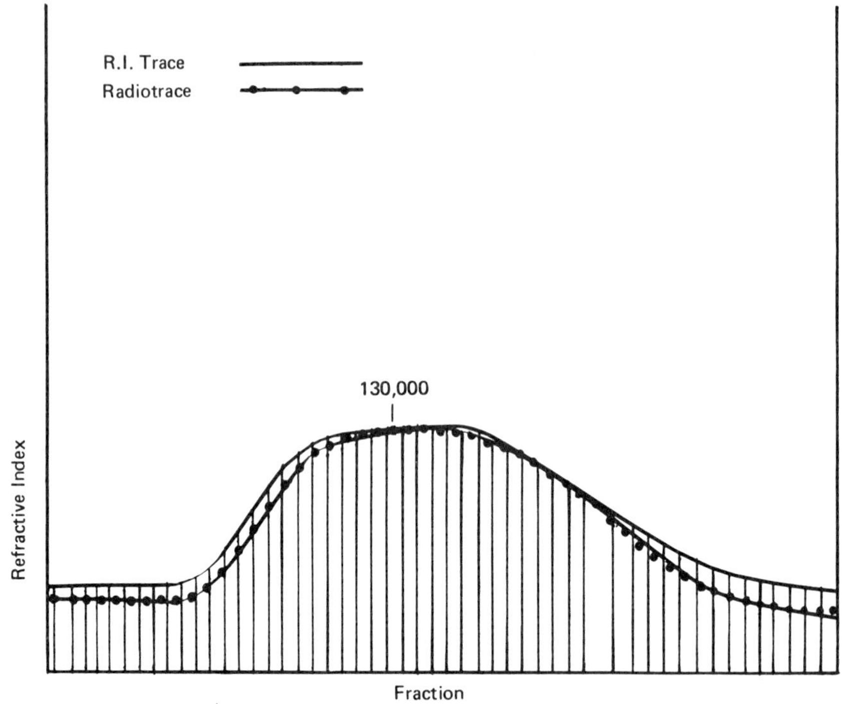

Figure 2 GPC molecular weight determination, [^{14}C]Poly Y-607 (I).

drink base, the 1% solution was placed in a dialysis bag and the bag placed in a reservoir of the soft drink (7-Up) at room temperature. Samples were removed from time to time and simply counted in a liquid scintillation spectrometer.

An even more complex system is represented by sewage sludge degradation and environmental fate studies in soil done with Dynapol's polymeric antioxidant Poly AO-79 anoxomer [3] labeled in the aromatic rings of the divinylbenzene units with ^{14}C (II, Fig. 6). These studies involved the measurement of labeled CO_2 or extractable labeled materials which could only have come from the labeled source. The results of some of the soil studies are shown in Table 3. In systems of this type, labeling is virtually the only way to carry out the study.

Sulfasalazine (III, Fig. 7) is a drug that is the most effective of the various sulfonamides in the treatment of ulcerative colitis [4,5]. Undesirable side effects result from absorption of the intact drug in the upper small intestine [6] and of sulfapyridine (IV) which results from reductive cleavage of the azo bond in the cecum [6,7] (Fig. 7). Poly ASA-171 (VI, Fig. 8) is a polymer designed to release the

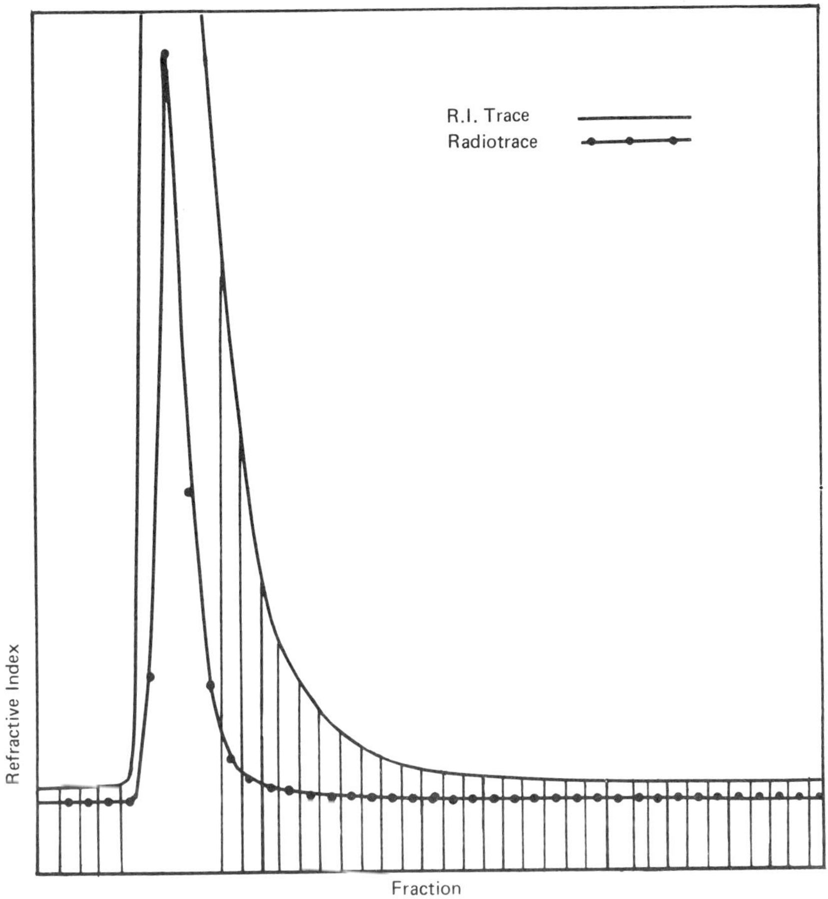

Figure 3 GPC % <2000 - [^{14}C]Poly Y-607 (I).

pharmacologically active agent 5-aminosalicylic acid (V) by reductive cleavage of the azo bond in the colon. Potential therapeutic advantages of the polymeric drug over the monomer include nonabsorption of both the intact drug and polymeric cleavage product and elimination of the side effects caused by the sulfapyridine produced when the monomeric drug is cleaved.

Figures 9 and 10 show the synthetic schemes used to label both the polymer and the pharmacologically active agent. With the label in the polysulfanilamide portion of the molecule (VII, Fig. 9) the metabolic fate of the polymer can easily be followed. On the other hand, with the label in the salicylic acid portion of the molecule (VIII, Fig. 10)

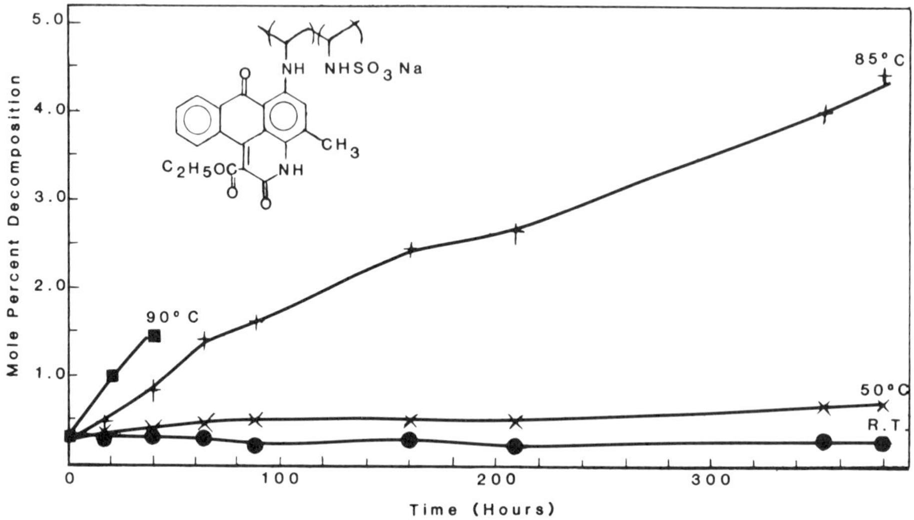

Figure 4 Stability study of a polymeric red dye temperature dependence at pH 7, H_2O.

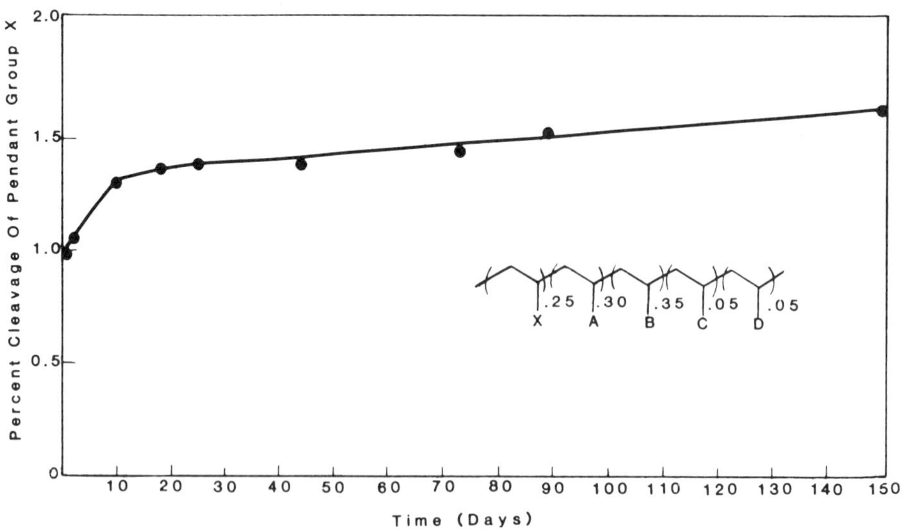

Figure 5 Rate of hydrolysis of group X, 1% solution in 7-Up at room temperature.

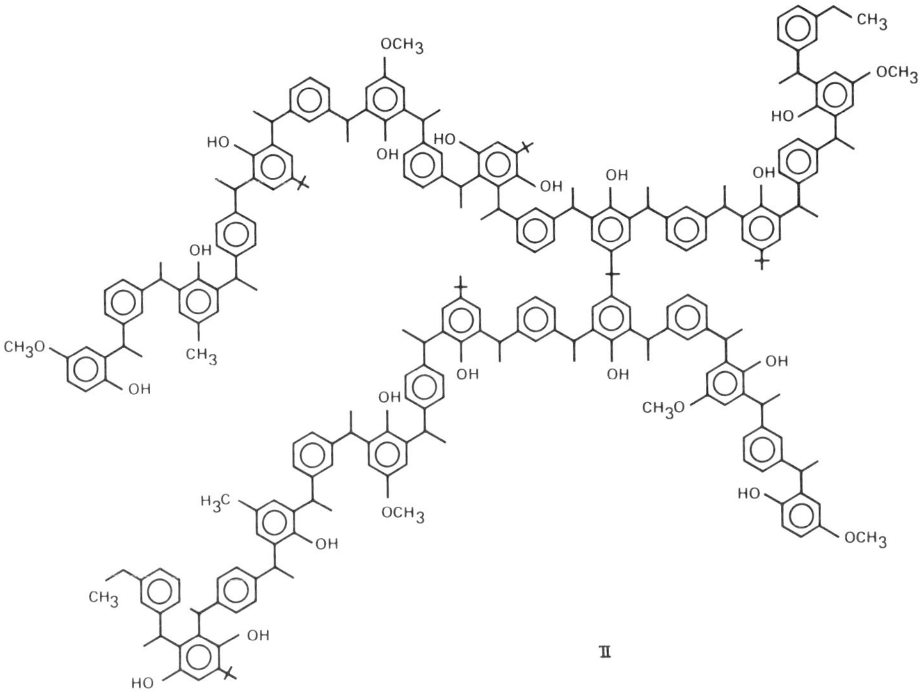

II

Figure 6 Poly AO-79 anoxomer (II).

the release rate and metabolic fate of the active part of the drug can be followed. In addition to the obvious uses for metabolic fate studies, the synthesis of the labeled compounds yielded valuable information about the degree of substitution and the amount of active 5-aminosalicylic acid the drug contained.

CONCLUSION

Such studies show that radioisotopes provide a powerful tool for obtaining very valuable information about the chemical and biological reactions of the functionalized polymers used as food additives, macromolecular drugs, herbicides, antifoulants, and so on (Table 4). Tracers may be applied to the study of total functionality, including the determination of limiting yields, the occurrence of side reactions, "fast" versus "slow" functional groups, polyelectrolyte effects on chemical reactivity, and so on. The rates of reactions involving attachment or cleavage of pendant groups on polymer chains are very conveniently determined by use of radiolabeled compounds, especially when the rates being

Table 3 Evolution of $^{14}CO_2$ from 50-g Samples of Garden Soil Supplemented with [^{14}C]Anoxomer (II)

		$^{14}CO_2$ Evolution as % of Dose 30 ppm [^{14}C]Poly AO	
Days of incubation (25-30°C), fluorescent light	DPM $^{14}CO_2$ recovered	$^{14}CO_2$ as percent of dose	$^{14}CO_2$ as cumulative percent of dose
11	1,189	0.01	0.01
13	807	0.007	0.017
19	695	0.006	0.023
27	1,558	0.013	0.036
39	16,800	0.144	0.180
46	2,699	0.023	0.203
54	2,478	0.021	0.224
67	4,267	0.037	0.261
81	11,307	0.096	0.357
90[a]	2,198	0.019	0.376
109[a]	125,657	1.07	1.45
125[a]	211	0.002	1.452
144[a]	278	0.0024	1.454
146	10,066	0.086	1.54

[a]20 ml of air added with change of CO_2 absorbant.

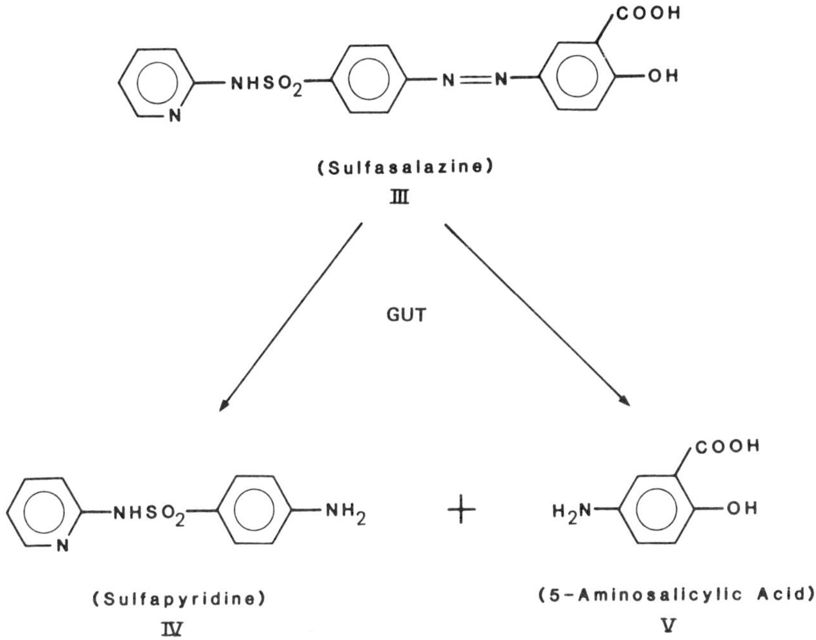

Figure 7 Metabolism of sulfasalazine.

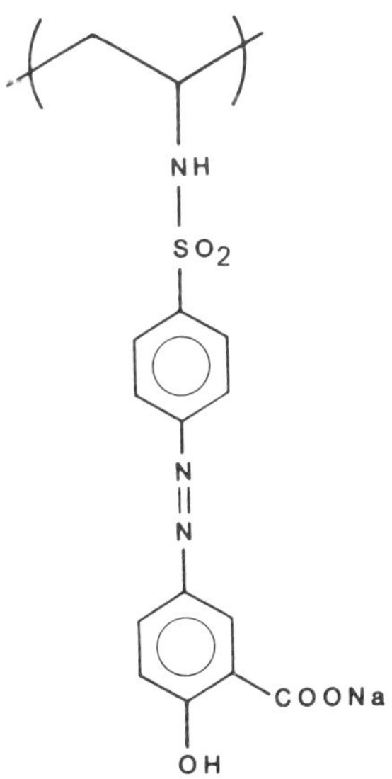

VI

Figure 8 Poly ASA-171 (VI).

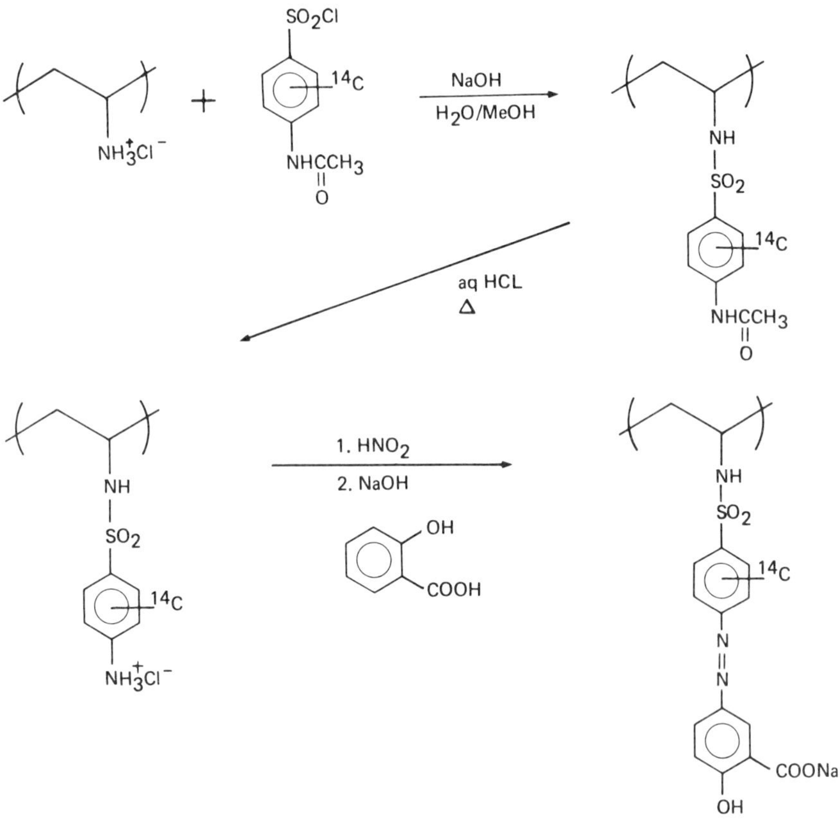

VII

Figure 9 Synthesis of [^{14}C-sulfanilamide ring]Poly ASA-171 (VII).

measured are very slow. In combination with gel permeation chromatography, information about the functionality distribution with respect to molecular weight can be readily obtained by use of labeled reagents. Studies of consecutive reactions on polymers are greatly aided by use of labeled materials. Although isotopes have already made some important contributions in the study of chemical reactions of polymers, their use has not been as widely exploited as it should be. We are in a period of widening horizons with regard to the ways in which chemically modified polymers are used to solve problems in the field of food, medicine, and environment. One can only expect that the use of isotopes will play an ever more important role in elucidating polymer chemistry in the future.

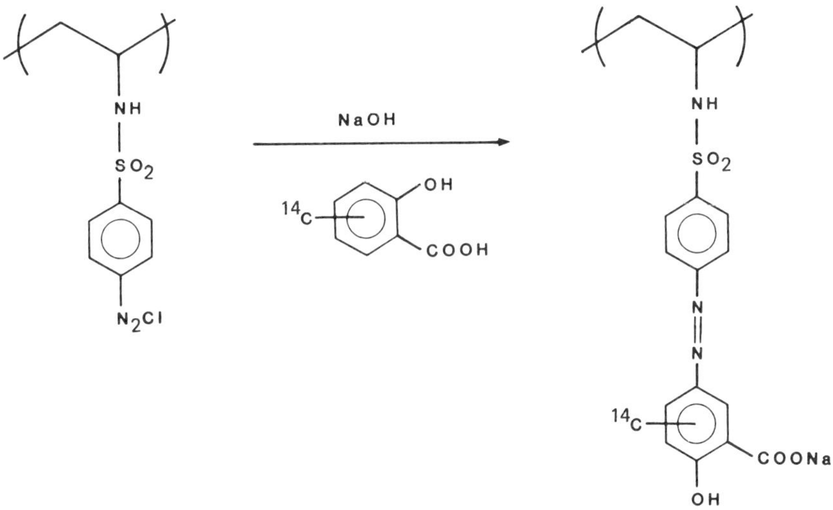

VIII

Figure 10 Synthesis of [^{14}C-salicylic acid ring]Poly ASA-171 (VIII).

Table 4 Radioisotopes in the Study of Chemical Reactions of Polymers

1. Distribution of functionality versus molecular weight
2. Accurate determination of degree of conversion and limiting yields
3. Composition of multiunit copolymers formed by consecutive chemical reactions
4. Rates of very slow reactions of polymers
5. Use of polymeric substrates in synthesis of radiolabeled compounds
6. Simple analysis of equivalency of polymeric reagents
7. Mechanism and reaction studies
8. Studies of the biological reactions of polymers

ACKNOWLEDGMENTS

The authors would like to acknowledge the contributions of David Matzinger, Steve Ng, Pat Scofield, Ynes Warren, and Dr. Ned Weinshenker.

REFERENCES

1. A. R. Cooper and R. G. Booth, *J. Appl. Polym. Sci.*, *23*:1373 (1979).
2. D. J. Dawson, *Aldrichim. Acta, 14*:23 (1981).
3. N. M. Weinshenker, Polymeric additives for food, in *Polymeric Drugs* (L. G. Donaruma and O. Vogl, eds.), Academic Press, New York, 1978, pp. 17-37.
4. P. Goldman and M. A. Peppercorn, *N. Engl. J. Med.*, *293*:20 (1975).
5. M. Windholz, ed., *The Merck Index*, 9th ed., Merck & Co., Rahway, N.J., 1976, p. 8090.
6. H. Schröder and D. E. S. Campbell, *Clin. Pharmacol. Ther.*, *13*: 539 (1972).
7. M. A. Peppercorn and P. Goldman, *J. Pharmacol. Exp. Ther.*, *181*:555 (1972).
8. T. M. Parkinson, T. Honohan, F. E. Enderlin, S. C. Halladay, R. L. Gale, S. A. de Keczer, P. L. Dubin, B. A. Ryerson, and A. R. Read, *Food Cosmet. Toxicol.*, *16*:321 (1978).

Chapter 15

A Sustained Release Ivermectin Implant for Livestock Pest Control*

J. ALLEN MILLER, R. O. DRUMMOND, and D. D. OEHLER
United States Livestock Insects Laboratory, United States Department of Agriculture, Kerrville, Texas

The need for improving the efficiency of pesticide usage and for prolonging the effectiveness of treatments in the control of livestock pests is well recognized. For several years, personnel of the U.S. Livestock Insects Laboratory have been interested in the application of controlled release technology to the problems of ectoparasite control in cattle [1]. The use of a sustained release implant to deliver systemic pesticides is one of several approaches under study [2].

Recently, a new family of potent anthelmintic agents called avermectins was discovered [3]. The avermectins are also active as animal systemic insecticides [4]. Ivermectin, Merck MK-933 [at least 80% of 22,23-dihydro-5-O-demethylavermectin A_{1a} and not more than 20% 22,23-dihydro-5-O-demethyl-25-de(1-methylpropyl)-25-(1-methylethyl)-avermectin A_{1a}], a member of this family of compounds, has been shown to be systemically active either orally or as an injection against ticks [5] and to be active as a larvicide against dung-breeding flies [6].

Because Ivermectin is active against these livestock pests at dosage rates in the range 1-10 μg/kg per day, there is an obvious potential for developing a sustained release implantable system for delivery of the drug over an extended period of time. Our studies toward the

---

*This chapter reports the results of research only. Mention of a pesticide does not constitute a recommendation for use by the U.S. Department of Agriculture (USDA) nor does it imply registration under FIFRA as amended. Also, mention of a commercial or proprietary product in this paper does not constitute an endorsement by the USDA.

development of such a system are presented in this report. The minimal sample sizes used in this series of tests were dictated by the limited availability of technical Ivermectin.

MATERIALS AND METHODS

In each study, Hereford steers were weighed and stanchioned indoors. They were fed a daily ration of alfalfa cubes and provided water ad libitum. Each group included an untreated steer as a control.

Implants were injected subcutaneously in the middle one-third of the outer ear slightly above center with a sterile Synovex Implanter. Before implantation, the injection site was scrubbed with a generous quantity of isopropyl alcohol to minimize the possibility of an infection.

Effectiveness of the treatments was determined by bioassays against adult Cayenne ticks, *Amblyomma cajennense* (F.), or adult lone star ticks, *Amblyomma americanum* (L.), feeding on the cattle and against larval horn flies, *Haematobia irritans* (L.), and stable flies, *Stomoxys calcitrans* (L.), developing in the manure. Ten pairs of unengorged adult ticks of the desired species were placed inside stockinette sleeves on treated and untreated cattle at various intervals after treatment. Females that had engorged and detached were collected daily and weighed. Later, the weight and estimated percentage hatch of egg masses were determined, and from these data we calculated the estimated larvae (EL). EL equals the grams of eggs times the estimated percentage hatch multiplied by 20,000 eggs per gram [7].

Manure samples were collected from each steer twice weekly and bioassayed to determine larvicidal activity against the horn fly and stable fly. These bioassays were conducted by placing 100 eggs of the desired species on each of several 100-g samples of manure. With the stable fly, 6 g of fish meal was added to each 100 g of manure to produce a suitable development medium. After the required incubation period, the pupae were washed from the samples, and adults were allowed to emerge in covered containers. Both number of pupae and number of adults that subsequently emerged were recorded. Abbott's formula was used to correct the observed mortality in the treated manure for the natural mortality in the manure from the untreated control.

Test 1

Microporous polypropylene (Accurel) pellets (3.75 mm diameter × 6 mm) were used to make the ear implants. Five 15-mg pellets were immersed in an acetonitrile solution of Ivermectin, and a vacuum was drawn in the system. The pellets were then removed, and the acetonitrile was allowed to evaporate from the pellets. Three of the pellets containing an estimated 53.5 mg of Ivermectin were implanted in the ear of one of the 300-kg Hereford steers (ca. 178 μg/kg). The remaining two pellets were analyzed for Ivermectin by a high-pressure liquid chromatography (HPLC) technique. A second steer was an untreated control.

Test 2

An implant containing 20% Ivermectin was formulated by dissolving technical Ivermectin in a melt of polyethylene glycol (PEG) (mol wt 15,000-20,000). The solution was then drawn by vacuum into a 3-mm-ID Teflon tube and allowed to cool. Upon cooling, the resultant solid rod (3-mm diameter) was removed and trimmed to the desired weight of 400 mg.

The implant was installed in the ear of a 310-kg Hereford steer to provide a dosage of 258 μg per kilogram of body weight. (The target dose was 200 μg/kg; however, an error in steer weight resulted in the higher actual dose.) A second steer was an untreated control during the first 4 weeks of the test. At the beginning of the fifth week, because of the slight swelling observed at the implant site, a 400-mg placebo (PEG without the Ivermectin) was implanted in the opposite ear of the treated steer and another in one ear of the control animal in an effort to determine the cause of the swelling.

Test 3

Of four Hereford steers (ca. 200 kg) used in this test, two were treated with ear implants identical to the one used in test 2 at a dose of 200 μg of Ivermectin per kilogram of body weight. A third steer was treated with a placebo and used as a control animal.

Alzet osmotic pumps (Model 1701) (Alza Corporation, Palo Alto, California) were used to treat the fourth steer. Because we were unable to determine directly the rate of release of drug from the PEG implants, the osmotic pump with its known, controlled rate of delivery was used as a standard upon which to gauge release from the implants. Pumps were surgically implanted, two at a time, subcutaneously, in the area between the brisket and the shoulder. Each pump delivered a nominal 1 μl/hr of a propylene glycol-glycerol formal formulation of Ivermectin (Merck Formulation B, 9.08 mg AI/ml). Therefore, while under treatment, this steer (174 kg) received 435 μl/day of solution for a dosage of 2.5 μg of Ivermectin per kilogram of body weight per day. In order to observe the residual activity of the compound, we installed two pumps each week for two consecutive weeks followed by a 3-week period without treatment. Two new pumps were then installed each week for three consecutive weeks. The decline in activity against larval horn flies and adult ticks was observed at the end of each treatment period.

Tick bioassays in this test were conducted with adult lone star ticks rather than Cayenne ticks. The lone star tick is more common in the United States and of greater economic importance than the Cayenne tick. A previous study [5] indicated about equal susceptibility of these species to Ivermectin.

RESULTS AND DISCUSSION

Test 1

Results of the manure bioassays showed that by the end of the first week posttreatment, mortalities of horn fly and stable fly larvae were 87% and 33%, respectively. During weeks 2-5, <50% horn fly mortality and no stable fly mortality could be attributed to the implant.

In addition, no effects of the implant were observed on survival, engorgement, and reproduction of the adult Cayenne ticks placed on the cattle at 6, 13, and 20 days posttreatment.

HPLC analysis of the two pellets not implanted indicated an average of 17.85 mg of Ivermectin per pellet. The three implanted pellets removed on day 41 postimplantation were found to contain 13.29, 16.8, and 16.06 mg AI. Therefore, an estimated 7.4 mg AI was released from the pellets over the 41 days in the ear. This release rate of about 0.6 μg/kg per day was insufficient for control of either larval flies in the manure or adult ticks on the steers.

Test 2

The results of the manure bioassay with horn fly larvae are shown in Table 1. Since the treatment appeared to have little effect on stable fly larvae (0-20% mortality), these data are not presented. Instead, the mortality of horn flies developing in the manure of an animal treated with a single 200-μg/kg injection (Merck formulation B) are presented for comparison [6]. Table 1 shows that the implant containing 258 μg AI/kg prevented horn fly development in the manure for up to 10 weeks, whereas the single injection of Merck formulation B of about the same dosage (200 μg/kg) was effective for only 4 weeks.

Effects on engorgement and reproduction of adult Cayenne ticks placed on the steers at nine intervals posttreatment are summarized in Table 2. In earlier studies (R. O. Drummond, unpublished data) conducted with identical conditions and techniques, in which a steer was injected with Merck formulation B at a rate of 200 μg/kg, the effect on ticks was evident for only 1 week postinjection. Drummond et al. [5] found that daily injections of 5 μg/kg resulted in 90% control of adult Cayenne ticks. The >70% control (average 86%) through 50 days posttreatment indicates that release rate from the implant was near this 5-μg/kg per day rate.

Table 1 Mortality of Larvae of Horn Flies in Manure of Steers Treated with Either a Single Injection (200 μg AI/kg) or an Implant (258 μg AI/kg) of Ivermectin

Weeks posttreatment	Corrected percent mortality[a] for indicated treatment	
	Injection[b]	Implant
1	99	100
2	93	100
3	100	100
4	98	100
5	74	99
6	25	100
7	0	100
8	0	100
9	—	100
10	—	98
11	—	62
12	—	63
13	—	4

[a]Corrected for control mortality by Abbott's formula.
[b]Data from Ref. 6.

In test 2, a slight swelling which persisted for 10-11 weeks was noted at the site of the implant containing Ivermectin. When placebos were installed in the opposite ear of the test steer and in one ear of the control steer, no swelling was observed. Therefore, either the drug was responsible for this slight inflammation or the initial implant caused an infection because of nonsterile technique. Because precautions were taken to avoid infection and since the swelling persisted for 10-11 weeks, the problem appears to have been with the drug.

Test 3

The results of the horn fly bioassays are shown in Table 3. The 20% Ivermectin implant at a dosage of 200 μg/kg body weight resulted in 98-100% mortality of the immature horn fly for 10-12 weeks. These

Table 2 Control of Adult *A. cajennense* on a Steer at Intervals After Single Implant (258 μg AI/kg) of Ivermectin

Animal	Number ♀	Average engorgement period (days)	Average weight (g) ♀	Average weight (g) Eggs	Average estimated percent hatched	Total EL[a]	Percent control of EL
Infested 7 days after implant							
Treated	5	16.2	0.345	0.136	80	8,785	83.4
Control	9	13.5	0.706	0.343	84	52,819	
Infested 14 days after implant							
Treated	0	–	–	–	–	0	100
Control	10	16.8	0.638	0.278	64	38,770	
Infested 21 days after implant							
Treated	0	–	–	–	–	0	100
Control	10	14.0	0.596	0.286	72	46,511	
Infested 36 days after implant							
Treated	6	20.8	0.211	0.079	73	6,147	72.1
Control	4[b]	13.5	0.552	0.280	98	22,009	
Infested 43 days after implant							
Treated	2	20.5	0.293	0.117	74	3,886	89.5
Control	7	9.4	0.635	0.335	80	37,210	
Infested 50 days after implant							
Treated	5	28.2	0.352	0.170	87	15,450	71.6
Control	9	13.9	0.622	0.323	93	54,427	

			Infested 64 days after implant				
Treated	8	15.8	0.503	0.267	78	34,540	28.9
Control	9	10.4	0.656	0.328	83	48,596	
			Infested 71 days after implant				
Treated	7	20.3	0.628	0.339	96	39,160	9.5
Control	10	18.5	0.592	0.280	77	43,257	
			Infested 78 days after implant				
Treated	9	13.3	0.606	0.317	82	41,403	0
Control	7	12.7	0.679	0.360	78	36,980	

[a]EL, estimated larvae = g eggs × estimated percent hatched × 20,000.
[b]Rest of ♀ crushed in sleeve.

Table 3 Mortality of Horn Fly Larvae in Manure of Steers Treated with Implants Containing Ivermectin (200 μg/kg)

Weeks posttreatment	Corrected percent mortality[a] for indicated treatment		
	Implant (200 μg/kg)		Osmotic pump (2.5 μg/kg/day)
	Steer 1650	Steer 1651	Steer 1499
1	100	99	100[b]
2	98	100	100
3	100	100	91[c]
4	100	99	100
5	100	100	86
6-10	100	100	100[d]
11	18	100	43
12	20	100	11
13	0	77	0
14	0	41	1
15-16	0	0	0

[a]Corrected for control mortality by Abbott's formula.
[b]Two-week treatment period.
[c]Three-week period without treatment.
[d]Three-week treatment period.

results are comparable to the 10-week duration observed in the previous test. Furthermore, the decline in effectiveness was quite rapid, with a drop from 100% mortality to 0% mortality in 3 weeks.

As in the previous study, a slight swelling was observed at the site of implantation in those animals receiving the Ivermectin implant. No swelling was observed in the control animal that received an identical implant minus the Ivermectin.

The continuous delivery of 2.5 μg/kg per day via the osmotic pumps resulted in 100% mortality of horn flies in the manure. The implanted pumps were active during weeks 1 and 2 and again during weeks 6, 7, and 8. The mortality (86-100%) observed during weeks 3, 4, and 5 is attributed to residual activity of the drug delivered in the first 2 weeks. The mortality observed during the 4 weeks following the second treatment period indicates that about a month is required for the manure to become suitable for horn fly survival after a continuous treatment of 2.5 μg/kg per day.

Results of the bioassays with the lone star ticks on the two animals given implants are presented in Table 4. In general, there was complete control of lone star ticks at 11-32 days posttreatment and >85% control through 46 days posttreatment. These data are similar to those for *A. cajennense*. Thus a single treatment with the PEG formulation does provide an extended period of tick control.

The delivery of 2.5 μg/kg per day via the osmotic pump did not afford complete control of the lone star tick (Table 5). A slight increase in effectiveness was observed during the second treatment period, although the dosage rate was identical to that of the first treatment period. These data are consistent with previous observations that about 5 μg/kg per day is near the minimum dosage necessary for complete control of ticks [5].

Despite the limited test group size, these results indicate that a PEG implant formulation of Ivermectin can be used to increase the efficiency of drug use. The 200-μg/kg dosage, when applied in the form of an implant, extended the period of horn fly control to about 77 days (11 weeks), compared with about 30 days of control for a single injection of Formulation B at the same dosage. It should be pointed out that the implant was designed for tick control but not specifically for horn fly control. Therefore, we sought to release about 5 μg/kg per day, a dosage considerably higher than the 0.5-1.0 μg/kg per day necessary for horn fly control [6]. It is conceivable that an implant with a lower release rate designed specifically to control horn flies in the manure could be effective for 6 months or more.

If 5 μg/kg per day is accepted as near the minimum effective dosage for control of adult Cayenne and lone star ticks, then the 200 μg/kg dosage could at best provide about 40 days of control. Therefore, the 40-50 days of control observed in our studies approached this theoretical limit of efficiency of drug usage. If additional supplies of technical Ivermectin can be obtained, improvements in duration will be sought by increasing the total dosage (400 μg/kg) while maintaining the daily release rate of about 5 μg/kg per day. In addition, we will pursue the quantification of levels of Ivermectin in the blood in order to more precisely study release rates.

ACKNOWLEDGMENT

All tables courtesy of U.S. Livestock Insects Laboratory, U.S. Department of Agriculture, Kerrville, Texas.

Table 4 Control of Adult *A. americanum* on Steers at Intervals After a Single Implant (200 μg AI/kg) of Ivermectin

Treatment (animal number)	Number ♀		Average engorgement period (days)	Average weight (g)		Average estimated percent hatched	Total EL	Percent control of EL
	Collected	Laid eggs		♀	Eggs			
			3 days pretreatment					
Treated (50)	9	9	14.5	0.349	0.192	70.5	25,626	47.4
Treated (51)	8	7	21.6	0.282	0.120	46.1	9,424	80.7
Control	10	10	12.5	0.546	0.264	93.6	48,789	—
			11 days posttreatment					
Treated (50)	3	1	23.3	0.136	0.008	0	0	100
Treated (51)	0	—	—	—	—	—	—	100
Control	10	10	14.0	0.392	0.218	95.8	41,905	—
			18 days posttreatment					
Treated (50)	0	—	—	—	—	—	0	100
Treated (51)	0	—	—	—	—	—	0	100
Control	8	8	15.2	0.584	0.344	89.9	49,222	—
			25 days posttreatment					
Treated (50)	0	—	—	—	—	—	0	100
Treated (51)	0	—	—	—	—	—	0	100
Control	9	9	15.0	0.520	0.280	83.4	46,573	—
			32 days posttreatment					
Treated (50)	0	—	—	—	—	—	0	100
Treated (51)	0	—	—	—	—	—	0	100
Control	9	9	16.7	0.654	0.373	73.7	52,830	—

			39 days posttreatment					
Treated (50)	0	—	—	—	—	—	0	100
Treated (51)	9	9	20.1	0.292	0.142	89.2	23,468	58.6
Control	9	9	13.0	0.586	0.322	98.2	56,759	—
			46 days posttreatment					
Treated (50)	1	1	27.0	0.223	0.123	95.0	2,337	95.3
Treated (51)	10	10	20.3	0.204	0.072	76.0	11,905	76.0
Control	10	9	15.0	0.471	0.285	96.2	49,659	—
			53 days posttreatment					
Treated (50)	8	8	16.5	0.308	0.155	89.5	21,889	0
Treated (51)	9	8	19.7	0.261	0.097	44.2	10,013	44.3
Control	5	4	13.2	0.605	0.361	66.2	17,974	—
			60 days posttreatment					
Treated (50)	10	10	16.7	0.288	0.140	88.3	25,794	53.0
Treated (51)	10	9	21.0	0.193	0.072	70.3	10,696	80.5
Control	10	9	21.4	0.532	0.320	95.4	54,908	—
			67 days posttreatment					
Treated (50)	8	8	13.2	0.408	0.222	93.0	33,466	34.5
Treated (51)	5	4	18.4	0.188	0.079	52.0	3,964	92.2
Control	9	9	12.1	0.537	0.290	97.1	51,081	—
			74 days posttreatment					
Treated (50)	Sleeve off		—	—	—	—	—	—
Treated (51)	8	8	18.6	0.300	0.118	47.5	10,056	74.5
Control	10	9	12.3	0.500	0.266	81.4	39,493	—
			81 days posttreatment					
Treated (50)	Sleeve off		—	—	—	—	—	—
Treated (51)	9	9	16.7	0.332	0.166	86.4	25,719	35.7
Control	10	9	13.6	0.535	0.281	70.9	39,986	—

Table 5 Control of Adult *A. americanum* on a Steer with Ivermectin Delivered by Osmotic Pump at a Rate of 2.5 μg/kg per Day

Treatment	Number ♀		Average engorgement period (days)	Average weight (g)		Average estimated percent hatched	Total EL	Percent control of EL
	Collected	Laid eggs		♀	Eggs			
First pump treatment, Jan. 26-Feb. 9 (2 weeks)								
Infested 3 days pretreatment								
Treated	5	3	18.0	0.147	0.043	66.0	3,110	93.6
Control	10	10	12.5	0.546	0.264	93.6	48,789	—
Infested 4 days after start of treatment								
Treated	3	3	17.0	0.278	0.142	96.0	8,142	80.2
Control	10	10	13.1	0.426	0.227	82.4	41,137	—
Infested 11 days after start of treatment								
Treated	6	3	16.2	0.181	0.077	97.0	8,959	78.6
Control	10	10	14.0	0.392	0.218	95.8	41,905	—
Infested 4 days after end of treatment								
Treated	9	9	15.9	0.300	0.152	74.2	23,971	51.3
Control	8	8	15.2	0.584	0.344	89.9	49,222	—
Infested 11 days after end of treatment								
Treated	9	8	17.5	0.229	0.112	81.4	14,388	69.1
Control	9	9	15.0	0.520	0.280	83.4	46,573	—
Infested 18 days after end of treatment (3 days before start of second treatment)								
Treated	8	3	21.5	0.100	0.054	55.0	2,225	95.8
Control	9	9	16.7	0.654	0.373	73.7	52,830	—

		Second pump treatment, March 2-22 (3 weeks)						
		Infested 4 days after start of treatment						
Treated	3	3	19.7	0.124	0.033	61.6	1,683	97.0
Control	9	9	13.0	0.586	0.322	98.2	56,759	—
		Infested 11 days after start of treatment						
Treated	4	3	26.5	0.245	0.156	91.0	8,775	82.3
Control	10	9	15.0	0.471	0.285	96.2	49,659	—
		Infested 18 days after start of treatment						
Treated	3	0	26.7	0.181	0	—	0	100
Control	5	4	13.2	0.605	0.361	66.2	17,974	—
		Infested 4 days after end of treatment						
Treated	7	4	21.7	0.272	0.169	60.0	7,976	85.5
Control	10	9	21.4	0.532	0.320	95.4	54,908	—
		Infested 11 days after end of treatment						
Treated	9	8	12.5	0.304	0.157	63.2	15,907	68.9
Control	9	9	12.5	0.537	0.290	97.1	51,081	—
		Infested 18 days after end of treatment						
Treated	2	0	16.0	0.130	0	—	0	100
Control	10	9	12.3	0.500	0.266	81.4	39,493	—
		Infested 25 days after end of treatment						
Treated	7	6	13.0	0.309	0.155	88.3	16,413	58.9
Control	10	9	13.6	0.535	0.281	70.9	39,986	—

REFERENCES

1. J. A. Miller, S. E. Kunz, and D. D. Oehler, in *Controlled Release of Pesticides and Pharmaceuticals* (D. H. Lewis, ed.), Plenum Press, New York, 1981, p. 311.
2. H. Jaffe, J. A. Miller, P. A. Giang, and D. K. Hayes, in *Controlled Release of Bioactive Materials* (R. W. Baker, ed.), Academic Press, New York, 1980, p. 237.
3. R. W. Burg, B. M. Miller, E. E. Baker, J. Birnbaum, S. A. Currie, R. Hartman, Y. L. Young, R. L. Monaghan, G. Olson, I. Putter, J. B. Tunac, H. Wallick, E. O. Stapley, R. Oiwa, and S. Omura, *Antimicrob. Agents Chemother.*, *15*(3):361 (1979).
4. D. A. Ostlind, S. Cifelli, and R. Lang, *Vet. Rec.*, *105*:168 (1979).
5. R. O. Drummond, T. M. Whetstone, and J. A. Miller, *J. Econ. Entomol.*, *74*(4):432 (1981).
6. J. A. Miller, S. E. Kunz, D. D. Oehler, and R. W. Miller, *J. Econ. Entomol.*, *74*(5):608 (1981).
7. R. O. Drummond, T. M. Whetstone, S. E. Ernst, and W. J. Gladney, *J. Econ. Entomol.*, *65*(6):1641 (1972).

Chapter 16

Design Parameters for Controlled Release Soybean Coatings

STEPHEN HONG-WEI WU and CLARENCE C. DANNELLY* Eastman Kodak Company, Kingsport, Tennessee

The demands of an increasing world population for food provided from a diminishing arable land base call for improved efficiencies in food production and utilization. Although we need increased agricultural productivity, excessive use of fertilizers and agrichemicals, even at present levels, in crop production can result in contamination of water supplies and environmental pollution from the runoff of such materials as phosphates and persistent pesticides [1-3]. The net effect of these factors is a need for improvements in agronomy practices that will increase yields, reduce costs, and prove environmentally acceptable. One approach to meeting this challenge is to improve the microenvironment of plant seeds by the use of controlled release coating systems [4-6].

Soybeans provide human food, animal feed, and material for many industrial uses. As a source of protein, oil, and fat, soybeans complement the contributions of most other major crops. Yet only in recent decades has significant progress been made in soybean production, in developing a scientific understanding of this crop, and in improving yields. However, the gain in yields has been smaller and less striking than the gains with other crops such as corn, wheat, rice, and sorghum [7,8]. For these reasons, and because soybeans have a shape and size that are ideal for encapsulation, we chose to study soybeans for the development of controlled release seed coating systems which may provide beneficial effects such as protecting the seeds from mechanical damage and deterioration, allowing precisely

**Present affiliation:* Retired

controlled delivery of agrichemicals in the microenvironment surrounding the seeds and improving seed germination, stand development, and yield.

The strategy undertaken in our study was to identify polymeric coating systems that could be applied by air-suspension coating technology, would not inhibit the rate or extent of soybean germination, and would serve as carriers for a variety of bioactive compounds to improve the seed environment and/or to achieve the precisely controlled delivery of active ingredients in the seed environment. Understanding of environmental factors such as water, oxygen, and heat requirements for soybean germination was crucial for the design of seed coatings. However, quantitative data about the relationship of soybean germination and the requirements of these environmental factors were limited in published reports [9-11]. Thus one objective of this work was to determine water-transport properties of natural seed coats and cotyledon tissues, and the temperature-dependent limiting requirements of water and total oxygen for germination of soybean seeds. The other objective was to utilize these parameters in the design of seed coating systems which would not interfere with the natural germination process but would provide beneficial effects.

EXPERIMENTAL

Seed Variety

Ransom soybean seeds (1977 and 1978) purchased from Jacob and Hartz Seed Company, Stuttgart, Arkansas, were used in all experiments. Seeds were stored at laboratory ambient conditions (ca. 25°C and ca. 55% rh) before use. The moisture content of seeds was less than 10%.

Water Imbibition of Soybeans

Individual seeds, or seeds with seed coats removed, were weighed and then immersed in distilled water or aqueous glucose solution, 5-30% (w/v), at room temperature from 1 min to 24 hr. Weight gains at various time intervals were measured to determine the water imbibition characteristics of soybeans in direct contact with water, and the effect of osmotic pressure on the water imbibition of soybean seeds.

The porosity of the natural seed coats was determined qualitatively by immersing soybean seeds overnight in aqueous solutions containing erythrosine (FD&C Red No. 3 dye, mol wt 879.9), poly(methyl methacrylate) latex particles dyed with methylene blue (0.1 to 0.5 μm), or both. The imbibed seeds were sectioned transversely to obtain thin-slice specimens for observation of the fine structures of seed coat and embryo tissues and the location of erythrosine molecules and latex particles.

The water vapor absorption of soybeans was determined by placing seeds in constant-relative humidity chambers (70-100%) at 25°C [12]. The percent weight gains after various periods of time up to 3 weeks were measured to plot absorption isotherms.

Water Requirements for Soybean Germination

The water requirement for soybean germination was determined in sand media. Natural sand was dried in an evacuated oven at 110°C and then stored in a desiccator. Saturation of 100 g of dry sand required 25 ml of water, which was defined as 100% water saturation. The moisture content of sand was measured by percent of the saturation value.

Soybeans (5 g, ca. 32 seeds) were planted approximately 1/2 in. deep in a 200-g sand bed in a flask open to the air. The moisture contents of the sand beds varied from 7.5 to 30% of the saturation value. After 5 days, the germinated and nongerminated seeds, measured by radicle emergence (>2 mm), were counted and weighed to determine the relationship of the degree of water imbibition and the rate of germination.

The effects of temperature on the water imbibition rate and the germination rate were determined by planting samples of 30-35 seeds in preequilibrated sand beds at 10 and 22°C in which the moisture levels in sand were controlled from 10 to 30% of the saturation value. After a period of 4 hr to 10 days, seeds were removed to determine the degree of water imbibition from ungerminated seeds and the germination rate from emerged seeds.

Oxygen Requirements for Soybean Germination

The germination of soybean seeds and the development of seedlings in a low-oxygen atmosphere at constant temperatures were determined by germinating individual seeds in Nessler test tubes which contained 20 g of sand, a controlled amount of water from 7.5 to 30% of the saturation value, and a known initial oxygen partial pressure from 0 to 2.4% (Fig. 1). The quantitative limiting total oxygen requirements were measured by germinating 5-20 seeds at different temperatures (20-35°C) in an Erlenmeyer flask which contained 100 g of sand, an optimal amount of water (ca. 20% of the saturation value), and a gas mixture of 6.46% oxygen and 93.54% nitrogen. The gas pressure inside the flask was adjusted to 1 atm. The gas compositions were analyzed by gas chromatography.

The percent germination, which was measured by the number of seeds with emerged radicles, and the oxygen availability, which was measured by calculating the initial available oxygen per gram of fresh seed weight, were plotted to obtain the limiting values of the total oxygen requirement for germination.

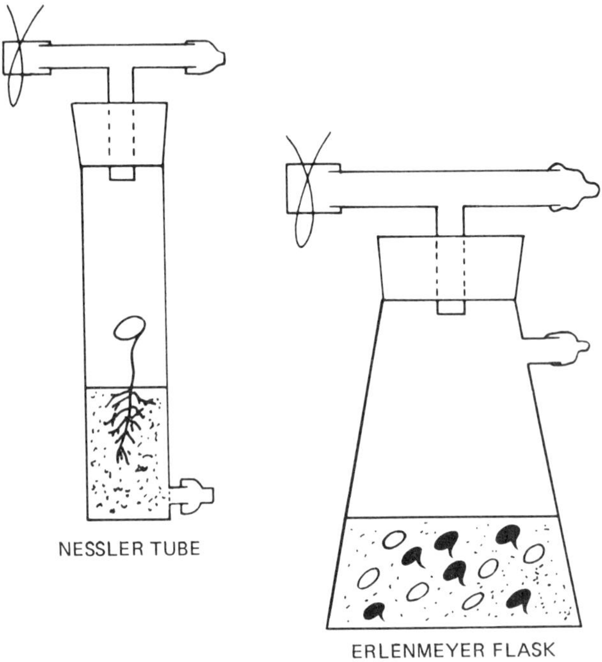

$$\text{MOL/g OF FRESH SEED WT} = \frac{PV \times \%\ O_2}{RT \times W_{SEED}}$$

Figure 1 Apparatus for the determination of O_2 requirements for seed germination.

Formulation of Coating Dispersions

The coating dispersions for the encapsulation of soybean seeds were composed of polymeric binders, pigments, active ingredients, and a solvent system. For the purpose of this chapter, typical compositions of coating dispersions were summarized in Table 1. When pigments or combinations of pigments and fillers were used in the formulation, they were ball-milled in acetone or methanol for 24 hr to ensure homogeneous mixing before use and then filtered through a 60-mesh screen to remove large particles.

The dispersions were prepared by adding the ball-milled pigments and agrichemicals to the polymer solution and then adjusted to a final solids content of approximately 4% (w/v).

Encapsulation of Soybean Seeds

A 4-in. air-suspension coater for spray-coating discrete particles was used for the encapsulation of soybean seeds. The detailed design of

Table 1 Composition of Seed Coatings

Polymer[a]		Pigment or active ingredient[b]	Polymer/pigment ratio (v/v)	Coating level (% of seed weight)	Solvent
1	PMMA	–	–	0.7-3.0	Acetone
2	PMMA	Talc	1:1	2-9	Acetone
3	PMMA	Talc/NaCl	1:1:2	4	Acetone
			1:2:1	4	Acetone
			1:3:0	4	Acetone
4	PMMA	Talc/$CaCO_3$	1:0.5:0.5	4	Acetone
			1:1:1	4	Acetone
			1:1.25:1.25	3.2	Acetone
5	EC	GA_3	–	0.5-3.0	Methanol

[a]Poly(methyl methacrylate) purchased from DuPont Co.; ethyl cellulose purchased from Dow Chemical Co.
[b]Talc purchased from Mallinckrodt; gibberellic acid (GA_3) purchased from Aldrich Chemical Co.

the apparatus and its distinctive features in comparison with other conventional fluidized-bed coaters were reported elsewhere [13]. In a typical operation, 250 g of soybean seeds was fluidized in the chamber with inlet air at 50-60°C and outlet air at 32-40°C. The coating dispersions were atomized at 20 psi through a nozzle (Fig. 2). Approximately 15 min was needed to spray-coat 250 g of seeds at 4% coating weight. Different coating dispersions could be applied subsequently to make multilayer coatings. For example, seeds were coated with an inner layer of cellulose ethyl ether (0.5% of seed weight), a middle layer of poly(methyl methacrylate) (PPMA)/talc/$CaCO_3$ (2% by weight), and then an outer layer of PMMA/talc (2% by weight).

Standard Laboratory Test for Seed Emergence

When both the emergence and the seedling development under normal conditions were required, a standardized test procedure was used for the laboratory evaluation of seed samples. Equal volumes of sand and Baccto potting medium were thoroughly blended and then placed in a rectangular plastic tray ($8\frac{1}{4}$ in. × $6\frac{1}{2}$ in. × 2 in.) bottomed-lined with a filter board. Five rows of five seeds each were positioned precisely on the surface, then covered with an additional amount of the blend so that the planted seeds were 1 in. under the surface. A controlled

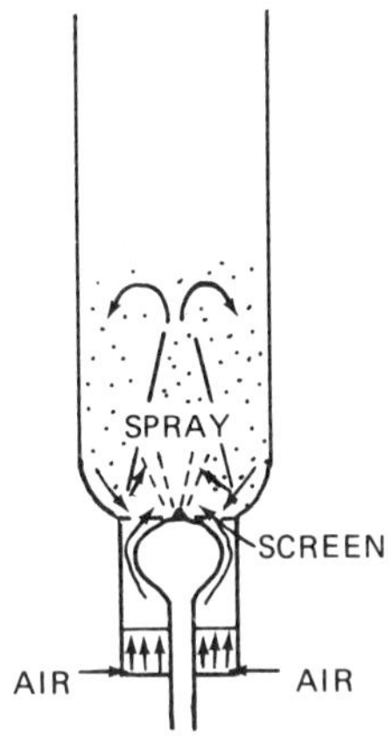

TEC AIR-SUSPENSION COATER

Figure 2 Air-suspension coater for the encapsulation of seeds. (Courtesy of C. C. Dannelly and C. R. Leonard, Eastman Kodak Company, Kingsport, Tennessee.)

amount of water (ca. 300 ml) was absorbed from the bottom of the tray. After the water was absorbed, the tray was placed into a polyethylene bag to prevent water loss. After 4 days, the bag was removed. Normal, abnormal, and dead plants were counted and recorded after 4 and 7 days.

RESULTS AND DISCUSSION

Water is a basic requirement for seed germination. It is essential for enzyme activation, thus permitting biochemical breakdown, translocation, and utilization of reserve storage of materials [14-16]. The water imbibition process is also an important transport mechanism for many nutrients or agrichemicals. Therefore, the transport properties of seed coats and cotyledon tissue, the temperature-dependent water imbibition rate of germinating seeds in various osmotic conditions, and the minimum water requirement for germination at certain temperatures are essential for the design of controlled release seed coating formulations.

Respiration increases rapidly during seed germination and is a function of temperature. Since respiration is essentially an oxidative process, an adequate supply of oxygen must be available. If the oxygen concentration is reduced substantially below that of air, germination and seedling development of most seeds are retarded. The rate of oxygen uptake during the early stages of germination and the total oxygen requirement for the emergence of radicles are two important parameters for the design of seed coatings. It was reported that the rate of oxygen uptake began to increase in an autocatalytic manner, reaching a rate of about 50 nmol of oxygen consumed per gram of fresh seed weight per minute after 5 hr of imbibition [17]. In this work, we determined the emergence of soybean seeds under a limited total oxygen supply at constant temperatures.

Water Imbibitions of Soybeans

Figure 3 illustrates the semipermeable property of natural seed coats. When soybeans were immersed overnight in aqueous solutions containing erythrosine and dyed-latex particles, it was observed from microscopic study that erythrosine molecules penetrated the epidermis, hypodermis, and inner parenchyma layers and ended up on the surface of cotyledon tissue; however, the latex particles penetrated the epidermis layer and partially entered the hourglass cells. Latex particles, particularly, accumulated on the interface of palisade and hourglass cells. These results provided evidence for the semipermeable character of soybean seed coats. The epidermal layer exhibits pore-like structures and allows penetration of micrometer-size particles. Other layers of seed coats permit permeation only by molecular-size particles. Thus the voids in the porous natural seed coat can be filled with agrichemical-pregnated particles of micrometer size as a means of controlled release.

The characteristic curve for water imbibition of soybean seeds as a function of time is shown in Fig. 4. About 15 hr was required for dry seeds to achieve a fully imbibed state. The average maximum weight gain was 130% of the initial seed weight. With the assumptions that seeds are approximately spherical and the diffusivity for water imbibition is independent of imbibed water concentration, the diffusivity was calculated to be 3.5×10^{-7} cm^2/sec, based on the Fickian diffusion model at short imbibition time periods. This result is particularly valuable as a reference for the selection and design of polymeric coatings for monitoring the water permeation rate. The Fickian diffusion model is inadequate over long time scales; however, an empirical model with an advancing relaxation front is able to fit data over the time range.

The effect of osmotic pressure on the water imbibition of soybean seeds within 2 hr of water-contact time is given in Fig. 5. The diffusivity of decoated soybean seeds in contact with liquid water was 7.7×10^{-7} cm^2/sec, approximately twofold higher than the value of intact seeds. The diffusivity of decoated seeds decreased linearly with increasing glucose concentration in water from 0 to 20% (w/v) in the semilog plot. When glucose concentration is higher than 20%, the

A

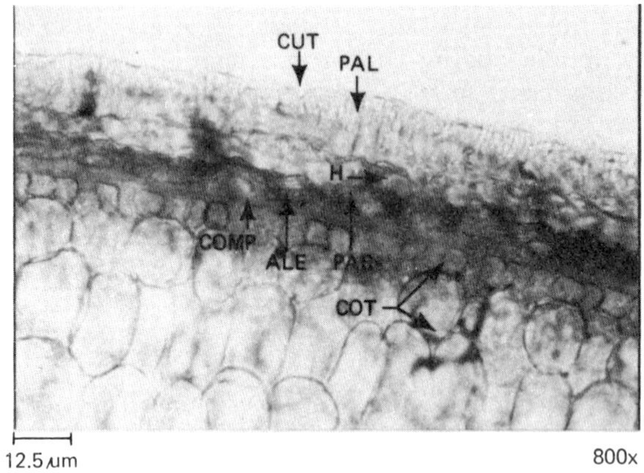

B

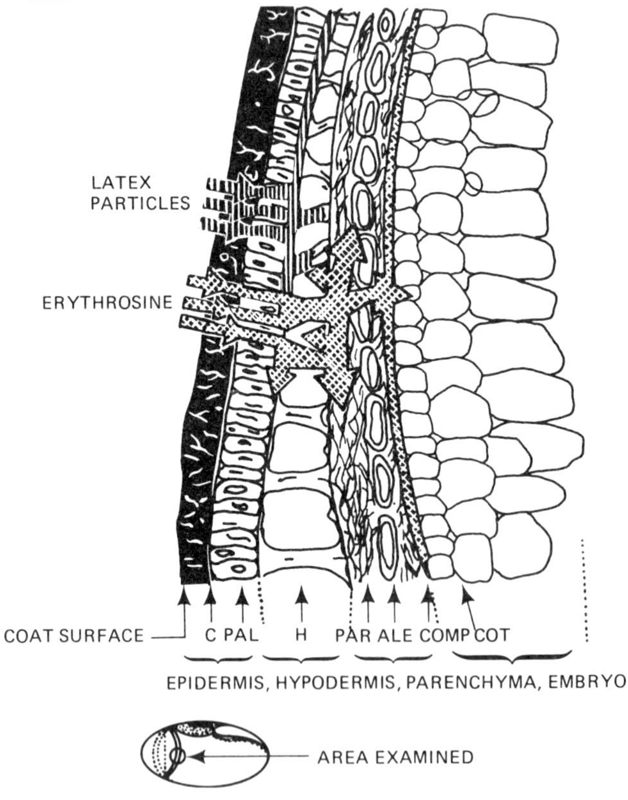

Figure 3 Cross section (A) and schematic diagram (B) of soybean seed coat immersed in aqueous solution containing erythrosine and latex particles. C, cuticle; pal, palisade; H, hourglass; par, parenchyma; Ale, Aleurone; COMP, compressed parenchyma; Cot, Cotyledon.

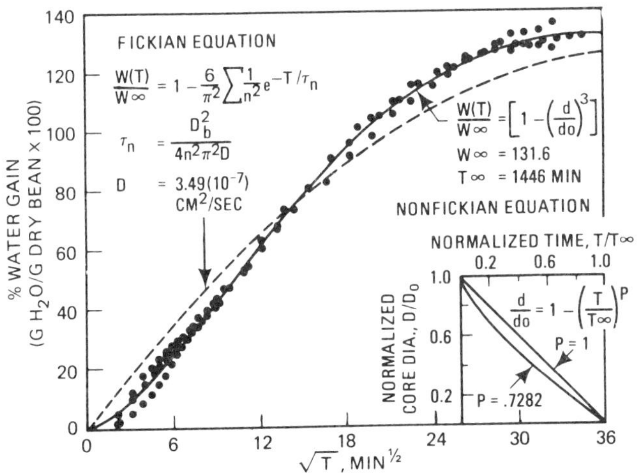

Figure 4 Water imbibition of soybean seeds at 25°C.

diffusivity decreases superexponentially. At 30% glucose concentration, the diffusivity was about 6% of the value of decoated seeds in pure water. These data are useful for the design of seed coatings which can modify the osmotic environment in the seed vicinity and thus monitor the imbibition and germination rates of seeds.

Water Requirement for Soybean Germination

Figure 6 illustrates schematically the effect of water content in sand on the germination and seedling development of soybeans.

Figure 7 shows the 5-day radicle emergence rate for soybean seeds under water-stressed conditions. The critical value of moisture uptake for the seeds to start radicle emergence was 60% of the initial seed weight, which was defined as 60% imbibition. The minimum degree of imbibition was 100% to achieve the maximum germination rate. The water vapor imbibition of soybean seeds placed in chambers of standard relative humidities is given in Fig. 8. The weight increase of uncoated seeds at 100% rh, 25°C, was less than 20% of the original weight, which is substantially lower than the critical amount of moisture needed to initiate the germination process at 25°C. These results are consistent with reported data [11,18].

Temperature-dependent water imbibition at different moisture levels is shown in Fig. 9. The percent radicle emergence as a function of time at three moisture levels is given in Fig. 10. The effect of temperature and moisture level in sand on the imbibition rate and the emergence rate of soybean seeds is summarized on Table 2. At 22°C, seeds

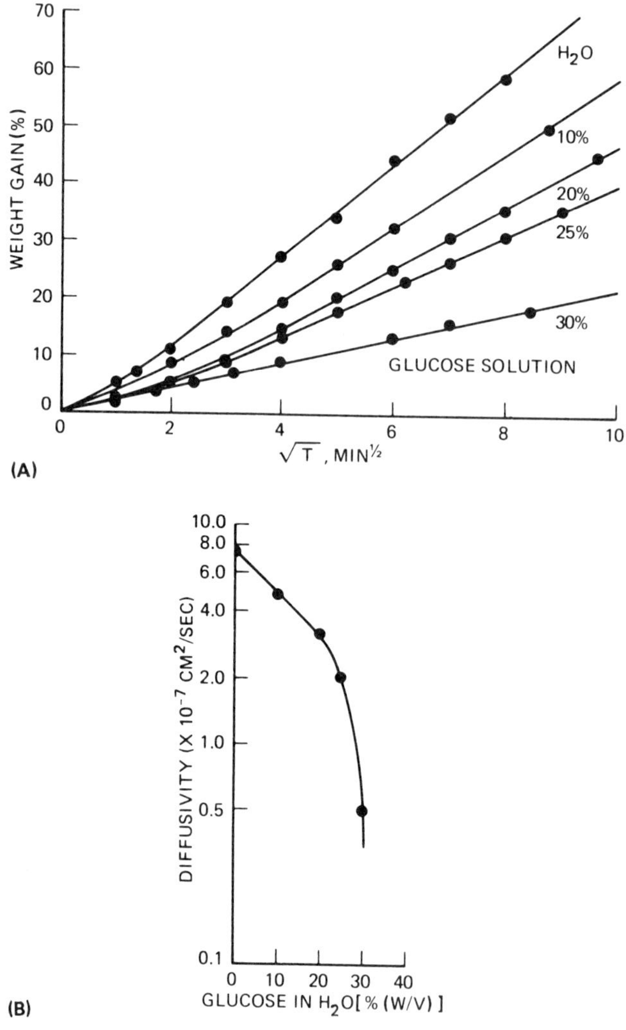

Figure 5 Water imbibition (A) and diffusivity (B) of decoated soybean seeds in glucose solution at 25°C.

in the 30% moisture saturated sand required only 8 hr to reach a moisture gain of 60% initial seed weight, which is the minimum requirement for germination, and reached 80% germination in 2 days. To reach the same germination rate at 20-15% moisture levels required 3.5-5 days. At 10°C, the germination rate was zero, even for fully imbibed seeds.

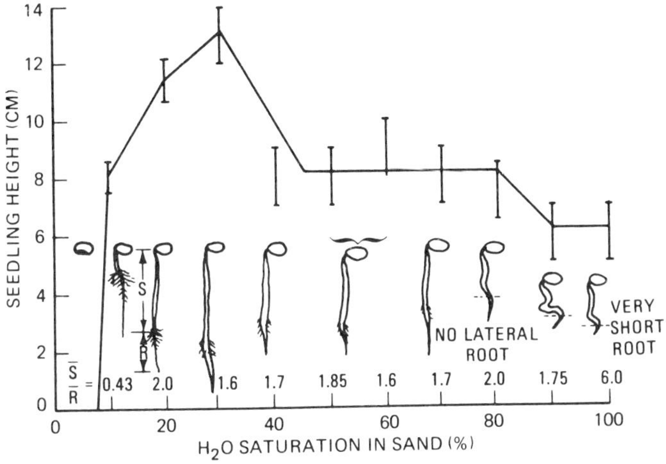

Figure 6 Effect of water availability in sand on soybean seedling development at 25°C for 7 days.

These results suggest that to achieve uniform high germination rate in the shortest time at 22°C, seeds require a rate of imbibition of about 60% weight gain in 8 hr. A seed coating that can regulate the water availability to seeds to protect soybean seeds from the adverse effects of excessive or subcritical soil moisture at times when soil temperature is sufficient for germination would be particularly valuable for farmers [19]. The possibility of such a coating can be demonstrated by a NaCl-containing seed coating in the later discussion of the germination of coated seeds.

Oxygen Requirement for Soybean Germination

The effects of total oxygen supply on the germination of soybean seeds in the environments of various water availabilities are shown in Fig. 11. Fully imbibed seeds kept in a nitrogen atmosphere without oxygen for 2 weeks did not have radicle emergence. With a limited total supply of oxygen, the growth rate of seedlings was reduced and completely stopped after oxygen was exhausted.

The semiquantitative minimum total oxygen requirement and the corresponding minimum percent water saturation of sand to observe the radicle emergence of soybean seeds in Nessler tubes kept at constant temperatures are given in Table 3. The limiting total oxygen requirement for radicle emergence was calculated to be 3-5 μmol per gram of seed. A more accurate measurement was obtained by using the Erlenmeyer flask method described earlier. The limiting total oxygen

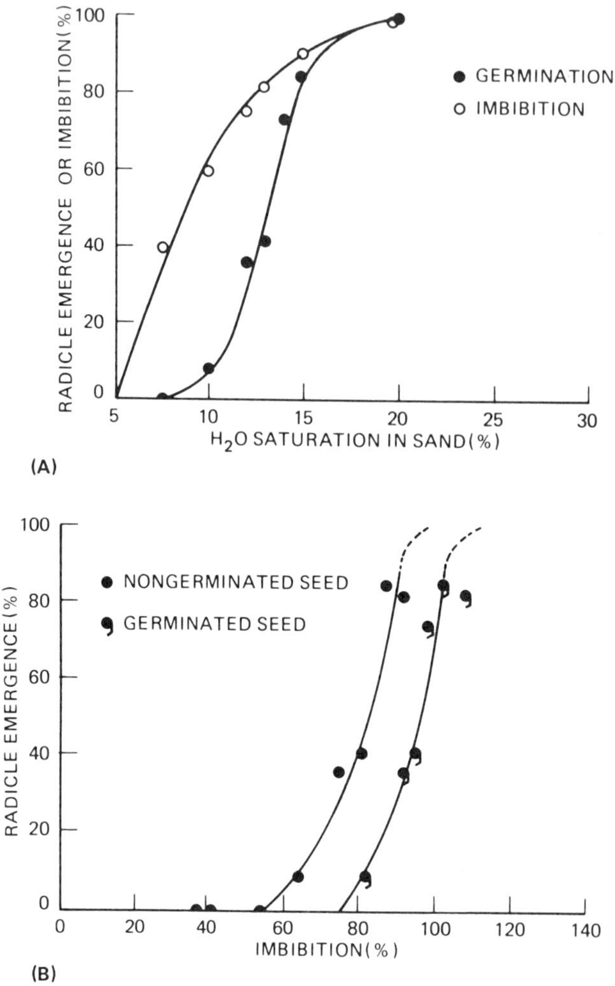

Figure 7 Germination of soybean seeds under water-stressed conditions at 25°C. (A) Degree of imbibition and 5-day emergence rate as a function of water availability in sand. (B) Relationship of 5-day emergence rate and degree of imbibition.

requirement for radicle emergence was determined to be 3.8 μmol per gram of seed at 25°C (Fig. 12). The effect of temperature on the oxygen requirement is shown in Fig. 12. Seeds required more oxygen for germination at 32°C than at 25°C, especially under a limited supply of oxygen.

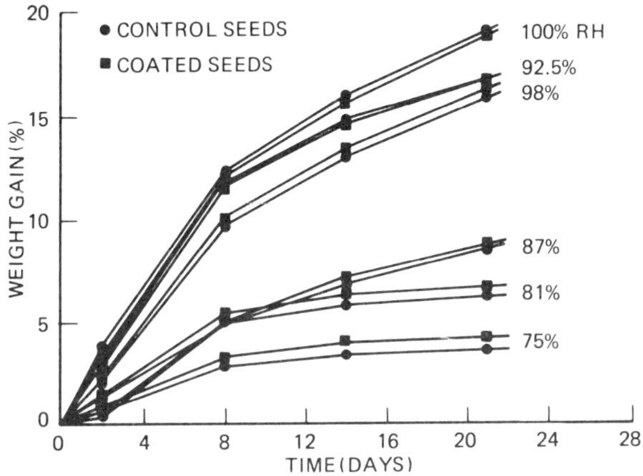

Figure 8 Water vapor absorption of uncoated and coated soybean seeds at constant relative humidities at 25°C. [Seed coating: 4% (w/w), PMMA/talc/$CaCO_3$ (1:0.5:0.5 by volume)]

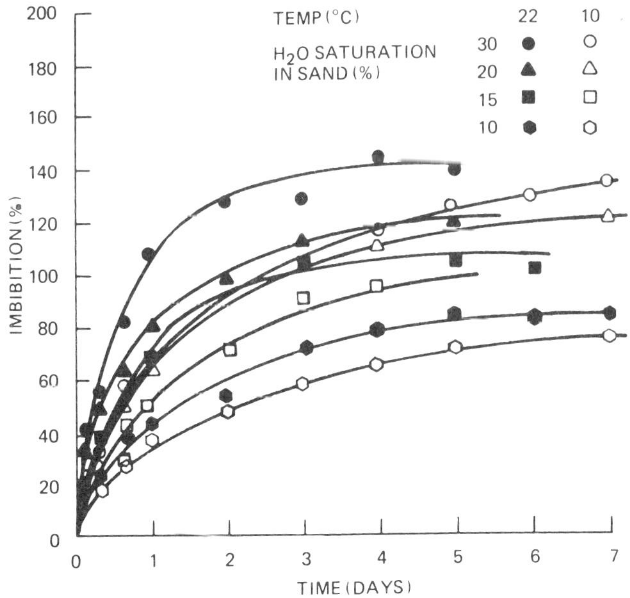

Figure 9 Soybean imbibition at various sand moisture levels as a function of time at 10°C and 22°C.

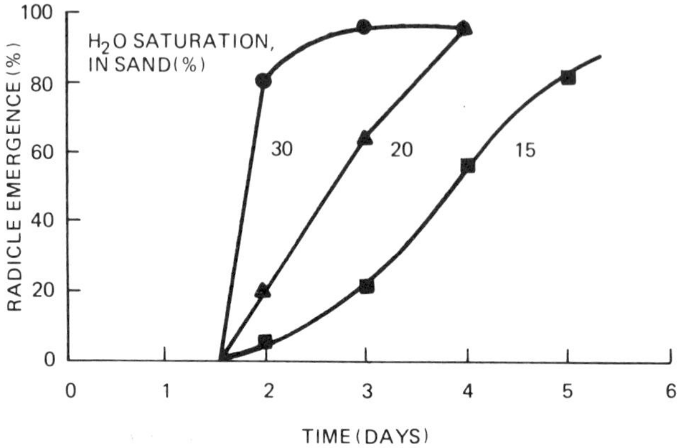

Figure 10 Soybean emergence at 22°C as a function of time at three moisture levels.

Germination of Coated Seeds

The ultimate objective for the determination of the requirements of water and oxygen at different temperatures for seed germination was to implement these important parameters in the design of seed coating systems which would not adversely affect the natural germination process but would provide beneficial effects to seeds or seed microenvironments through certain controlled release mechanisms.

The coating systems listed in Table 1 will be discussed to illustrate the design principle and the effects of polymeric coatings on the germination of coated soybean seeds.

Seeds coated with cellulose ethyl ether (Ethocel) at 0.5 to 3% of seed weight were tested for emergence at two levels of watering (300 ml and 450 ml) by using the standard laboratory test described earlier.

Table 2 Effect of Temperature and Moisture Level in Sand on the Imbibition Rate and the Germination Rate of Soybean Seeds

H_2O saturation (%)	30		20		15		10	
Temperature (°C)	22	10	22	10	22	10	22	10
Time (hr) (60% imbibition)	8	19	12	22	16	32	48	88
Time (days) (80% germination)	2	—	3.5	—	5	—	—	—

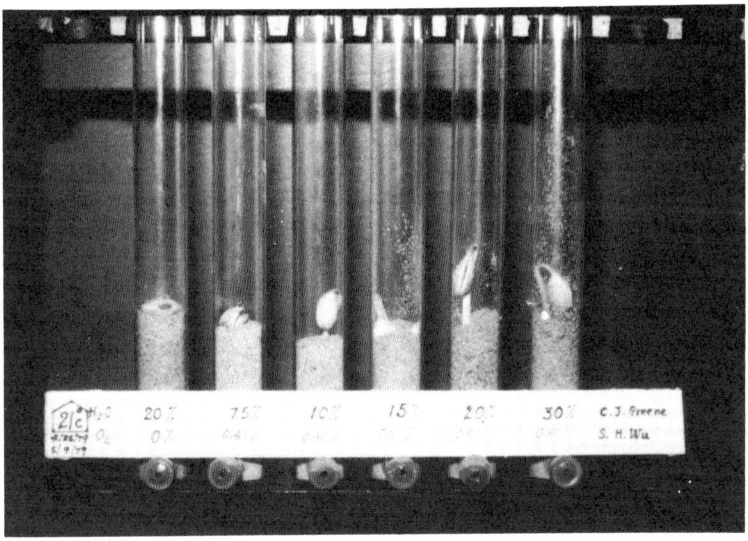

(A)

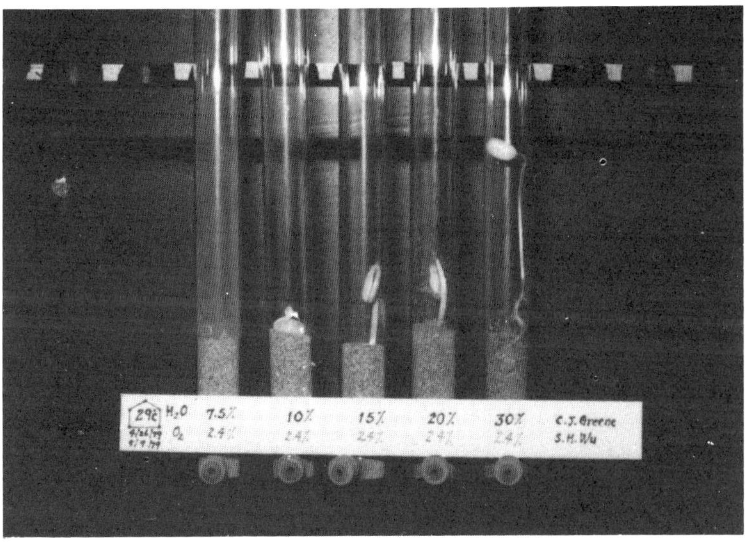

(B)

Figure 11 Effect of total O_2 supply on the germination of soybean seeds at various water availabilities and temperatures. (A) At 21°C, initial oxygen: 0.41%; water: 7.5-30% saturation in sand. (B) At 29°C, initial oxygen: 2.4%; water: 7.5-30% saturation in sand. Time: 14 days.

Table 3 Minimum Total O_2/H_2O Requirements for the Germination of Single Soybean Seeds in Nessler Tubes

Temperature (°C)	O_2 (% v/v)	H_2O (% of saturation values)
21	0.3	7.5
25	0.4	7.5-10
30	0.6	10-15
35	2.4	15-20

Ethocel coatings at all four coating levels and at both watering levels delayed the emergence for 3 days relative to the control (Fig. 13). The magnitude of the delay increased with increased coating level and was greatest at the high watering level. Only at the 3% level did the coating adversely affect final emergence.

These results can be explained partly by the Ethocel coating-induced retardation of oxygen transport for seed germination. In Fig. 12, the emergence rate of the control seeds increased steadily with the initial total oxygen availability in the range 4-15 μmol per gram of fresh seed weight. However, the emergence rate of Ethocel-coated seeds leveled off at 60% in the same range.

Similarly, seeds coated with PMMA at 0.73% or 2.82% had substantially fewer normally developed radicles and more short radicles than did the control with PMMA (B. L. Kirkpatrick, private communication).

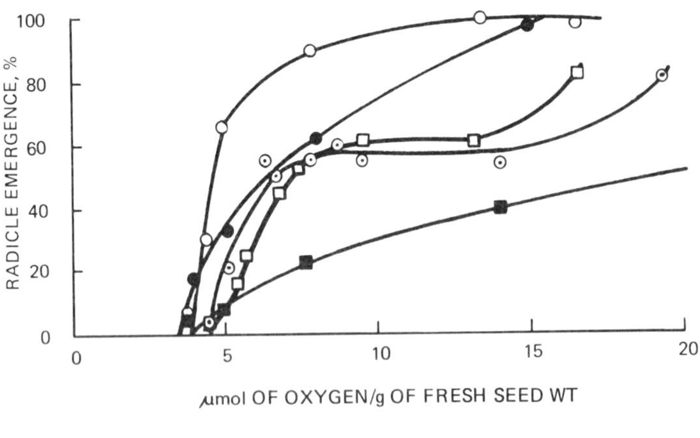

Figure 12 Total oxygen requirement for soybean germination at two temperatures. Control at 25°C (O), at 32°C (●); EC-coated seeds at 25°C (ʘ); GA_3-containing coated seeds at 25°C (□), at 32°C (■).

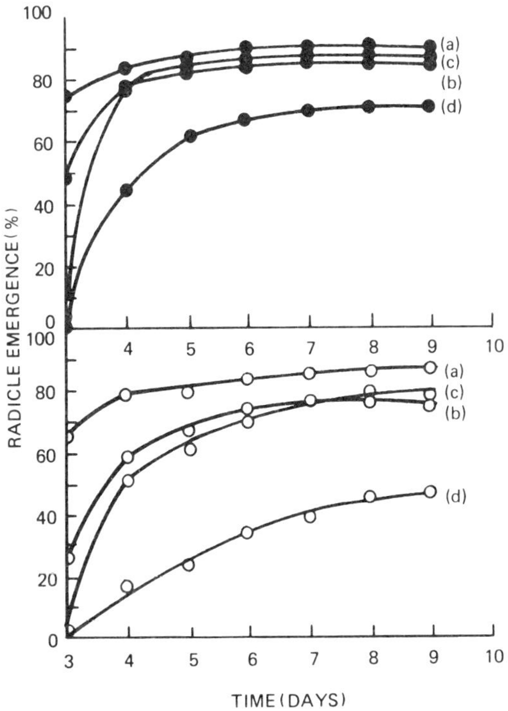

Figure 13 Effect of Ethocel coatings on soybean germination at two watering levels: ●, low; O, high. EC coating: (a) control, 0%; (b) 0.5%; (c) 2%; (d) 3% coating (w/w).

Thus the Ethocel and the PMMA coatings delayed the onset of the natural germination process. To overcome the problem of delayed germination induced by polymeric coatings, we found that when a large percentage of pigments was incorporated in the seed coating formulation, the porosity of the coating could be increased to the extent that the coating did not inhibit the natural imbibition and germination process. The first evidence is as shown in Fig. 8. Soybean seeds (control) and seeds coated with 4% (by weight) PMMA/talc/$CaCO_3$ (1:0.5:0.5 by volume) were placed in chambers with standard relative humidities from 75 to 100% at room temperature for 21 days. The total weight increase after 21 days and the rate of weight gain for coated and uncoated seeds were virtually identical. Thus the coating did not interfere with the water vapor transport to seed tissues.

The next evidence was observed from the effects of polymer/talc seed coating thickness on germination of soybean seeds under oxygen tension (Fig. 14). Soybean seeds were coated with a layer of 3, 6, and

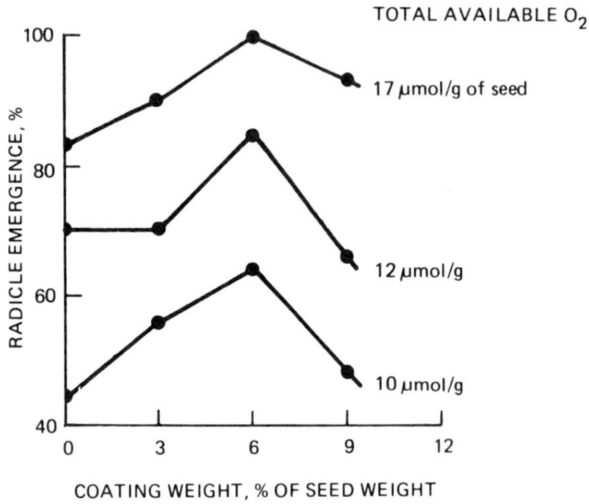

Figure 14 Effect of PMMA/talc (1:1 v/v) coating thickness on soybean germination under limited total O_2 supply at 25°C. Time: 5 days.

9% by weight) PMMA/talc (1:1 by volume). Emergence was measured by germinating a sample of 30-50 coated seeds in a sealed flask which contained 200 g of sand, sufficient water for 100% seed imbibition, and a limited amount of initial oxygen. The three oxygen levels were calculated to be 10, 12, and 17 μmol per gram of coated seed weight. From Fig. 14, germination improved with all coatings as oxygen availability increased. At each of these three levels of oxygen, seeds with 6% coating exhibited the highest emergence among the coated seeds and the 5-day emergence data were approximately 20% higher than the control. This result suggests that highly pigment-loaded polymeric coatings do not interfere with the natural germination process. Furthermore, an optimum coating thickness may enhance the emergence of soybean seeds. A possible explanation for the enhancement of germination could be that the seed coatings modified the water transport rate and provided a means for homogeneous wetting of seed tissues. Thus the slower hydration may allow the restoration of membrane integrity to occur relatively quickly and before much leakage of solutes from seeds occurs [20].

Many electrolytes and minerals can be incorporated in polymer/pigment seed coating systems to alter the water imbibition rate or to deliver micronutrients to the seed vicinity.

The effects of NaCl-containing coatings on the germination of soybean seeds under water-stressed growth conditions are shown in Fig. 15. Seeds were coated with a layer of 4.2% (by weight) PMMA/talc/NaCl. The coating compositions for three samples were (a) 1:3:0,

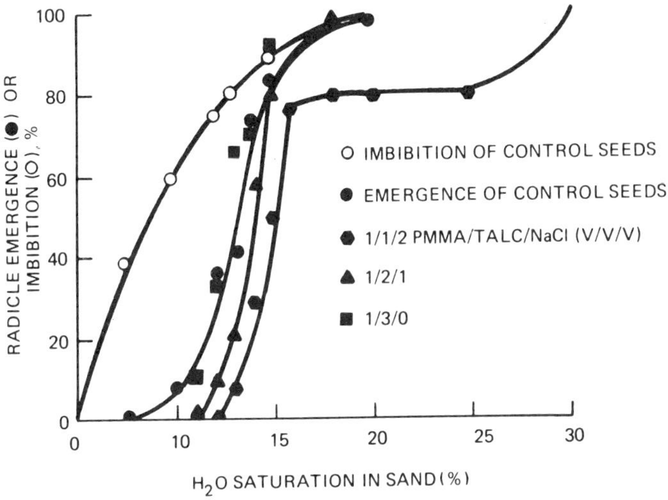

Figure 15 Germination of NaCl-containing coated soybean seeds under water-stressed conditions at 25°C.

(b) 1:2:1, and (c) 1:1:2 (by volume). The emergence rate was measured by germinating a sample of 5 g of coated seeds in a sand bed in which the moisture level ranged from 7.5 to 25% of the saturation value. Sample (a), without NaCl in the coating, exhibited the same germination rate as the control seeds at all moisture levels. But the germination rates of samples (b) and (c) decreased within the crucial range of moisture level (10-15% of the saturation value). At 13% moisture level, the germination rate was 45% for (a) but <10% for (c).

One of the problems facing the grower of soybeans is that the soil moisture at planting time may be high enough to induce some germination but not to support vigorous seedling growth. This result demonstrated the possibility that an appropriate amount of electrolyte in the coatings could delay germination until sufficient soil moisture is available.

Bioactive materials can also be delivered to the seed microenvironment and cause observable effects through a combination with seed coatings discussed above. An experimental design was evaluated to determine the effects of gibberellic acid (GA_3) containing seed coatings on soybean germination under various supplies of oxygen. Seeds were coated with an inner Ethocel layer (0.5%) containing varying amounts of GA_3 (0-12.5 ppm of seed weight) and an outer layer consisting of PMMA/talc/$CaCO_3$ (1:1.25:1.25 by volume, 3.2% seed weight). Coated and uncoated seeds did not differ in their minimum total oxygen requirements for germination (Fig. 12). With a sufficient supply of

Table 4 Crushing Strength for Coated and Uncoated Soybean Seeds (Ransom Seeds, 1978)

	A	B	C
Coating	Uncoated	4% Talc/PMMA (1:1 v/v)	6% Talc/PMMA/$CaCO_3$ (1:1:1 v/v)
Number of seeds	20	20	20
Crushing strength (kg)	10.73	11.39	15.39
Standard deviation	1.22	1.16	0.86

oxygen in open air, seeds treated with GA_3 emerged earlier than uncoated seeds or coated seeds without GA_3. However, with a limited total supply of oxygen, seeds treated with GA_3 exhibited a lower 5-day emergence rate than coated seeds without GA_3 (Fig. 12). A possible explanation is that GA_3-treated seeds might require higher oxygen uptake for the initial germination process. These results demonstrated the effect of the coating system on the oxygen requirement for seed germination and the ability to deliver an agrichemical in the microenvironment of the seed.

The coating systems discussed so far serve not only as controlled release layers for the modification of seed imbibition and the delivery of agrichemicals in seed microenvironment, but also as layers to prevent mechanical damage. This can be seen from the increase of the crushing strength for coated seeds compared with the uncoated seeds in Table 4.

CONCLUSIONS

The requirements of water and total oxygen and the effects of temperature on these requirements were determined for soybean germination. These parameters are essential to an understanding of the soybean germination process and crucial for the design of controlled release seed coating systems. It was found that heavily pigmented polymeric coatings do not interfere with the natural germination process. These coatings can be used as controlled-release coating systems for the delivery of micronutrients, minerals, and agrichemicals in the microenvironments of seeds to cause desirable effects during the germination process or seedling development. These coatings may also be used to prevent mechanical damage to seed during storage and handling.

ACKNOWLEDGMENTS

The authors are very grateful to Ms. C. J. Greene for her excellent technical assistance and to Dr. Bruce L. Kirkpatrick and A. R. Gamble for the experimental results in Fig. 13. Thanks are also given to Dr. M. A. Pollock, Dr. M. A. Sandhu, and Dr. C. H. Benton for helpful discussion and to Ms. H. H. V. Le and Mr. B. W. Oliver for assistance in obtaining coated seeds.

REFERENCES

1. H. B. Scher, ed., *Controlled Release Pesticides*, ACS Symp. Ser. No. 52, American Chemical Society, Washington, D.C., 1977.
2. N. Cardarelli, *Controlled Release Polymeric Formulations*, ACS Symp. Ser. No. 33, American Chemical Society, Washington, D.C., 1976, p. 208.
3. G. G. Alan, et al., *Chemtech*, 171 (March 1973).
4. F. E. Porter, *Chemtech*, 284 (May 1978).
5. W. Heydecker and P. Coolbear, *Seed Sci. Technol.*, *5*:353 (1977).
6. D. G. Jones, R. G. Druce, and G. Williams, *J. Appl. Bacteriol.*, *30*(3):511 (1967).
7. B. E. Caldwell, ed., *Soybeans: Improvement, Production and Uses*, Agron. Ser. No. 16, American Society of Agronomy, Madison, Wis., 1973, p. IX.
8. R. Shibles, I. C. Anderson, and A. H. Gibson, *Crop Physiology* (L. T. Evans, ed.), Cambridge University Press, Cambridge, 1975, p. 151.
9. L. G. Heatherly and J. W. Russell, *Agron. J.*, *71*:980 (1979).
10. A. R. Grable and R. E. Danielson, *Soil Sci. Soc. Am. Proc.*, *29*: 12 (1965).
11. J. R. Hunter and A. E. Erickson, *Agron. J.*, *44*(3):107 (1952).
12. D. S. Carr and B. L. Harris, *Ind. Eng. Chem.*, *41*:2014 (1949).
13. C. C. Dannelly and C. R. Leonard (to Eastman Kodak Co.), U.S. Patent No. 4,117,801 (1978).
14. A. M. Mayer and A. Poljakoff-Mayber, *The Germination of Seeds*, Pergamon Press, Elmsford, N.Y., 1975, p. 21.
15. L. O. Copeland, *Principles of Seed Science and Technology*, Burgess, Minneapolis, Minn., 1976, p. 55.
16. J. D. Bewley and M. Black, *Physiology and Biochemistry of Seeds in Relation to Germination*, Vol. 1, Springer-Verlag, New York, 1978, p. 106.
17. J. N. Siedow and M. E. Girvin, *Plant Physiol.*, *65*:669 (1980).

18. R. Peters, *Kans. Univ. Sci. Bull.*, *13*:23 (1920).
19. H. C. Wien, E. J. Littleton, and A. Ayanaba, *Stress Physiology in Crop Plants* (H. Mussell and R. C. Staples, eds.), Wiley, New York, 1979, p. 283.
20. E. W. Simon, *Pestic. Sci.*, *9*:169 (1978).

Chapter 17

The Role of Silvex Herbicide Residues in the Environment*

EDWARD O. GANGSTAD Office Chief of Engineers, Washington, D.C.

The concept that there is no threshold below which a chemical agent does not induce a biological interaction is one theory of residue toxicology which has received widespread attention. This concept is theoretically true in that, when one atom or molecule enters the reactive region of another, a chemical interaction will result. This would imply that the entrance of even one molecule into the protoplast might produce a biological effect that is probably deleterious. If the word *effect* is used in a strict sense, the probability is that the interaction of one xenobiotic molecule with another molecule of a cell component could result in an "effect." It is more probable, however, that stochastic determinants impose a lower limit on the dose-response relationship between molecules within the homogeneous mass of the protoplast. In terms of mass action, if a chemical is administered near its toxic level, the interaction is cumulative, the reaction will move to the right, and the plant or animal will slowly die. This also implies that there is a threshold of response to toxic materials.

AQUATIC HERBICIDE CHRONICITY

Acute Toxicity

The toxic effect of a herbicide depends on many complex factors. Although no single way of expressing the potential effect is completely

*Findings in this report are not to be construed as an official Department of the Army position unless so designated by other authorized documents.

reliable, the most rapid and convenient indicator for most chemicals is the acute toxicity (the single dosage necessary to produce death). The usual way of expressing acute toxicity is by means of an LD_{50} (median lethal dosage) value. The LD_{50} is a statistical estimate of the dosage that would be lethal to 50% of a large population of the test species. Although LD_{50}s give no information on the dosage that would be lethal to every individual of the species, or to treatment given in some other way than in the test, the LD_{50} value, with its confidence limits, is probably the most convenient and reliable means available for comparing the inherent toxicity of chemicals.

Even though the LD_{50} nomenclature is commonly applied to animal species only, there is enough similarity between cases to establish rules of thumb relating lethal levels for a species in laboratory toxicity tests to potential effects from field exposure [5-7,67]. Thus if herbicide X has a LD_{50} of 10 mg/kg, and is known to kill plants in the field when applied at 2.24 kg/ha, herbicide Y with a LD_{50} of 5 mg/kg might be expected to kill plants in a similar environment at 1.12 kg/ha [3,4].

Subacute Toxicity

An empirical value that represents the minimum repeated dosage (mg/kg) that is lethal may be defined as subacute or chronic toxicity. Quinn et al. [5] determined these values for diquat, 2,4-D BEE, and silvex. Test plants were treated at geometrically spaced dosage levels until test dosage levels were found that produced 25, 50, and 90% mortality. This program to establish a subacute dosage or treatment from which the plant could not recover is defined as the dosage that would be suitable for slow-release herbicide application. Test levels within the mortality range 25-90% are approximately straight-line functions [1,2,5].

It is observed that differences related to percent mortality, concentration of herbicide, specific herbicide applied, method, and time of exposure do exist. Matrix analysis of the data indicated that those differences due to plant species as such are relatively small. The amount of toxicant (i.e., rate of application), the concentration and specific herbicide, and the method and time of exposure are highly significant. For 90% mortality, the estimated days of exposure ranged from 10 to 31 days (Table 1). Under laboratory conditions, it was possible to demonstrate the chronic effects of herbicides at levels of 1, 0.1, and 0.01 ppm concentration. It is thought that a field application of 0.1 ppm would represent a level feasible for operational control. The exposure time required is estimated at 19, 23, and 27 days for diquat, 2,4-D BEE, and silvex, respectively, under accumulative treatment conditions. However, suitable field trials would be necessary to determine more exactly the levels required under an operational program [5].

Table 1 Estimated Time to 90% Mortality for Herbicide Chronicity Treatments as the Mean Effect of the Plant Species Studied

Exposure[a]	Herbicide	Concentration (ppm)	Time[b] (days)
Constant	Diquat	1.00	10
Constant	Diquat	0.10	15
Constant	Diquat	0.01	16
Cumulative	Diquat	1.00	15
Cumulative	Diquat	0.10	19
Cumulative	Diquat	0.01	24
Constant	2,4-D BEE	1.00	15
Constant	2,4-D BEE	0.10	19
Constant	2,4-D BEE	0.01	24
Cumulative	2,4-D BEE	1.00	19
Cumulative	2,4-D BEE	0.10	23
Cumulative	2,4-D BEE	0.01	27
Constant	Silvex	1.00	18
Constant	Silvex	0.10	23
Constant	Silvex	0.01	28
Cumulative	Silvex	1.00	23
Cumulative	Silvex	0.10	27
Cumulative	Silvex	0.01	31

[a]Constant: herbicide added daily and test water changed; cumulative: herbicide added daily without change of test water.
[b]Mean of Eurasian watermilfoil (*Myriophyllum spicatum* L.), wild celery (*Vallisneria americana* Michx.), and waterweed (*Elodea canadensis* Michx.) treatments.
Source: Ref. 5.

CONTROLLED RELEASE HERBICIDES

Controlled release herbicide-elastomer formulations that extend the control of aquatic weeds have been developed. In other formulations the herbicide is physically incorporated in a polymeric matrix and release occurs by diffusion. Controlled release formulations may also be obtained by synthesis of polymers that contain herbicides as pendant side chains [10,11]. Herbicide release occurs by the slow, sequential hydrolysis of the herbicide-polymer chemical bonds. This provides a sustained release of herbicide over an extended period of time. The actual rate of release depends on the nature of the herbicide-polymer bond and the dimensions and structure of the resultant macromolecular combination. Unsaturated herbicide monomers were prepared by the reaction of the appropriate acids and alcohols in the presence of dicyclohexylcarbodiimide. This method is superior to preparations employing the reaction of a herbicide acid chloride with an alcohol. The herbicide release rates of polymers containing herbicides as pendant substituents are extremely slow in water with pH 7 at 30°C. However, the herbicide release rates can be increased by incorporating hydrophilic groups along the polymer's "backbone" [6-11].

Preliminary hydrolysis studies of poly(vinyl 2,4-dichlorophenoxyacetate), poly(2-acryloyloxyethyl 2,4-dichlorophenoxyacetate), poly (2-acryloyloxyethyl 2-(2,4,5-trichlorophenoxy) propionate, poly(2-methacryloyloxyethyl 2,4-dichlorophenoxyacetate), and a series of copolymers containing units which increase the hydrophilicity of the polymer's backbone (aminimides, acrylic acid, and 2-hydroxyethyl acrylate) have been carried out. The herbicide release rates increased as the hydrophilicity of the copolymer backbone increased. Hydrolysis studies of poly(vinyl 2,4-dichlorophenoxyacetate), poly(2-acryloyloxyethyl 2,4-dichlorophenoxyacetate), and poly(4-acryloyloxybutyl 2,4-dichlorophenoxyacetate) under carefully controlled conditions have been completed to give approximate release rates.

While the actual field application remains to be determined by detailed study, it is presumed that when controlled release data are properly coupled with chronicity data, it will be possible to formulate controlled release herbicides that are environmentally superior to standard herbicide formulations for particular weed problems in certain sites under a specified set of conditions.

TOXIC THRESHOLD RESPONSE

Dinman [12], in a review of approximately 400 studies in vitro of enzymatic toxic inhibition, determined that the threshold concentration of these substances was approximately 1 in 10,000. He states that concepts concerning response toxicities over a lifetime are absolutely inadequate in the absence of quantitative data. In the Bionetics Study [13], the method of evaluation was to use concentrations of 1000-10,000 times the level found in the environment. These data and subsequent data are indeed open to question, because the dosage level is a nearly lethal insult to the physiology of the test animal, and the animals selected for test are strains which have many more genes for tumor mutability than do normal animals.

Kenaga [14], in a detailed study of the toxicities of 75 different insecticides and herbicides for 10 different test species, found highly significant relationships between acute and chronic no-effect toxicities, with a correlation coefficient between 0.53 and 0.82 and a predicted value within a magnitude of 0.98-1.99.

The Scientific Committee of the American Industrial Health Council (AIHC) has reviewed the Occupational Safety and Health Administration (OSHA) proposal for the regulation of chemicals posing a potential occupational carcinogenic risk [*Federal Register, 42*:54147-54247 (October 4, 1977)] [15]. OSHA identified principles alleging to represent the relationship of chemicals to cancer. However, AIHC declares that OSHA's principles, taken collectively, present an erroneous concept for sound regulatory policy decisions. AIHC has developed the following points as a guide to policy decisions relating to chemicals as potential human carcinogens.

1. *Epidemiology.* Although "environmental" factors may account for 60-90% of all cancer, only a small fraction of these are related to occupational exposure to industrial chemicals or substances in the workplace. Furthermore, the incidence of cancer is not increasing when rates are adjusted to account for increased life expectancy and cancers attributable primarily to cigarette smoking. Thus inferences of an impending cancer epidemic from occupational exposure to industrial chemicals are misleading, and drastic action such as imposition of emergency standards is not warranted.

2. *Acceptable Risk.* Since absolute safety is an impossible goal, attention should be focused on "socially acceptable risks" from exposure to suspect carcinogens. This concept is supported by logic and by numerous federal statutes, including the Occupational Safety and Health Act. Emphasis should be on relative risk and on risk above background levels. Risks associated with occupational exposure to suspect carcinogens must be related to other occupational and non-occupational risks.

3. *Dose-Response; Threshold; No-Effect Level.* Modern toxicology is based on experimental evidence demonstrating that a dose-response relationship exists for toxic substances. These relationships have been demonstrated for many substances and should be used for risk analysis.

4. *Validity of Data from Animal Bioassays for Carcinogenicity.* The results of studies indicating chemicals as confirmed or suspect carcinogens must be evaluated for validity based on accepted scientific principles. Since many conclusions on carcinogenicity have been based on subjective observations, the decisions should be delegated to a panel of experts in this field assisted by decision makers to resolve differences of opinion (i.e., Dispute Resolution Conferences).

5. *Extrapolation from Animals to Humans.* Scientific judgment is required in evaluating data from bioassays in animals as indicative of what might happen in humans exposed to the same chemicals in the workplace. Consideration must be given to validity of the data to humans and the specific environment.

6. *Relative Potency and Time to Tumor.* The classification scheme proposed by OSHA blurs distinctions between carcinogenic substances. Regulatory policy should be based on the carcinogenic risk posed by a particular substance under a set of observed conditions of the environment [64,65].

Societal Decision

Kraybill [16], in a detailed analysis of the proper perspective for the risk assessment of cancer, suggests that there are a number of factors that must be taken into account: (1) body retention or accumulation, (2) threshold level or safe dose, (3) margin of safety between a measurable effect and "no-adverse effect," (4) the time interval required to produce the adverse effect, and (5) the level or metabolic overloading in the bioassay used to produce the adverse effect.

Jukes [66], in a detailed discussion for the American Industrial Health Council on risks that are acceptable, says that the remarkable thing about the current negative attitude toward acceptable risks is that this atmosphere of public concern has been created by imagination rather than measurable effects. A few years ago we used to point out that there was not a single case of any consumer having been injured by a pesticide that had been applied in accordance with the regulations. There have, of course, been cases of industrial accidents from pesticides, including injury to applicators, but not to consumers. Today, such reassuring statements count for nothing. We are told that it is impossible to connect cause and effect, especially since cancer may take 30 years to develop following the original exposure.

Natural Threshold

Truhaut [17], in a discussion of possible levels of carcinogenic compounds in the environment, points out that we do live in a world whose environment does contain natural carcinogens from which there is no escape. It is very difficult to evaluate the environmental dose-effect relationships of these natural carcinogens because low-level exposure data are very limited. It is argued that since a no-effect level cannot be presently determined, no tolerance level can be established. However, we can say that nature itself does have a threshold occurrence "ground zero" or tolerance level that can readily be established for risk assessment from simple hospital records [18] (i.e., the vital statistics of actual cases).

Models for Risk Analysis

It is established that natural laws in biology are as determinate as those of the physical world. Risk analysis of these effects have been made with different models (i.e., for single-hit and multihit) using different mathematical functions. As illustrated in Table 2, these models are not in good agreement among themselves, differing more than 1 million-fold. From the generally known (established) information it is reasonable to assume that there is a good deal of scatter, that there are many factors which act to prevent carcinogenesis, and that the single-hit models do not reflect the actual case [64].

Table 2 Estimated Human Risks from Saccharin Ingestion of 0.12 g/Day[a]

	Lifetime cases per million exposed	Cases per 50 million persons per year
Rat dose adjusted to human dose by surface area rule		
Single-hit model (Hoel, 1977)	1200	840
Multistage model (with quadratic term) (Hoel, 1977)	5	3.5
Multihit model (Sci. Comm. Food Safety Council, 1978)	0.001	0.0007
Mantel-Bryan probit model (Brown, 1978)	450	315
Rat dose adjusted to human dose by mg/kg/day equivalence		
Single-hit model (*Saccharin and Its Salts*, 1977)	210	147
Multihit model (Sci. Comm. Food Safety Council, 1978)	0.001	0.0007
Mantel-Bryan probit model (Brown, 1978)	21	14.7
Rat dose adjusted to human dose by mg/kg/lifetime equivalence		
Single-hit model (Brown, 1977)	5200	3640
Multihit model (Sci. Comm. Food Safety Council, 1978)	0.001	0.0007
Mantel-Brown probit model (Brown, 1978)	4200	2940

[a]For complete reference information, see bibliographic data within Ref. 64.
Source: Ref. 64

TOXICOLOGICAL STUDIES OF SILVEX RESIDUES

The herbicide silvex [2-(2,4,5-trichlorophenoxy) propionic acid] has been found to be effective for control of certain aquatic weeds. After introduction into the environment for aquatic plant control, silvex could persist unchanged or be converted to certain metabolites as a result of biological or nonbiological transformation. Similarly, the herbicide metabolites could persist and accumulate in the water and hydrosoil as well as in the food chain and could possibly constitute a health hazard if aquatic organisms from the treated waters were to be used as human food. Therefore, the identification and measurement of residue levels of silvex and its metabolites was necessary in order to evaluate fully the potential effect of this chemical on the aquatic environment and thus indirectly on humans [2,19-27,30,46,47].

Rice Samples of rough rice and rice straw from Arkansas, Louisiana, and Texas were analyzed by Syracuse University Research Corporation (SURC) using the gas chromatographic method recommended by the U.S. Food and Drug Administration (FDA), reported by SURC to be sensitive to 0.01 ppm silvex. The data indicated that the residues will not exceed 0.1 ppm in rice and 0.5 ppm in rice straw from two silvex treatments of growing rice at rates of 0.75 lb/acre plus 1.5 lb/acre.*

Sugarcane Samples of raw sugarcane from Louisiana were analyzed by Wisconsin Alumi Research Foundation (WARF) for residues of silvex using a gas chromatographic method verified to 0.05 ppm. Residues decreased to 0.05 ppm by mid-August, 10-16 weeks after the last of two applications of silvex at 2.4 lb/acre as the PGBE ester formulation. Milling and processing studies were also conducted with sugarcane containing residues of silvex from an additional late summer application of silvex 8 weeks prior to harvest in late October. The data indicate that if any residue should occur in sugarcane at harvest, it would remain largely with the bagasse.*

Samples of various sugarcane fractions and factory by-products were also obtained from sugarcane given an additional late season treatment to commodities. Data on mill fractions from mature cane showed that most of the residue remained in the bagasse rather than in the juice. The residues in bagasse and juice were roughly 2.5 and 0.2 times as high as in the cane from which they were derived. Factors obtained from residues in other by-products compared in whole raw cane were 1 for factory syrup, 2 for first molasses, and 0.1 for raw sugar. Therefore, theoretical residues of 0.05 ppm in raw sugarcane would be equivalent to 0.13 ppm in bagasse, 0.01 ppm in juice, 0.05 ppm in syrup, 0.001 ppm in molasses, and 0.005 ppm in raw sugar.

Grass Samples of grass were collected at intervals after treatment with silvex at rates up to 12 lb acid equivalent (ae) of silvex per acre for brush control in California, Michigan, North Carolina, and Texas. Residues of silvex (and of other phenoxy herbicides) were determined by International Research and Development Corporation (IREC) in Mattawan, Michigan, using a gas chromatographic method similar to

*Abstracted from the National Agricultural Chemicals Association, Industry Task Force Pesticide petition 8F0675, with permission.

that used for sugarcane. The residues declined to 10 ppm/lb per acre of treatment within 4-12 weeks after application depending on physical factors such as rainfall, sunlight, and rate of growth of the grass.*

Forage Legumes A residue study on silvex in birdsfoot trefoil and grasses was reported in 1963 from Cornell University. Established trefoil treated with 1.5 lb of silvex on May 2, 1960, and harvested 36 days later, contained silvex residues of 0.9-3.6 ppm, while treatment with silvex at 0.75 lb/acre ae contained 0.19 ppm when harvested 6 weeks after treatment. Timothy regrowth contained 1.74 ppm in plots treated originally with 3 lb/acre ae.*

Milk Feeding studies were conducted by the Dow Chemical Company at increasing levels from 10 to 100 ppm silvex in the total diet of dairy cows for 2-3 weeks at each level. Samples of milk and cream were analyzed for residues of silvex and of 2,4,5-trichlorophenol using a gas chromatographic method verified to 0.05 ppm silvex and its corresponding phenol. A level to 1000 ppm caused residues of 0.05-0.23 ppm in milk and cream. No 2,4,5-trichlorophenol was detected at any feeding level.*

Meat and Meat By-products of Cattle and Sheep Preliminary data on residues of silvex and of 2,4,5-trichlorophenol in muscle and kidney of cattle were presented in December 1970. Analyses of fat and liver of cattle and of muscle, fat, liver, and kidney of sheep were completed by the Dow Chemical Company in 1971. Tissue samples were also analyzed for silvex by U.S. Department of Agriculture (USDA) personnel at College Station, Texas.

Groups of three cattle were slaughtered the day following the last of 28 consecutive days on a complete ration containing 300, 1000, or 2000 ppm silvex, and 7 days after replacing the 2000-ppm diet with untreated feed (2000 + 0). Similarly, two groups of three sheep were fed 2000 ppm silvex for 28 days and were slaughtered the next day or 7 days after withdrawal.

Analysis for silvex and 2,4,5-trichlorophenol in muscle and kidney samples were made, using a gas chromatographic method verified to 0.05 ppm silvex and its corresponding phenol. Average residues of 0.6, 1.2, and 1.7 ppm silvex were found in muscle at feeding rates of 300, 1000, and 2000 ppm, and residues of 18, 14, and 24 ppm were found in kidney at the same feeding rate. No 2,4,5-trichlorophenol was detected in any samples of muscle or kidney at any feeding rate. The residues of silvex decreased to 0.01 ppm in muscle and 1.8 ppm in kidney at 7 days after withdrawal from an ingested level of 2000 ppm silvex.*

---

*Abstracted from the National Agricultural Chemicals Association, Industry Task Force Pesticide petition 8F0675, with permission.

The data indicate that residues of silvex are likely to occur in tissues of animals ingesting forage containing 300 ppm silvex, such as immediately after application of this herbicide at rates of 2 lb/acre ac or more. The residues in tissues of such animals would be less than 1 ppm in muscles and fat, approximately 4 ppm in liver, and 18 ppm in kidney. Data on tissues of animals fed at the exaggerated level of 2000 ppm silvex in the total diet indicated that the residues will decrease approximately 10-fold if the animals are given untreated feed for 1 week before being slaughtered, after grazing on freshly treated areas.*

Apples and Plums. The residues of silvex in apples were determined in December 1967. Samples of Macintosh and Delicious apples were harvested in Michigan, New York, and Massachusetts 0, 1, 13, or 33 days after application of a 20-ppm spray to prevent preharvest drop. No residue was detected when the apples were analyzed by a colorimetric procedure which indicated 0.1 ppm silvex equivalent in untreated apples.

Data on residues in plums were presented in December 1967 indicating 0.1 ppm silvex in or on ripe fruit. Based on the data for apples, one can assume that no detectable residue will remain in or on plums harvested 60 days after application of a 20-ppm spray according to the registered use.

Bound Residues. No indication for the presence of "bound" residues of phenoxy herbicides was obtained when samples of many agricultural commodities were subjected to special extraction and hydrolysis procedures in 1971. This corroborated the opinion that bound or conjugated residues are intermediates in the breakdown and elimination of phenoxy herbicides by plants and animals.*

Fish and Related Aquatic Organisms

Silvex and related phenoxyalkyl herbicides are relatively nontoxic to fish and related aquatic organisms. In general, silvex is quite similar to other phenoxyalkyl acid herbicides in the range of toxicity and relationship between various esters, salts, and amines (Table 3). The isoctyl ester is the least toxic of the various esters of silvex and other phenoxyalkyl acid herbicides. No significant effect of herbicide activity from tests made on hardness ranging from very soft to very hard water have been found. Both the propylene glycol butyl ether esters and the potassium salt of silvex applied to farm ponds at concentrations (3-5 ppm) may kill some fish and cause adverse physiological effects on redar sunfish. No adverse effect could be ascertained on plankton and on fish-food organisms [31-35].

---

*Abstracted from the National Agricultural Chemicals Association, Industry Task Force Pesticide petition 8F0675, with permission.

Table 3 Silvex Toxicity to Experimental Animals

	Sex	LD_{50} (mg/kg)	Range
Kuron			
Rats	F	1070	700-1150
Mice	F	2140	1540-2990
Guinea pigs	M	850	600-1190
Rabbits	M	850	600-1190
Chicks	M,F	2000	1350-2960
Na salt			
Albino rats	–	500	390-650
Mixed butyl esters			
Rats	F	600	250-1000
Rabbits	F	750	500-1000
Chicks	M,F	1190	707-2000
Mono-, di-, and tripropylene glycol butyl ether ester			
Rat	F	621	473-814
Guinea pigs	M	1250 (est.)	500-2000
Mice	F	1410 (est.)	1000-2000
Rabbit	F	819	610-1070
Chicks	M,F	1190	847-1670

Source: Ref. 26.

Wildlife and Experimental Animals

Studies were made on the effects of silvex acid and silvex butoxyethanol ester on bobwhite quail, ring-necked pheasant, and mallard ducks. Tests were designed to determine LD_{50} values (defined as ppm toxicant in a dry diet calculated to produce 50% mortality in 8 days on treated diet followed by 3 days on untreated diet). The LD_{50} values for silvex acid on ring-necked pheasant was 3000; Japanese quail, 5000; mallard ducks, 5000; and bobwhite quail, about 3000. Although silvex (acid and ester) is irritating to the skin and eyes, it does not appear to be hazardous to game birds and mammals when properly applied.

When administered orally to dogs, silvex has produced only weak signs in the forms of ataxia and stiff movements of the hindlegs. Repeated doses may or may not eventually lead to death, produce loss of appetite, loss of weight, vomiting, depression, roughness of coat, general tenseness and muscular weakness, and interference with carbohydrate metabolism. Two cases of a transitory diabetiform condition observed in spraying personnel following work with chlorinated phenoxy herbicides point in the same direction. However, hyperglycosuria could not be reproduced with certainty in rabbits; only one out of five animals responded in this way in exploratory experiments, where the doses ranged from 125 to 500 mg/kg and the period of administration from 6 to 50 days [26-29].

Residues in Water and Hydrosoil

Bailey et al. [36] simulated experiments in three ponds according to the current recommendation for control of alligatorweed by the U.S. Corps of Engineers. Silvex was applied as the propylene glycol butyl ether esters at the rate of 8 lb ae per surface acre. A second application was made during a summer to kill plants missed in the first application. Almost complete hydrolysis (99%) occurred within 33-49 hours and the water concentration of silvex acid decreased to zero by the third week. Silvex absorbed onto hydrosoil sediment disappeared by the fifth week following treatment.

A field study of silvex persistence was carried out in a creek having very little water movement. After the first application, concentrations ranged from 83 ppb 1 day after spraying to 1.1 ppb after 21 days. Silvex was not detectable after 35 days. After the second application, concentrations ranged from 19 ppb 1 day after spraying to 0.48 ppb after 70 days. Following the third application, concentrations decreased from 73 ppb immediately after spraying to 2 ppb after 38 days, and to 0.1 ppb after 6 months. Silvex could not be detected 1 year after application. Another field test was carried out in a fast-flowing stream which provided maximal opportunity for dilution and interchange of water. Residues of silvex were not detected except during the first few hours following treatment. The maximal level found in this study was 0.05 ppb [37,38].

ENVIRONMENTAL DEGRADATION AND PERSISTENCE

A number of workers have investigated the metabolism of silvex by terrestrial plants and microorganisms [34-45]. Alexander and Aleem [39] and Burger et al. [48] reported that silvex was very resistant to microbial degradation. They suggested that the recalcitrant nature of the molecule resulted from the number of chlorine atoms attached to the aromatic nucleus and from the presence of chlorine on the meta position of the ring. However, Horvath [49] demonstrated that certain m-chloroaromatic compounds such as 2,4,5-trichlorophenoxyacetic acid and 2,3,6-trichlorobenzoic acid, which have a chlorine in the meta position, are cometabolized to 3,4-dichlorocatechol by a *Brevibacterium* species isolated from lake water.

Ou and Sikka [50], showed that silvex is extensively degraded to the extent of ring cleavage by cometabolism of selected aquatic microorganisms. These findings are in contrast to those of other workers [1,8] who reported that silvex, as well as other phenoxy herbicides which also have a chlorine in the meta position on the aromatic nucleus, were highly resistant to microbial degradation in soil. The failure to show microbial degradation of these chemicals is attributed to the use of pure cultures which excluded the possibility of cometabolsim.

Although Ou and Sikka [50] clearly showed biodegradation of silvex, no metabolites, except a trace amount of 2,4,5-trichlorophenol (identified on the basis of thin layer chromatography), could be found. The intermediate compounds were probably degraded as rapidly as they were formed, so that subsequent concentrations were too small to be detected. This suggestion is supported by the finding that 2,4,5-trichlorophenol and 3,5-dichlorocatechol, the two possible silvex metabolites, were degraded quite readily by the mixed culture without a lag period. The appearance of 2,4,5-trichlorophenol in the culture fluid, together with the capacity of the cells for assimulation, suggest that it forms part of the pathway of the silvex degradation. The cells also extensively degraded 3,5-dichlorocatechol, suggesting that it is a likely intermediate in the pathway of silvex degradation. On the basis of these finds, it is postulated that silvex metabolism by the mixed culture involved a cleavage of the ether linkage to give rise to 2,4,5-trichlorophenol, which was then dehalogenated and hydroxylated, resulting in the formation of 3,5-dichlorocatechol. The latter may then be degraded by the pathways described by Bollag et al. [51].

Dioxin (TCDD)

Under present conditions of manufacture this contaminant is usually present in silvex at less than 0.1 ppm, thus ensuring that very little TCDD is inadvertently applied [52]. Like silvex, any contaminating TCDD would be deposited on the leaves of treated vegetation or on soil and water in the vicinity, although as indicated for silvex, small amounts could enter air or water and be carried some distance from the site of application. Water transport, however, is sharply limited by the fact that the solubility of TCDD in water is only 0.2 ppb [54]. As a consequence, it would tend to remain on the surface of plants and soil at the site of application.

Photochemical decomposition of TCDD has been studied at Dow Chemical Co. [53] and the U.S. Department of Agriculture [55]. Exposure of 1.02 mg of TCDD in 100 ml of water-saturated chloroform to ultraviolet light at 35°C caused 50-100% degradation in 2.5 hr. Using a sunlamp with a peak emission at 310 nm, irradiated TCDD dissolved in methanol and was found to have a half-life of 3.5 hr. Rapid decomposition was also reported in natural sunlight when approximately 5 ml of a 24-ppm methanol solution of TCDD was sealed in glass tubes and exposed to 7000-9000 footcandles of sunlight, with a half-life of approximately 5 hr, virtual disappearance in 48 hr, and none detectable after

72 hr. Similar rates of decomposition, however, were not observed when the TCDD was placed on the surface of dry soil, where irradiation for 96 hr with a sunlamp (maximum energy at 310 nm) did not cause any significant loss by either photodecomposition or volatilization.

Interactions of TCDD with soil have also been studied. When TCDD was placed on the surface of five very different soils and subject to leaching with water, the TCDD did not move into any of the soils, probably because of its very low water solubility. Similarly, in leaching experiments using soil thin-layer chromatographic techniques, no TCDD moved from the spot of origin in either a Hagerstown silty clay loam or a Norfolk sandy loam. It would thus appear that most of the chemical falling on the soil surface would remain there [55].

The fate of TCDD mechanically incorporated into soil has also been investigated. Radiolabeled TCDD was mixed into soil at the rates of 1, 10, and 100 ppm and soil extracts radioassayed 20, 40, 80, and 160 days after application. The amount of radioactive material (probably TCDD) in the soil decreased 15-20% in 160 days, indicating that this compound was very slowly degraded in the soil and could persist for more than a year [55].

The possibility that TCDD incorporated in the soil might be absorbed by plants has been studied. Soybean and oat plants were grown on lake-land sand containing 0.06 ppm radiolabeled TCDD, which is 40,000 times the amount that would appear in soils treated with 20 lb/acre of silvex containing 0.1 ppm TCDD. Less than 0.2% of the available TCDD was absorbed by either type of plant, with radioactivity reaching a peak at 10 days, at which time it measured about 0.12 ppm in oats and 0.05 ppm in soybeans on a dry weight basis; then it declined to an insignificant level at 40 days [55].

SILVEX RESIDUE TOLERANCE

Industry Task Force Petitions

Amendments to the Industry Task Force petitions for silvex (PP8F0675) were submitted to the U.S. Environmental Protection Agency (EPA) in December 1970 and October 1971 with a revised list of tolerance. The amendments were prepared by Dow and included residue data obtained by Dow from feeding studies with these herbicides in dairy cows, beef cattle, and sheep.

The tolerances proposed for silvex by the Industry Task Force were 300 ppm in or on grass; 0.5 ppm in or on rice straw and sugarcane bagasse; 0.1 ppm (negligible residue) in or on apples, plums, rice, and sugarcane, and in meat and meat by-products of cattle, goats, and sheep; and 0.05 ppm (negligible residue) in milk [57-62].

Negligible Residue Tolerances

Calculations of the permissible daily intake for silvex are presented in item 10 of the letter from Dow to EPA, dated December 30, 1970. These were based on a no-effect level of 0.9 mg/kg per day as found for male dogs given 0.0056% Kurosal SL* in the total diet continuously for 2 years. This level was chosen because minor pathological changes were reported for male dogs but not for female dogs or rats at 0.019% equivalent to 2.6 mg/kg per day for 2 years.

Regulations published in 1967 [*Federal Register*, *32*(73):6059 (April 15, 1967)] indicated that negligible residue tolerances can be based on 1/2000 of the no-effect level found in 90-day feeding studies in two species of animals. On the other hand, permissible tolerances for human foods are generally based on a safety factor of 100 over a no-effect level found in 2-year feeding studies and in the multigeneration reproduction study.

Tolerances of 0.1 ppm silvex are at the negligible level, as proposed in the petition pp 1E1012 submitted by the U.S. Corps of Engineers [58] and by the Industry Task Force on Phenoxy Herbicide Tolerances [53,54]. Calculations based on 1/2000 of a no-effect level of 7 mg/kg per day in 90-day feeding studies in rats and dogs and on a daily intake of 1.5 kg of food by a 60-kg human show that the entire diet could contain (7/2000) × (60/1.5) + 0.14 ppm silvex without exceeding the 2000-fold safety factor for negligible residues.

It is apparent that the effects produced in these and subsequent teratogenic studies were due to the very high dose administered to pregnant animals by injection in the penetrating solvent DMSO, which is toxic in itself and which enhances the toxicity of the test compounds by affecting the phospholipids of the cell wall membranes. Gas chromatographic analyses have shown no trace (0.1 ppm) of TCDD, an impurity in Dow silvex [53-56].

Data obtained by Dow indicated a no-effect level of approximately 7 mg/kg per day in 90-day feeding studies in rats and dogs. Three studies were done, one with the propylene glycol butyl ether ester, one with the sodium salt of silvex, and one with a potassium salt formulation in rats and dogs, which showed no significant toxicological effect at a dose level of 2.6 mg/kg per day [53-56].

Silvex Brush Killer

According to Section A of the Control of Engineers petition (pp 1E1012) for Silvex Aquatic Herbicide, the Dow product Kuron* Brush Killer (PGBE esters of silvex) is included as silvex ester, local procurement, USDA Reg. No. 464-162, Dow Chemical Co., as described in Federal Specification O-H-215a. On November 4, 1970, the Pesticides Regulation Division requested Dow to furnish additional fish toxicity data to

*Dow Chemical Company registered trademark.

demonstrate conclusively the safety of this product to bluegill fry, largemouth bass fry, yellow perch, and walleyes. By letter of June 29, 1971, Dow submitted available fish toxicity data on silvex derivatives, plus arguments in support of continued registration of this product for use in aquatic sites. EPA concurred and approved the revised labeling for Kuron, outlining special precautions for use in aquatic weed control, August 5, 1971 [53-56].

Special Precautions

Silvex should be applied only in accordance with state and local laws and regulations governing chemical treatment of bodies of water for control of weeds.

To avoid injury, silvex should not be used in ponds supplying water for irrigation (including rice production), for agricultural sprays, for domestic purposes, or for livestock.

Silvex should not be applied to water containing valuable fish unless some fish kill can be tolerated; kill may occur in shallow coves if application is not uniform or in shallow areas not diluted by fresh water. Therefore, it is recommended that pond edges or lake shoreline be treated first so that fish will not be trapped in shallow pockets or inlets. When used as recommended, silvex is not ordinarily harmful to aquatic animals.

To minimize the exposure of desirable vegetation along the shoreline, silvex should be applied only when water levels are low.

Algicides such as copper sulfate should not be applied for 3 days before or after applying silvex, since they may interfere with the action of the herbicide.

Control Alternatives

When immediate solutions are demanded by the public, chemicals provide a predictable response on almost all problem species. In recent years, biological control methods have been used successfully for some problem species, such as alligatorweed. However, this method often takes several years to reach the desirable level of control, and the effectiveness is often unpredictable. Integrated control techniques permit management decision trade-offs that take into account predictability, control effectiveness, costs, and environmental compatibility. With no exception, each of the present control methods alone is inadequate for the control of all aquatic pest plants.

SILVEX HAZARD AND RISK EVALUATION

Hazard or Risk

The hazard of a herbicide is the chance that harm will come to the applicator or bystanders or consumers or livestock or wildlife or crops and so on from the use of the herbicide. Hazard is often confused with toxicity. They are not the same. A highly toxic herbicide is usually considered "hazardous" because of the risk that the applicator, bystanders, and so on, can be injured. However, safe and careful handling of a highly toxic herbicide can make it a low risk or low hazard. Many factors besides toxicity can make a herbicide hazardous. These include the target involved, the formulation chosen, the concentration and dosage used, the type of herbicide, and the skill of the applicator [63].

Concentration and Dosage A highly toxic herbicide which is very dilute can be fairly safe. A moderately toxic herbicide which is very concentrated can be hazardous. Using a gallon per acre of a slightly toxic herbicide can be as hazardous as a pint per acre of a moderately toxic herbicide because of the concentration effect.

Amount Used It is estimated that 300,000 lb ae of silvex are used for aquatic application per year, as shown in Table 4. The greatest amount (200,000 lb) is used for ditchbank and shoreline application to control saltcedar, alligatorweed, and various other woody and semi-woody species. About 100,000 lb is estimated for control of submersed and emersed aquatic weeds in lakes, ponds, and canals.

Method of Application About 100,000 lb ae of silvex is applied by air, roughly 50,000 lb by fixed wing and an equal amount by helicopter. About 100,000 lb is applied by ground rigs—a standard tractor-mounted boom spray—but a minor amount is applied as a directed single nozzle spray from a boat. In most of these operations, a crew of two is used,

Table 4 Estimated Pounds per Year, Concentration, and Exposure Time for Aquatic Use Pattern of Silvex According to Site and Method of Application

Site of application	Pounds per year ($\times 10^3$)	Concentration (lb/100 gal)	Exposure (hr/yr/person)
Ditchbank and shoreline			
Fixed wing	50	4-8	100
Helicopter	50	4-8	100
Ground	100	4-8	150
Ponds and lakes			
Ground	100	4-8	150

Source: USDA-States-EPA Silvex RPAR Assessment Team, *The Biologic and Economic Assessments of Silvex*, Government Printing Office, Washington, D.C.

one person to pilot the aircraft or boat, and one person to load and/or spray chemicals.

Formulations The silvex esters are used for ditchbank, shoreline, or canal applications. Lake and pond applications are generally made with the granular potassium salt.

Time of Application Silvex is generally applied during the early spring for ditchbank and shoreline application but may be applied in the late winter to avoid any hazard to field crops in the area. Canals, lakes, and ponds are generally treated in the early summer.

Concentration of Treatment Air application is made at rates of 2-4 gal of concentrate in 10-30 gal of water per acre. Ground application is generally made at rates of 2-4 gal of concentrate in 100 gal of water per acre.

Treatment Exposure Air applicators make 5-10 runs per day and treat 50-100 acres/day. Ground applicators spray 4-6 hr/day and treat 10-30 acres/day. The period of spray activity is not commonly more than 2 months per year. The bystander population is generally less than 10 people per square mile in the area of treatment during the time of treatment. The relative exposure times for sites and methods of application for aquatic use of silvex are summarized in Table 4 and the estimated dermal and inhalation exposure hazard for silvex aquatic use are given in Table 5.

Operator Hazard Based on dermal exposure experiments, human absorption of 2,4,5-T (silvex) is estimated to range from less than 0.001 mg/kg per hour to a maximum of 0.095 mg/kg per hour when exposed skin is wet with spray for the entire application period. An operational monitoring study showed human absorption of 0.001-0.03 mg/kg per hour. Addition of a long-sleeved shirt and gloves to work apparel in place of a short-sleeved shirt reduces exposure by 91%.

DISPUTE RESOLUTION*

A dispute reolution conference held on the toxicity of 2,4,5-T was held in Arlington, Virginia, June 4, 5, and 6, 1979, as an attempt to devise a mechanism by which disputes can be resolved. While recognizing that sociopolitical aspects of controversial issues must be considered in the resolution of disputes, a credible interpretation of the body of available scientific data must be a primary requirement for decision makers. Without such an interpretation, decision making would rest solely on value judgments, which vary with individuals and change

*Scientific Dispute Resolution Conference on 2,4,5-T, American Farm Bureau Federation, Park Ridge, Illinois, 1979, with permission.

Table 5 Estimated Dermal and Inhalation Exposure Hazard for Silvex Aquatic Use

	Margin of safety			
	Silvex		TCDD	
Exposure[a]	PD-1[b]	AT[c]	PD-1[b]	AT[c]
1. Dermal exposure—backpack sprayer	3	5.6×10^3	43	4.1×10^4
2. Dermal exposure—tractor	11	1.1×10^6	167	8.8×10^6
3. Dermal exposure—aerial application	312	3.9×10^8	6.0×10^3	3.0×10^8
4. Inhalation—aerial application	870	7.2×10^5	1.5×10^4	1.2×10^7

[a]Order of criteria of exposure of risk.
[b]Margin of safety.
[c]Adjusted margin of safety using the factorial method.
Source: Exposure analysis according to the methods of the working group of the USDA-States-EPA 2,4,5-T RPAR Assessment Team, *The Biologic and Economic Assessment of 2,4,5-T*, Government Printing Office, Washington, D.C.

with time. Accordingly, this conference was deliberately designed to test a mechanism by which the differences among scientists might be resolved. Experience in that aspect of dispute resolution would then provide guidance for future conferences in which sociopolitical aspects could be addressed as well.

In planning the Dispute Resolution Conference, the use of a specific controversial issue was judged to be necessary. The herbicide 2,4,5-T became an obvious choice as a model because of its controversiality and its having been in dispute for many years without resolution. Because the herbicide was also in the RPAR process (Rebuttable Presumption Against Registration—EPA's decision-making procedure for the re-registration of pesticides), the conference was specifically timed to occur during the 1-month public comment period following EPA's issuance of Position Document Number 3. The first week of June was selected for the conference after discussions with the Deputy Assistant Administrator for Pesticide Programs, because late April or early May seemed most probable for issuance of PD-3. Unfortunately, PD-3 had not yet been issued at the time of the conference and it was not yet available at the time this report went to press. Nevertheless, it is important to make the point that the time for the conference was selected so that it would fit into the sequence of decision-making events in the RPAR process.

Selection of participants for the conference began in February. Since the conference was to be an attempt to resolve disputes on the interpretation of the scientific data available, participants were to be scientists who had conducted research with 2,4,5-T or its contaminant TCDD, or were recognized as being expert in a specific field related to one of the disputatious issues about 2,4,5-T. Individuals who had conducted research on 2,4,5-T and TCDD were identified by a review of the published literature. In an attempt to assure that each of the six workshops had participants who represented different points of view about the issues at controversy, letters were sent in March 1979 to six environmental organizations requesting the identification of scientists who should participate in a discussion of the data. The six organizations were: (1) Environmental Defense Fund, (2) Friends of the Earth, (3) Health Research Group, (4) National Audubon Society, (5) Sierra Club, and (6) John Muir Institute. The National Audubon Society responded to the request by suggesting that the Environmental Clearing House might be able to identify participants. None of the environmental organizations suggested participants for the conference.

CARCINOGENESIS

A review of the published literature reveals no evidence that 2,4,5-T is a carcinogen (Table 6). TCDD is carcinogenic for rats and mice. The following tabulation provides an estimate of lifetime excess lung cancer per million female rats continuously exposed to TCDD.

Continuous lifetime daily exposure (pg TCDD/kg body wt[a])	Excess lung cancer incidence per million rats exposed
10	40
1	4
0.1	0.4
0.01	0.04

[a]pg, picograms; 1 picogram = 10^{-6} μg = 10^{-12} g.

The tabulation is to be interpreted on the basis of the following criteria:

Table 6 Summary of Animal Data Available to Assess Potential Oncogenicity of 2,4,5-T

Species	Strain	Route administration	Results	References
Mouse	F_1 hybrid of C57B1/6 and C3H/Awf (strains X and A)	Diet	No increase in tumors due to ingestion of 2,4,5-T	Innes et al., *J. Natl. Cancer Inst.*, 1969
Mouse	F_1 hybrid of C57B1/6 and AKR (strain Y or B)	Diet	No increase in tumors due to ingestion of 2,4,5-T	Innes et al., *J. Natl. Cancer Inst.*, 1969
Mouse	Strain X or A of above	Subcutaneous injection	No increase in tumors due to injection of 2,4,5-T	Bionetics Res. Lab. report to the National Cancer Institute, August 1968
Mouse	Strain Y or B of above	Subcutaneous injection	No increase in tumors due to injection of 2,4,5-T	Bionetics Res. Lab. report to the National Cancer Institute, August 1968
Mouse	XVII/C	Diet	No increase in tumors due to ingestion of 2,4,5-T	Muranyi-Kovacs et al., *Br. J. Cancer*, 1976
Mouse	C3Hf	Diet	Statistical increase in overall incidence of tumors[a]	Muranyi-Kovacs et al., *Br. J. Cancer*, 1976
Mouse	XVII/C	Subcutaneous injection	No increase in tumors due to injection of 2,4,5-T	Muranyi-Kovacs et al., *Eur. Assoc. Cancer Res.*, 1977
Mouse	C3Hf	Subcutaneous injection	No increase in tumors due to injection of 2,4,5-T	Muranyi-Kovacs et al., *Eur. Assoc. Cancer Res.*, 1977
Rat	Sprague-Dawley	Diet	No increase in tumors after lifetime ingestion of 2,4,5-T	Kocibs et al., 1979
Rat	Sprague-Dawley	Diet	No increase in tumors based on preliminary data available at this time	Status Report Laboratory for Pharmacology and Toxicology, Hamburg, Germany, 1978

[a]Attempts by the EPA to validate this study have been unsuccessful (EPA Carcinogenic Assessment Group Statement of February 23, 1979.

1. Lung cancer was selected as the most significant neoplasm induced in the Kociba study, but the tabulation would not be changed if the heptocellular carcinoma was selected.
2. Extrapolations were based on the single-hit model, which produces a projected greater tumorgenic effect than other mathematical models for carcinogenicity extrapolation.
3. The tabulation gives risk estimates for the upper 99% statistical confidence limits (again projecting higher tumor incidence at low dose levels).
4. Quantitative extrapolation of animal data to the human situation was not performed because
   a. The mechanism of carcinogenesis is unknown.
   b. Potentiation or inhibition of TCDD by other chemicals can occur.
   c. Humans are genetically heterogeneous.
   d. Humans have a longer life span.
   e. Humans have heterogeneous environmental exposures.
   f. Humans may be more or less sensitive to TCDD-induced carcinomas, and so on.

MUTAGENESIS

Effect of 2,4,5-T

Numerous studies of the mutagenicity of 2,4,5-T have been conducted with submammalian and mammalian assays (Table 7). The results of these tests have been negative or inconclusive. The types of tests employed measured primary DNA damage, gene mutations, and chromosome effects. Thus one can assume that reasonably adequate experimental data have been generated for 2,4,5-T and that these data are not suggestive of mutagenic activity, but these data cannot be considered definitive evidence for no effects in humans.

Effect of TCDD

TCDD has been shown to be a potent inducer of P-448 enzymes of the liver, lung, and kidney in mice and rats. The inducing effect in rats was observed at doses as low as 0.002 μg/kg.

Direct assessment of the mutagenicity of TCDD (based on published reports) is rather limited. Studies have been conducted in bacteria, both *Salmonella* and *Escherichia coli*, and mammals. The results from rodent dominant lethal and cytogenetic evaluations were negative. These two tests measure chromosome observations and do not provide for an assessment of TCDD to induce gene mutations in mammalian cells.

Results from several microbial studies have shown that TCDD increases the frequency of gene mutations. The response was observed in both *E. coli* and *Salmonella*. These data may be assumed to establish

TCDD as a potential mammalian mutagen via gene mutation. Confirming in vivo studies of in vitro studies using cultured mammalian cells have not been reported.

The microbial data suggested that DNA repair processes were involved in the mechanism of action since no mutagenic effects were obtained in studies with repair-defective bacteria strains.

The type of molecular event induced by TCDD may be important in developing an appreciation of the carcinogenic mechanism of this agent. The bacteria data suggest that TCDD acts as a direct initiator of malignant transformation since most mutagenic carcinogens are of the initiator class. Few promoters or co-carcinogens show mutagenic activity.

Chromosome observation analysis of humans exposed accidentally or occupationally to TCDD have been negative. However, these data are insufficient to be considered definitive evidence for no effects in humans.

In summary, the mutagenicity studies conducted on 2,4,5-T and TCDD are consistent with the reported carcinogenic responses and suggest that the carcinogenic activity of TCDD is via initiation.

TERATOGENICITY

Effect of 2,4,5-T on Reproductive Parameters in Animals

A review of early studies in animals revealed that high doses of 2,4,5-T containing 0.1 ppm TCDD or less produced cleft palate (mouse only) or embryo lethality in a number of experimental species (mouse, rat, hamster, sheep, monkey, rabbit). A recent three-generation reproduction study in rats was available for examination by this group. Neonatal survival was decreased in a dose-related manner, and the no-adverse-effect dose level in the species most sensitive to 2,4,5-T, the mouse, was 20 mg/kg per day.

Effect of TCDD on Reproductive Parameters in Animals

Studies in rats and mice for teratogenic and embryo-toxic effects revealed the highest no-effect dose level in rats to be 0.03 μg/kg per day (teratogenicity). At higher doses, cleft palates, intestinal hemorrhage, kidney changes, and embryo-fetal lethality were observed.

In studies conducted in rats and monkeys an apparent no-effect level in rats was 0.001 μg/kg per day, a level 10 x below the demonstrated no-effect level in rhesus monkeys.

Effects of 2,4,5-T and TCDD on Reproductive Parameters in Humans

Analysis of available data leads this group to the conclusion that no adverse effects on human reproduction have yet been demonstrated after exposure to 2,4,5-T or TCDD.

Table 7 Summary of Mutagenesis Tests with 2,4,5-T

Species and type of test	References	Results
Microorganisms		
Salmonella typhimurium	Anderson et al., 1972, *J. Agric. Food Chem.*, *20*:649; Ercegovich and Rashid, 1977, *174th ACS Meet.*	Negative
Saccharomyces cerevesiae	Siebert and Lemperle, 1974, *Mutat. Res.*, *22*:111; Fahrig, 1974, *IARC Publ.* *10*:161	Negative
Bacillus subtilis	Shirasu et al., 1976, *Mutat. Res.*, *40*:19	Negative
Senatia subtilis and Escherichia coli	Fahrig, 1974, *IARC Publ.* *10*:161	Negative
Drosophila		
Sex-linked recessive lethals	Majamdur and Golia, 1974, *Can. J. Genet. Cytol.*, *16*:465	Slight increase
Sex-linked recessive lethals	Vogel and Chandler, 1974, *Experientia*, *30*:621	No increase
Somatic cell mutations	Rasmusen and Svahlin, 1978, *Ecol. Bull.*, *27*:190	No increase
Mammalian systems		
Mice dominant lethal and micronucleus	Buselmaier et al., 1972, *Biol. Zbl.*, *91*:311; Jenssen and Renberg, 1976, *Chem. Biol. Interact.*, *14*:29	Negative
Cytogenetic effects—gerbils	Majamdur and Hall, 1973, *J. Hered.*, *64*:213	Inconclusive
Cytogenetic effects—mice	Davring and Hultgren, 1977, *Hereditas*, *85*:123	Inconclusive
Human data		
Cytogenetics—workers	Kilian, 1975, NYAS Workshop, March 28; Johnson, 1971, *Bioscience*, *21*:899	Negative

Microorganisms		
Escherichia coli	Hussain et al., 1972, *Ambio, 1:32*	Increased mutations
Salmonella typhimurium TA-1530	Hussain et al., 1972, *Ambio, 1*:32	Negative
Salmonella typhimurium TA-1532	Hussain et al., 1972, *Ambio, 1*:32	Increased mutations
Salmonella typhimurium TA-1532	Seiler, 1972, *Experientia, 29*:622	Increased mutations
Salmonella tester strains	Communication of B. Ames to USDA, March 1974	Negative
Mammalian systems		
Dominant lethal, rats	Khera and Ruddick, 1973, *Adv. Chem. Ser. 120*	Negative
In vivo cytogenetics, rats	Green, 1975, unpublished report	Negative
Human data		
Seveso plant workers, cytogenetics	Rohrborn et al., 1978, *Mutat. Res.*, in press	Inconclusive
Seveso, fetal-fetal material	Reggiani, 1978, *Arch Toxicol.*, *40*:161	Inconclusive

Source: Ref. 64.

Effects of the Test Substances on Reproductive Parameters in Animals

2,4,5-T Neonatal survival in three-generation studies in rats (through the 21-day suckling period) was decreased in a dose-related manner in the groups that received 10 and 30 mg 2,4,5-T per kilogram per day from their diet. In the group that received 3 mg/kg per day, no adverse effects were seen. The dosage of TCDD contained in the amount of 2,4,5-T consumed by the 3-mg/kg per day group was 0.000001 μg/kg per day.

TCDD Adverse effects seen after ingestion of TCDD in three-generation studies in rats from the diet at 0.01 and 0.1 g/kg per day were decreased fertility, decreased number of pups per litter, and decreased survival of pups through the 21-day suckling period.

In the 0.001-μg/kg per day group, no adverse effects were noted in fertility, number of pups per litter, or in postpartum body weight gain. No consistent effect was noted in postnatal survival. In this experiment, no toxicologically significant effect was noted at the 0.001-μg/kg per day level, but this finding may have been due to variability observed in the control groups. Therefore, this conclusion should be reevaluated after results from additional experimentation are available in which less variation is obtained in the control groups. Until the experiment is repeated, the 0.001-μg/kg per day dose level should be considered as the no-effect level.

Effects of 2,4,5-T and TCDD on Reproductive Parameters in Humans

Alsea Study The miscarriages reported in this study were not demonstrated to result from the spraying of the forests with 2,4,5-T because:

1. The depth of the search for abortions was not uniform among the groups being compared, especially since the physicians in the control area and the urban area were, since the investigators did not have direct access to hospital records in each area but had to rely on data analysis conducted by the hospital staff.
2. Only a portion of the spontaneous abortions occurring in the three areas were taken into account.
3. The incidence of abortions was increased in the study area only in June 1976, when 14 of the 24 abortions occurred, even though spraying was conducted from 1972 to 1977. The spontaneous abortion rates in the study area for the remaining 5 years were comparable with those in the urban and control areas (personal communication between Sune Larsson and Robert Brown, acting Deputy Director, Special Pesticide Review Division).

4. The level of exposure was not determined in the study area; for example, a number of the women who had abortions resided near the western edge of the study area, where the prevailing wind would have minimized exposure (transcript from the 2,4,5-T Suspension Order Hearing, U.S. District Court, Bay City, Michigan, April 1979).

Swedish Study The workshop participants concluded that:

1. Analysis of possible 2,4,5-T exposures in 10 women from Varmland County who had infants with neural tube defects revealed that exposure did not occur during pregnancy (report from the Swedish National Board of Health and Welfare, September 1977).
2. In addition, a similar increase of neural tube defects was seen in this area before 2,4,5-T spraying was conducted in Sweden.
3. Other clusters of neural tube defects were identified in Sweden at the same time in areas not sprayed with 2,4,5-T. Hence the teratology work group did not view these data as demonstrating a teratogenic response in humans that could be realted to 2,4,5-T exposure.

New Zealand Data reported by a physician in three cases of neural tube defects, and the 18 cases reported on television were considered by the work group. It concluded that there was no evidence to suggest a relationship to spraying with 2,4,5-T.

Yarram District (Victoria, Australia) The workshop group did not review the data in detail and accepted the conclusions expressed in the relevant 1978 report. These were:

1. The cluster of babies with birth defects born in Yarram in 1975-1976 was not such as to suggest that a specific local cause was operative.
2. Analysis of all information available showed no evidence that these birth defects were caused by exposure to 2,4-D or 2,4,5-T.
3. The normal agricultural use of 2,4-D and 2,4,5-T has not been shown to cause birth abnormalities in domestic animals, nor is there evidence to connect such use with human birth abnormalities.
4. Victoria lacks organized research on the epidemiology of defects and lacks an adequate system of surveillance of those birth defects which are not rapidly lethal (report of the Consultative Council on Congenital Abnormalities in the Yarram District, 1978).

Vietnam These data were previously reviewed by the Advisory Committee on 2,4,5-T and no causal relationship was found between 2,4,5-T and any effect on human reproduction. Additional data were not available and therefore possible exposures in Vietnam were not addressed by this work group.

Arkansas The work group examined the data and concurred with the conclusions drawn by the authors that there was no correlation between the incidence of cleft lips and/or palates and the use of 2,4,5-T. (See Ref. 64 for bibliographic data.)

Seveso (based on data presented by Drs. L. Sanchioni and H. Rehder and evaluated by the Advisory Committee):
and evaluated by the Advisory Committee):

1. Twenty-eight of the 35 induced abortions were represented by products of conception that were partially fragmented during curettage and incomplete for morphologic evaluation. The only abnormality detected was in one fetus for the RT zone, which was trisomic. No morphologic malformations were noted in any of these fetuses.
2. A slight increase in the incidence of spontaneous abortions was determined in the B zone. These increases might have been due to improved registration (some of the abortions might have been self-induced). Fourteen of the 57 cases of spontaneous abortuses and perinatal mortality examined were malformed structurally (24.6%). This incidence was within the range that might be expected generally, but could not be compared to the rate in this particular area prior to the accident, as no data are available. The types of malformations seen were consistent with those that would be expected spontaneously. All the reported malformations were in the R and RT zones, where the soil concentrations of dioxin were below detectable limits.

HUMAN EXPOSURE WORKSHOP

The probability of human exposure to even transitory toxic concentrations of silvex is limited largely to application personnel. These effects are known and do not represent a serious problem when label precautions are followed. The group agreed that:

1. Sufficient evidence exists to date to conclude that chloracne in humans is the most frequently manifested consequence of exposures to TCDD and may occur without other evidence of toxicity.
2. The group found no evidence for an abortifacient effect of TCDD in humans.

3. The group considered the Alsea, Oregon, data and reached the consensus that such serious deficiencies existed in the data that no conclusions were possible regarding possible abortifacient effects of 2,4,5-T.
4. With regard to the data on TCDD exposure in Seveso, the group concluded that no evidence exists of manifest teratogenic effect in Seveso over the time period of observation.
5. The group concluded that there was no evidence of an association between birth defects of the neural tube and exposure to 2,4,5-T in either the New Zealand or Victoria, Australia, investigations.
6. The group agreed that the available data cannot be interpreted as providing either positive or negative evidence of a carcinogenic effect in humans.
7. TCDD was not found in the urine of personnel who applied 2,4,5-T sprays in the forest. Based on a TCDD concentration of 0.04 ppm in the formulated product, 2.9×10^{-6} μg/kg per workday is the maximum amount that could have been absorbed.

REFERENCES

1. N. F. Cardarelli, *Proc. Int. Controlled Release Pestic. Symp.*, Wright State University, Dayton, Ohio, 1975, pp. 344-357.
2. Corps of Engineers, *Silvex Aquatic Herbicide*, Pesticide Petition 1E1012, Office of the Chief of Engineers, Washington, D.C., 1970.
3. J. Hayes, *Clinical Handbook on Economic Poisons*, U.S. Dept. of Health, Education and Welfare, Communicable Disease Center, Atlanta, Ga., 1963.
4. J. Hayes, *Toxicol. Appl. Pharmacol.*, *2*:327 (1967).
5. S. A. Quin, N. F. Cardarelli, and E. O. Gangstad, *J. Aquat. Plant Manage.*, *15*:74 (1977).
6. K. K. Steward and L. L. Nelson, *Hyacinth Control J.*, *10*:35 (1972).
7. R. A. Elliston and K. K. Steward, *Hyacinth Control J.*, *10*:38 (1972).
8. E. O. Gangstad, R. H. Scott, and R. G. Cason, *Controlled-Release Herbicides*, Aquatic Plant Control Program, Tech. Rep. 1, U.S. Army Eng. Waterways Exp. Sta., Vicksburg, Miss., 1972.
9. F. W. Harris, L. K. Post, and W. A. Feld, Factors Influencing the Release of Herbicides from Polymer Matricies: The Ethylcellulose Matrix, Wright State University, Dayton, Ohio, 1972.
10. F. W. Harris, W. A. Feld, and B. Bowen, Investigation of Factors Influencing Release of Herbicides from Polymers Containing Herbicides as Pendent Side Chains, Part I, Wright State University, Dayton, Ohio, 1974.

11. F. W. Harris, W. A. Feld, and B. Bowen, Investigation of Factors Influencing Release of Herbicides from Polymers Containing Herbicides as Pendent Side Chains, Part II, Wright State University, Dayton, Ohio, 1975.
12. B. D. Dinman, *Science, 175*:495 (1972).
13. National Cancer Institute Studies of Pesticides, Congressional Record—Senate, Washington, D.C., 1969, pp. 4412-4417.
14. E. E. Kenaga, *Down Earth, 35*:25 (1979).
15. American Industrial Health Council, Scientific Statement and Bibliography on OSHA's Generic Carcinogen Policy, Scarsdale, N.Y., 1978.
16. H. F. Kraybill, *Pest Control, 43*:9 (1975).
17. R. Truhaut, *Exotoxicol. Environ. Safety, 1*:31 (1977).
18. U.S. Department of Health, Education and Welfare, *Mortality Trends for Leading Causes of Death, United States 1950-1969*, Department of Health, Education and Welfare Publ. No. (HRA) 74-1853, 1974.
19. M. M. Baschetti, *Proc. Northeast. Weed Control Conf., 13*:315 (1959).
20. B. C. Cowell, *Trans. Am. Fish. Soc., 94*:371 (1965).
21. E. O. Gangstad, *Aquatic Use Pattern for Silvex*, Aquatic Plant Control Program, Tech. Rep. 5, U.S. Army Eng. Waterways Exp. Sta., Vicksburg, Miss, 1973.
22. J. Gaylor and A. Houser, *Down Earth, 18*(3):2 (1962).
23. A. Houser and J. Y. Gaylor, *Proc. South. Weed Conf., 15*:244 (1962).
24. F. B. McGilvrey and J. H. Steenis, *Weeds, 13*:66 (1965).
25. M. E. Pierce, *Proc. Northeast Weed Control Conf., 16*:435 (1962).
26. M. L. Leng, *Down Earth, 28*:12 (1972).
27. M. L. Leng, in *Fate of Pesticides in Large Animals* (G. W. Inie and H. W. Dorough, eds.) Academic Press, New York, 1977, pp. 53-76.
28. W. R. Mullison, *Proc. South. Weed Conf., 19*:426 (1966).
29. W. R. Mullison, *Weed Sci., 18*:738 (1970).
30. J. D. Pope, W. S. Cox, and A. R. Grezenda, *Adv. Chem. Ser. No. 160*:200-206 (1966).
31. J. S. Hughes, *Proc. South. Weed Conf., 15*:265 (1962).
32. J. S. Hughes and J. T. Davis, *Weeds, 11*:50 (1963).
33. C. R. Walker, Univ. Mo. Bull. 64(24), *Eng. Ext. Ser. No. 2*:17 (1965).
34. C. R. Walker, *Water Sewage Works, 3*:113 (1969).
35. C. R. Walker, *Hyacinth Control J., 1*:5 (1971).
36. G. W. Bailey, A. D. Thurston, Jr., J. D. Pope, Jr., and D. R. Cochrane, *Weed Sci., 18*:413 (1970).
37. D. R. Cochrane, J. D. Pope, Jr., H. P. Nicholson, and G. W. Bailey, *Water Resources Res., 3*:517 (1967).

38. E. W. Whitney, R. D. Estes, R. O. Smitherman, and E. O. Gangstad, *Hyacinth Control J.*, *12*:20 (1974).
39. M. Alexander and M. I. Aleem, *J. Agric. Food Chem.*, *9*:44 (1961).
40. L. J. Audus, ed., *The Physiology and Biochemistry of Herbicides*, Academic Press, New York, 1964.
41. C. H. Fitzegerald, C. L. Brown, and E. C. Beck, *Plant Physiol.*, *42*:459 (1967).
42. R. H. Hamilton, J. Hurter, J. K. Hall and C. D. Ercegovich, *J. Agric. Food Chem.*, *19*:480 (1971).
43. R. Hendrickson and W. R. Meagher, *J. Agric. Food Chem.*, *17*: 601 (1969).
44. M. A. Loos, J. M. Bollag, and M. Alexander, *J. Agric. Food Chem.*, *15*:585 (1967).
45. M. A. Loos, R. N. Roberts, and M. Alexander, *Can. J. Microbiol.*, *13*:679 (1967).
46. M. A. Loos, Phenoxyalkanoic acids in *Degradation of Herbicides* (P. C. Kearney and D. D. Kaufman, eds.), Marcel Dekker, New York, 1969, p. 1049.
47. W. R. Meagher, *J. Agric. Food Chem.*, *14*:599 (1966).
48. K. Burger, I. C. MacRae, and M. Alexander, *Soil Sci. Am. Proc.*, *26*:243 (1962).
49. R. S. Horvath, *Bull. Environ. Contam. Toxicol.*, *5*:537 (1971).
50. L. Ou and H. C. Sikka, *J. Agric. Food Chem.*, *25*:1336 (1977).
51. J. M. Bollag, G. G. Briggs, J. E. Dawson, and M. Alexander, *J. Agric. Food Chem.*, *16*:829 (1968).
52. E. A. Woolson, R. F. Thomas, and P. O. J. Enson, *J. Agric. Food Chem.*, *20*:351 (1972).
53. Dow, Silvex Petition, Part III, Item 19: The degradation of 2,3,7,8-tetrachlorodibenzo-p-dioxin by ultraviolet light, The Dow Chemical Co., Midland, Mich., 1970.
54. Dow, Silvex Petition, Part III, Item 20: Solubilities of 2,4,7,8-tetrachlorodibenzo-p-dioxin. The Dow Chemical Co., Midland, Mich., 1970.
55. P. C. Kearney, E. A. Woolson, J. R. Plimmer, and A. R. Isensee, *Residue Rev.*, *29*:137 (1969).
56. A. L. Young, J. A. Calcognia, J. W. Thaken, and J. W. Trembley, *The Toxicology, Environment Fate and Human Risk of Herbicide Orange and Its Associated Dioxin.* USAF Occupational and Enviornmental Health Laboratory TR-78-92, Brooks Air Force Base, Tex., 1978.
57. T. R. Bartley and E. O. Gangstad, *J. Irrig. Drainage Div., ASCE*, *100*:231 (1974).
58. P. A. Frank and R. D. Comes, *Weeds*, *15*:210 (1967).
59. E. O. Gangstad, *Hyacinth Control J.*, *9*:46 (1971).
60. E. O. Gangstad, *J. Sanit. Eng. Div., ASC*, *98*:397 (1972).

61. E. O. Gangstad, *Aquatic Use Pattern for Silvex,* Aquatic Plant Control Program, Tech Rep. 5., U.S. Army Waterways Expt. Sta., Vicksburg, Miss., 1973.
62. University-EPA-USDA Ad Hoc Subcommittee, The Development of Data for Registration of Pesticides for Specialty and Small Acreage Crops and Other Minor Uses, Department of Entomology, Michigan State University, East Lansing, Mich., 1973.
63. USDA-States-EPA 2,4,5-T RPAR Assessments Team, *The Biologic and Economic Assessments of 2,4,5-T*, Washington, D.C., Tech. Bull. No. 1671, U.S. Department of Agriculture, 1982.
64. American Farm Bureau Federation, *Sci. Dispute Resolution Conf. on 2,4,5-T*, American Farm Bureau Federation, Park Ridge, Ill., 1979.
65. J. A. Zack and R. R. Suskind, *J. Occup. Med.*, *22*:11 (1980).
66. Thomas H. Jukes, *Naturwissenschaften*, *61*:6 (1974).
67. Stanislaw Krawiec and J. D. Morre, *Down Earth*, *24*:7 (1968).

Chapter 18

The Use of Controlled Release Herbicides in Waste Burial Sites

FREDERICK G. BURTON, DOMINIC A. CATALDO, JOHN F. CLINE, and W. EUGENE SKIENS Pacific Northwest Laboratory, Richland, Washington

Controlled release formulations of herbicides have been applied to the soil in the manner traditional for herbicides: on the surface or mixed into the top few inches of soil. The controlled release formulation allows another option that we propose to use to place herbicides, contained in controlled release formulations, in a layer at least 1 ft below the surface of the soil, in order to prevent root penetration below that level. Ideally, the herbicide will prevent root tip cell division but will not translocate within the plant, thus assuring that the plant will survive, preserving the ground cover. Trifluralin is one of the herbicides that does not translocate and was chosen for use in this study. A number of applications for this technology are possible, particularly in waste management.

For example, 25 inactive sites in the United States have extensive uranium mill tailings which release radioactive radon gas. The Uranium Mill Tailings Control Act of 1978 directed the Secretary of the U.S. Department of Energy to take steps to provide for "the stabilization, disposal and control in a safe and environmentally sound manner of such tailings in order to prevent or minimize radon diffusion into the environment and to prevent or minimize other environmental hazards from such tailings." Initial studies have been carried out at a Grand Junction, Colorado, tailings site to develop sealing techniques for radon flux attenuation. These include a multilayer clay/aggregate barrier [1] and an asphalt emulsion coating [2]. In the case of the asphalt coating, a soil cover is essential for protection against degradation of the asphalt by oxidation and ultraviolet radiation. However, both the asphalt and the clay/aggregate barrier can be penetrated by the roots of plants growing in the soil cover, creating the possibility of breaking the radon seal.

A second alternative in which the buried layer of controlled release herbicide might be applicable is in shallow land-disposal facilities [3] such as those containing low-level radioactive wastes or, in some cases, toxic chemical wastes. The controlled release system will prevent root intrusion into the buried materials and the subsequent translocation of potentially hazardous materials into the plant shoots with resulting environmental dispersion. Such applications require slow release of herbicide for extended periods on the order of 100 years. Methods described in current publications for controlling release of herbicides extend their effectiveness by, at most, a few weeks [4-6]; only one publication [7] discusses effective periods of a few years.

METHODS AND MATERIALS

In the present studies, two different forms of polymeric carrier/ delivery (PCD) systems were used to investigate the controlled release of herbicides. In the initial study, a sheet was made of homogeneous mixtures of an individual polymer and trifluralin. Several of these sheets, using a different polymer each time (with trifluralin) were used to compare release rates from the various polymers. Cylindrical pellets in two sizes from mixtures of Profax* PS-1600 polypropylene and trifluralin were fabricated and formulated to determine the interaction of PCD systems with soil.

In these systems the initial release rate from the PCD device will be comparatively high until the herbicide on and near the surface of the device has been released. This will permit rapid attainment of the minimum effective level (MEL) of herbicide in the soil surrounding the device. When surface herbicide has been released, the release rate from the system will be determined by Fick's laws of diffusion. Herbicide in the immediate vicinity of the device reduces the concentration gradient, reducing the release rate and prolonging the period of subsequent release.

In the absence of information on the concentration of herbicide in the environment at the surface of the device (and thus its effect on the release rate), the extreme was chosen in which the concentration of herbicide at the surface of the device (in the soil or in vitro) is nearly zero. Thus we will be able to obtain an estimate of the minimum effective lifetime of the device.

*Registered trademark of Hercules, Inc., Wilmington, Delaware.

In Vitro Release Rates

The device (sheet or pellet) to be tested was placed in a flow cell (Fig. 1) at a temperature of 13 ± 1°C. This temperature was chosen as representative of the temperature in arid areas at 1-2 m below ground level. The extracting solution (water containing 10% methanol and 0.1% Triton X-100, to enhance the solubility of the herbicide) was pumped through the flow cell at a rate of 800 ml/day, and collected in a glass container. All lines exiting from the flow cell were glass or metal to avoid absorption that occurs with plastic lines. The herbicide was extracted from the flow-cell effluent by twice shaking duplicate aliquots (usually, 100 ml) of the effluent with 5 ml of chloroform. Approximately 4 g NaCl was added to the aqueous solution before shaking to achieve complete extraction of the herbicide by a salting-out effect. For each aliquot, the combined chloroform extract was brought up to volume in a 10-ml volumetric flask, and the concentration of trifluralin measured at 420 nm on a Cary 219 spectrophotometer. (The blank was a chloroform extract of fresh extracting solution.) The daily release rate was calculated from the concentration of herbicide in the aliquot, the length of time over which the sample was collected, and the volume of sample collected in that period.

Pellet Size

The first functional pelletized PCD system was fabricated with 10% trifluralin in Profax PS-1600 polypropylene. Each pellet, 1-3 mm in diameter and 2-7 mm long, weighed approximately 10 mg. When tested in the flow system previously described, the release rate was 19.8 μg/day per gram of pellets (±2.4 SD).

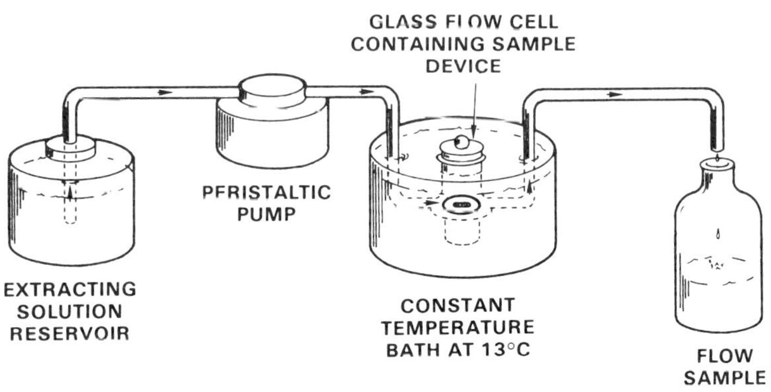

Figure 1 Continuous flow system for studying release rates of herbicides from polymeric carrier delivery systems. (From Ref. 8.)

Since these small pellets contained insufficient trifluralin for long-term (100 year) release, larger pellets were fabricated to take advantage of their increased volume-to-surface area. A practical upper limit on pellet size is imposed by the means available (mechanical seeders) to distribute the pellets uniformly over the ground. Cylindrical pellet dimensions of 9 mm diameter and 9 mm length were determined to be optimal for the uses proposed.

Phytotoxicity and Degradation Studies

The objective of these studies was to determine the MEL of trifluralin sufficient to restrict basipetal root growth while compensating for reductions in concentration resulting from microbial decomposition, chemical degradation, and diffusion from the chemical biobarrier zone created by the PCD system.

Laboratory-scale screening studies employed 5-cm (ID) × 35-cm lysimeters containing 120 g of Ritzville silt-loam (18% moisture). A 2-cm zone, located 25 cm from the surface, was established to simulate in situ releases from a PCD device in trifluralin-amended soil, and to test diffusion of herbicide from PCD devices. Each lysimeter was equipped with a series of longitudinally placed sampling ports, spaced at 2-cm intervals, which provided a means of determining (1) trifluralin concentrations in the soil column at the point at which roots ceased to elongate, (2) rates of trifluralin diffusion from the treatment zone, and (3) release rates of the PCD devices and subsequent longitudinal diffusion rates. Microbial and chemical degradation rates were determined by batch soil incubation. The trifluralin content was determined by assay of random soil cores.

RESULTS AND DISCUSSION

To prevent disruption of physical barriers by roots from vegetation, chemical biobarriers require (1) the presence of a sustained MEL of herbicide/antimetabolite, and (2) a phytotoxin which prevents elongation of a wide variety of roots, but with minimal effect on plant growth so that it will not significantly affect revegetation efforts. After preliminary evaluation of a series of commercially available herbicide/antimetabolite formulations, trifluralin was selected for detailed examination because it prevented longitudinal root growth but did not significantly affect root and shoot dry-matter production.

The steady-state release rates of trifluralin from a variety of polymer sheets were determined to make a preliminary evaluation of their suitability for use in the proposed application (Table 1). Based on these results, as well as other parameters (physical characteristics, loading ability, and polymer cost), filled polyethylene and polypropylene polymers appeared to be the best choices. These polymers

Table 1 Release Rates (±SD) of Trifluralin from Polymeric Carrier/Delivery Systems (Sheets)

Polymer type	Release rate (μg/day/cm^2)
Poly(ether)urethane[a]	3.4 ± 1.0
Ethylene vinyl acetate[b]	9.3 ± 3.3
Silicone rubber[c]	91.7 ± 16.8
Polyester[d]	7.3 ± 1.7
Polyethylene[e]	1.5 ± 0.2
Polypropylene[f]	4.2 ± 0.4

[a]Estane 5714-F, B. F. Goodrich, Cleveland, OH 44131.
[b]Microthene 763, U.S.I. Chemicals, New York, NY 10016.
[c]MDX4-4515, Dow Corning, Midland, MI 48640.
[d]Hytrel 5525, DuPont, Wilmington, DE 19898.
[e]Microthene MN 711-20, U.S.I. Chemicals, New York, NY 10016.
[f]Shell 520, Houston, TX 77002.
Source: F. G. Burton, D. A. Cataldo, J. F. Cline, and W. E. Skiens, in *The State of Waste Isolation in the U.S. and Elsewhere. Advocacy Programs and Public Communications*, Vol. 2 (R. G. Post, ed.) Proc. Symp. Waste Manage., Tucson, Ariz., February 23-26, 1981, The University of Arizona, Tucson, Ariz., pp. 1009-1021.

combine low release rates (therefore long lifetimes for a given loading) with slow polymer degradation rates when in contact with soil. In addition, their relatively low cost make them suitable for the proposed application.

Using laboratory-scale lysimeters and a 2-cm zone of soil amended with 0, 10, or 20 ppm trifluralin, MELs for individual plant species were determined by analysis of trifluralin concentration in soil at the point at which root elongation ceased. Seeds of 13 different species were planted; after which 12-24 days elapsed until roots contacted the trifluralin-treated zone or ceased longitudinal growth. The MEL of trifluralin varied with plant species, ranging from 0.3 to 6.4 ppm at the point of root growth cessation. Table 2 summarizes results for the species studied. Since it is essential that the chemical biobarrier be of minimal toxicity, root and shoot dry matter production was determined in our experiments. With the exception of Winter Fat and Four-wing Saltbush, trifluralin had little effect on dry matter production; no symptoms of toxicity were observed. The weight reductions observed may have resulted from a substantial loss (40-60%) in rooting volume, caused by the presence of the trifluralin-loaded soil layer.

Table 2 Minimum Effective Levels of Trifluralin Required to Inhibit Longitudinal Root Growth, and Effects on Shoot and Root Dry Weight

Plant	Time for root to reached treated zone[a] (days)	Duration of study (days)	Minimal effective concentration[b] (ppm)	Effect on shoot/root dry weight[c] (% of control)
Russian thistle	17	31	0.3	92/82
Tansy mustard	21	45	4.7	90/85
Fourwing saltbush	15	45	4.0	72/77
Gardner saltbush	16	45	3.1	115/94
Winter fat	18	55	1.9	57/50
Crown vetch	14	45	6.4	94/115
Rocky mountain penstemon	24	45	0.9	99/101
Palmer penstemon	20	45	1.5	102/97
Whitmar wheatgrass	13	45	0.8	97/85
Thickspike wheatgrass	21	59	0.7	71/67
Russian wildrye	14	56	0.5	86/82
Lewis blue flax	13	56	2.5	83/101
Bitterbrush	14	54	1.2	95/96

[a]Roots grew from 18 to 24 cm below surface; 2-cm treated zone located 25 cm from surface.
[b]Plugs for analysis removed from soil just below root zone.
[c]Mean of three replicates.
Source: F. G. Burton, D. A. Cataldo, J. F. Cline, and W. E. Skiens, in *The State of Waste Isolation in the U.S. and Elsewhere. Advocacy Programs and Public Communications*, Vol. 2 (R. G. Post, ed.), Proc. Waste Manage., Tucson, Ariz., February 23-26, 1981, The University of Arizona, Tucson, Ariz., pp. 1009-1021.

Deep placement of the PCD devices in soil should result in a loss of trifluralin primarily by microbial decomposition and chemical degradation (hydrolysis). To maintain the MEL this loss must be compensated by an equivalent release of the herbicide from the PCD device. A Ritzville silt-loam amended with 2 or 10 ppm trifluralin, and maintained at 18% moisture, resulted in a calculated half-life of approximately 50 days for trifluralin (Fig. 2). Although half-life will vary with soil type and field moisture conditions, this calculation provides an indication of the long-term, sustained, in situ release rate of trifluralin required from a PCD system in order to maintain the MEL.

In the initial studies we used sheets because of the simplicity of determining release rates; however, for application in the field, pellets are much more practical.

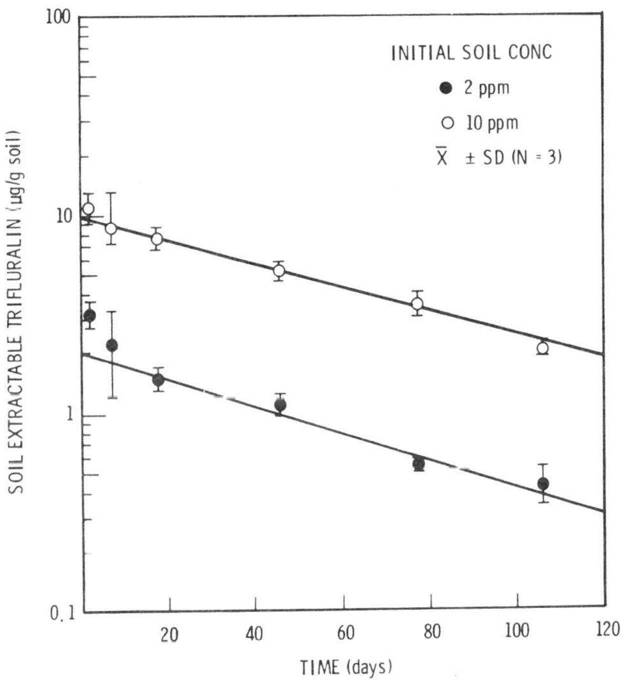

Figure 2 Degradation rate of trifluralin in Ritzville silt-loam, 18% moisture, 21°C. From F. G. Burton, D. A. Cataldo, J. F. Cline, and W. E. Skiens, in *The State of Waste Isolation in the U.S. and Elsewhere. Advocacy Programs and Public Communications*, Vol. 2 (R. G. Post, ed.), Proc. Symp. Waste Manage., Tucson, Ariz., February 23-26, 1981, The University of Arizona, Tucson, Ariz., pp. 1009-1021.

To test the suitability of PCD devices for maintaining a required concentration of trifluralin in soil, polypropylene (Profax PS-1600) PCD devices (measured in vitro flow rate, 19.8 μg/day per gram) loaded at three different concentrations (0.5-, 1.0-, and 3.0-g pellets per 400 g of soil) were placed in soil, and soil trifluralin levels were measured over time (Fig. 3). In each case, near-equilibrium levels were attained within 30 days.

Based on the in vitro release rate and the amount of trifluralin in the pellet, these devices would last only 14 years (because of their small size) at a zero-order release rate. However, taking into account the degradation rate and the equilibrium levels that were determined for these devices, it appears that the in vivo release rate in soil is approximately half the rate determined in vitro, possibly indicating a reduced concentration gradient of the herbicide between the environment and the polymer under field conditions. It is therefore possible

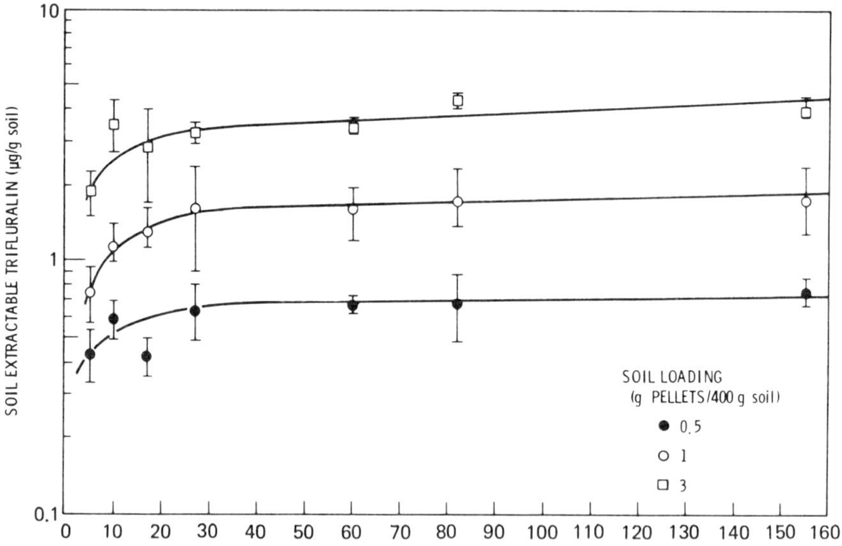

Figure 3 Trifluralin concentration in Ritzville silt-loam with time, resulting from the presence of a trifluralin-releasing PCD system supplied at three loading rates. From F. G. Burton, D. A. Cataldo, J. F. Cline, W. E. Skiens, in *The State of Waste Isolation in the U.S. and Elsewhere. Advocacy Programs and Public Communications*, Vol. 2 (R. G. Post, ed.), Proc. Symp. Waste Manage., Tucson, Ariz., February 23-26, 1981, The University of Arizona, Tucson, Ariz., pp. 1009-1021.

that the potential lifetime of the devices in the field may be increased by a factor of approximately 2.

Because the theoretical lifetime of these devices was insufficient for the proposed application, larger devices (9 mm in diameter and 9 mm long) were fabricated to take advantage of the extended release rate possible. In vitro release rates after 70 days were about 25-30 μg/day per device. This release rate (on a surface area basis) is actually somewhat higher than that of the smaller devices, possibly because these devices were molded (leading to randomly arranged polymer chains) while the smaller devices were extruded (leading to more organized polymer chains).

These 9 mm × 9 mm pellets have also been used in studies to determine their suitability in preventing root penetration. A layer of soil was placed in a lysimeter, the pellets were added in densities from 1 to 4 pellets per square inch, and the lysimeter was filled with soil and seeded with a test plant. At the end of the study the lysimeters were taken apart and the density of pellets necessary to prevent root penetration was determined. Using barley as the test plant, roots ceased to elongate in the treatment zone at all densities tested.

Studies on these devices have been extended to determine the characteristics of trifluralin release under various conditions. Initial analyses indicate that the concentration of trifluralin recovered from the soil after diffusion from the device is inversely proportional to a soil moisture content of 6-18%. Diffused trifluralin is strongly sorbed by the soil (Ritzville silt-loam), reaching a concentration of approximately 2 ppm at 2 cm from the pellet after 30 days, while at 8-10 cm from the pellet, concentrations were undetectable.

SUMMARY

Based on the information cited, a trifluralin-releasing device was developed with a theoretical effective lifetime approaching 100 years. When placed in soil, the PCD system will prevent root penetration through the soil layer without harming the overlying vegetation. Equilibrium concentrations of trifluralin in soil can be adjusted (together with the theoretical life of the device) to suit specific needs.

Our system was designed specifically to protect the asphalt layer or clay/aggregate barriers in uranium mill tailings piles. PCD devices composed of pellets could also be implanted over burial sites for radioactive and/or toxic materials, preventing translocation of those materials to plant shoots, and therefore into the biosphere.

ACKNOWLEDGMENT

This work was supported by the U.S. Department of Energy under Contract DE-AC06-76RLO 1830.

REFERENCES

1. R. W. Nelson, G. W. Gee, and C. A. Oster, *3rd Symp. Uranium Mill Tailings Manage.*, Colorado State University, Ft. Collins, Colo., November 24-25, 1980, pp. 79-88.
2. J. N. Hartley, P. L. Koehmstedt, D. J. Esterl, and H. D. Freeman, *Waste Management 80*, Tucson, Ariz., March 10-14, 1980. PNL-SA-8414, Pacific Northwest Laboratory, Richland, Wash., 1980.
3. J. F. Cline, D. A. Cataldo, W. E. Skiens, and F. G. Burton, *Nuclear Technology*, *58*:150-153.
4. W. A. Gentner and L. L. Danielson, *Proc. Int. Controlled Release Pestic. Symp.*, University of Akron, Ohio, September 1976, pp. 7.27-7.32.
5. G. G. Allan, J. W. Beer, and M. J. Cousin, *Controlled Release Pesticides* (H. B. Sher, ed.), ACS Symp. Ser. No. 53, American Chemical Society, Washington, D.C., 1977, p. 94.
6. C. L. McCormick and M. Fooladi, *Controlled Release Pesticides* (H. B. Sher, ed.), ACS Symp. Ser. No. 53, American Chemical Society, Washington, D.C., 1977, p. 112.
7. G. G. Allan, J. W. Beer, M. J. Cousin, and R. A. Mikels, *Controlled Release Technologies: Methods, Theory, and Applications*, Vol. 2 (A. F. Kydonieus, ed.), CRC Press, Boca Raton, Fla., 1980, p. 7.
8. F. G. Burton, W. E. Skiens, N. R. Gordon, J. T. Veal, D. R. Kalkwarf, and G. W. Duncan, *Contraception*, *17*:221 (1978).

Chapter 19

Controlled Release for Suppression of Rice Storage Pests

BRUCE L. PARKER University of Vermont, Burlington, Vermont

NORMAN L. GAUTHIER Chittenango, New York

AGIS KYDONIEUS Health-Chem Corporation, New York, New York

Of the world food consumed, grains represent the major bulk of calories and protein. As population grows, increasing food supplies becomes more and more important. One vital and neglected step toward this end is to reduce the food losses that occur between harvest and consumption. Postharvest losses of major food commodities in developing countries are in the tens of millions of tons per year and valued at billions of dollars [1]. Loss factors vary tremendously depending, among other things, on the crop stored, year, location, length of storage, and pest or pest combination [2].

In West Malaysia in past years, up to 10% of the total rice harvest has been lost due to storage pests [3]. Singh [4] estimated that the government of this small country annually spent about $52,000 for control of rice storage pests in their few storehouses. Many different insect species are involved and *Sitophilus oryzae* (L.) is considered to be the most damaging [5-7].

S. oryzae is a common storage pest in the tropics. It thrives under warm climatic conditions, but infestations in insulated or protected stores in temperature regions is not uncommon. Adults can live for 4-5 months and each female can lay between 300 and 400 eggs. The female weevil makes a small hole in the kernel of grain with her mandibles, then with her ovipositor inserts an egg directly into this hole. The egg hole is sealed with a plug which she produces from a gelatinous fluid. This protects the egg. The larva feeds and develops within a single kernel, consuming its contents. Because the pest spends most of its life cycle inside the individual kernel, it is extremely difficult to control.

By the year 2000 it is projected that world population will increase from 4 billion to 6 or 7 billion. Presently, between 450 million and 1 billion people do not have enough food to eat, and this number will increase in the future.

Food production must increase to meet demands, and concurrently, problems associated with grain storage are expected to multiply. This will be confounded by the fact that governments will probably be forced to stockpile more grains locally. The need for safe and effective chemicals for use in protecting food commodities from damage by stored product insects has made the search for new innovative methods very important. The expansion of controlled release technology has the potential to bridge this gap. The objective of the research described herein was to determine if controlled release formulations of chlorpyrifos and malathion were efficacious for control of *S. oryzae* in stored rice in Malaysia.

EXPERIMENTAL

In large and small warehouses in West Malaysia rice is commonly stored in polyethylene bags of various thicknesses and sizes. These packages are preferred by sellers and consumers in southeast Asia because of their convenience and ease of handling. Unless the contents of these bags are insect free at heat-sealing time, infestations will build rapidly and significant grain damage occurs. An extensive series of experiments were conducted in Malaysia beginning March 1, 1979, to demonstrate the efficacy of chlorpyrifos and malathion for control of *S. oryzae*. Each of the compounds was formulated by Herculite Products, Inc. (Hercon Division of Herculite Protective Fabrics Corp., a subsidiary of Health-Chem Corporation, 1107 Broadway, New York, N.Y. 10010) in the form of laminated delivery systems.

Approximately 900 kg of local rice variety MAT Candu was obtained from a government storehouse at Tanjung Karang, Selangor. The rice was sifted on a screen (36 holes per 100 mm^2) to remove broken grains, dust, and frass. Next it was placed in a freezer and held for 48 hr at -10°C. This storage period killed the indigenous insect infestation. The rice was then removed from the freezer, allowed to come to ambient temperature, air dried, and weighed into plastic bags. Each plastic bag measured 15 cm × 23 cm, was made of 0.12-mm polyethylene, and contained 500 g of rice.

Twenty adult lab-reared *S. oryzae* were placed in each bag. Prior to heat-sealing the bags, small controlled release dispensers of varying areas and concentrations were prepared and placed inside (Table 1).

Table 1 Controlled Release Dispensers Tested for Efficacy in West Malaysia, 1979

Laminated dispenser reservoir concentration (%)	
Chlorpyrifos	Malathion
4.60	6.05
5.50	6.30
6.30	6.40
8.20	10.74
10.85	10.87
12.00	11.46

Each device tested was replicated in four bags. Bags with rice and insects but without controlled release material were sealed as controls. All bags were stored at ambient temperature (the mean daily temperature was approximately 27°C) for 7-7.5 months. Following the storage period each bag was opened and the following data recorded for comparative purposes:

1. Number of living and dead *S. oryzae*
2. Number of other arthropods present
3. Weight of whole grain
4. Weight of dust, frass, and other waste materials
5. Percentage of broken grains

In addition to these data, each bag was visually assessed for quality using the following scale:

Rating	Criterion
1	No damage visible; mostly dead adult insects
2	Light damage; a few living adult insects seen
3	Moderate damage; obvious insects present
4	Heavy damage apparent; a lot of living insects present
5	Product unacceptable; many, many insects seen

Following analysis of the grain for insects present, quality, and weight measurements, random samples were taken from each treatment and shipped to Herculite Products for residue analysis.

Essentially, the Hercon process enables us to implant active chemicals protectively sealed in a layer between outer plastic layers. A schematic cross section of a typical delivery system is shown in Fig. 1. The specially formulated inner layer is actually an active agent reservoir. In this instance, it contains dissolved insecticide. An almost unlimited range of other active agents can be used. The agent migrates continually, due to the imbalance of chemical potential, through one or more initially inert outer layers to the surface, where it is rendered biologically or physiochemically active. At the surface, the insecticide is removed by volatilization, thermal or ultraviolet degradation, alkaline or acid hydrolysis, or mechanically by humans, insects, rainfall, wind, or other agents.

The factors that affect the control of release rates are the varying of the concentration of the diffusant, or the composition or construction of the plastic that makes up the multilayered structure, or both. Taking these factors and combining them with proprietary technology, a dispenser can be programmed to deliver an active agent to the surface at calculated rates and levels. Thus we can obtain the most desirable release rates for the period of time required by the end-use application.

RESULTS AND DISCUSSION

Rice in this experiment stored for 7 months without insecticides and infested with *S. oryzae* was heavily damaged, with a high percentage increase in insect population and the resultant quality poor, with a lot of broken kernels. The mean visual quality was 3.8 with 570% population increase of *S. oryzae* (Figs. 2,3).

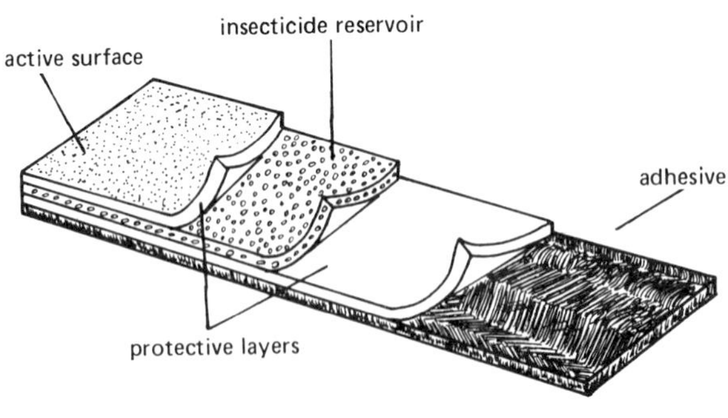

Figure 1 Schematic illustration of the controlled release delivery system used in this study. (Courtesy of Hercon Technology, New York, New York.)

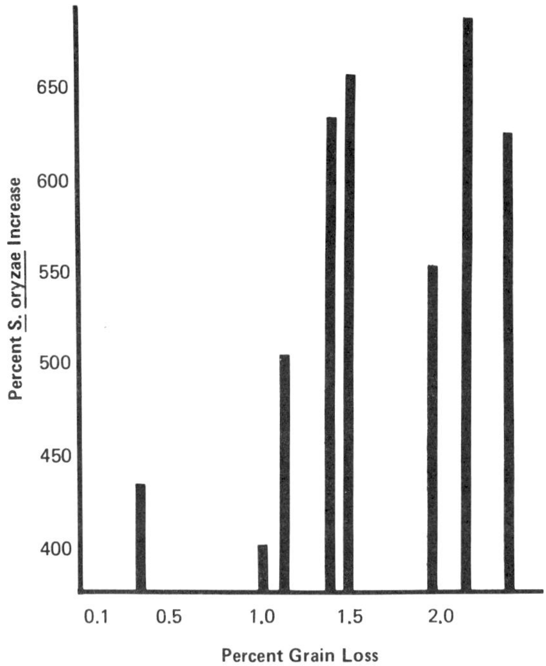

Figure 2 Population increase of *S. oryzae* and resultant percent grain loss after 7 months of storage in West Malaysia. The rice was stored without protection by insecticides (checks).

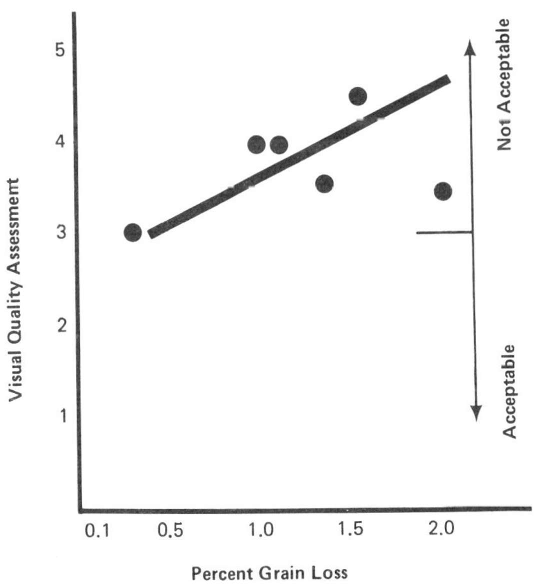

Figure 3 Relationship between visual quality of rice stored for 7 months without insecticide protection and percentage grain lost by *S. oryzae* feeding.

Rice stored with controlled release dispensers containing chlorpyrifos or malathion appeared quite different from the controls mentioned above. The percentage increase of populations of *S. oryzae* decreased as the area of the controlled release dispenser, which was exposed to *S. oryzae* in each bag, was increased (Table 2, Figs. 4,5). There is a positive correlation between the population increase of *S. oryzae* and the percentage of grain lost due to feeding. This relationship is influenced by the insecticide in the controlled release dispensers present in the bags. In general, in the treatments, the higher the population of rice weevils the more grain is consumed (Figs. 6-8). This is consistent with population increases in the checks.

The effects of insect feeding in the treatments as observed by the percent of grain loss is also related to the visual quality assessment made at the termination of storage. The trend was: the higher the percentage grain loss, the poorer the visual quality assessment gradient (Figs. 9,10). However, the quality rating in our treatments was

Table 2 Population Response of *S. oryzae* in Treated Rice Held in Storage for 7 Months

Controlled release dispenser concentration in reservoir	Controlled release area exposed (cm^2)	Percent increase in *S. oryzae*
Chlorpyrifos, 4.6%	0.98	856
	3.92	229
	7.90	175
	31.40	61
	50.00	14
Malathion, 10.74%	1.96	781
	12.50	681
	37.50	216
	50.00	90
	62.50	14
Chlorpyrifos, 10.85%	12.50	140
	15.70	123
	31.00	53
	36.00	35
	100.00	12
Malathion, 6.4%	12.50	533
	25.10	172
	31.40	103
	40.00	78
	80.00	32

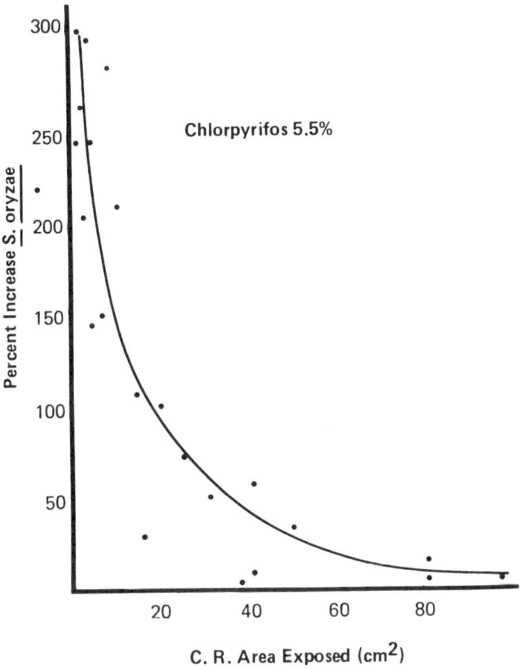

Figure 4 Graphic representation of the relationship of the percentage of population increase of *S. oryzae* and the controlled release area with chlorpyrifos exposed in rice stored for 7 months.

consistently in a range of light to insignificant damage, rendering the rice completely acceptable.

Quality of rice was also related to the total area of the controlled release dispenser exposed to the insects in the bag. The larger the area used, the better the resultant quality of the rice after 7 months of storage (Table 3).

Data in Table 3 also show the size (expressed as area) of the controlled release device needed to obtain a quality rating of 1.75 or 1.50 (good-quality grain). Both ratings were considered perfectly acceptable.

Results of the laboratory analysis of insecticides on rice samples are given in Table 4. Variability in residues found is attributed, in part, to the different concentrations of toxicant in the laminate, to different construction of the dispensers, and to the area of the dispensers exposed within the individual rice bags. Certain trends were apparent. All the dispensers used in this experiment were still active and contained sufficient insecticide in the laminate reservoir to effect

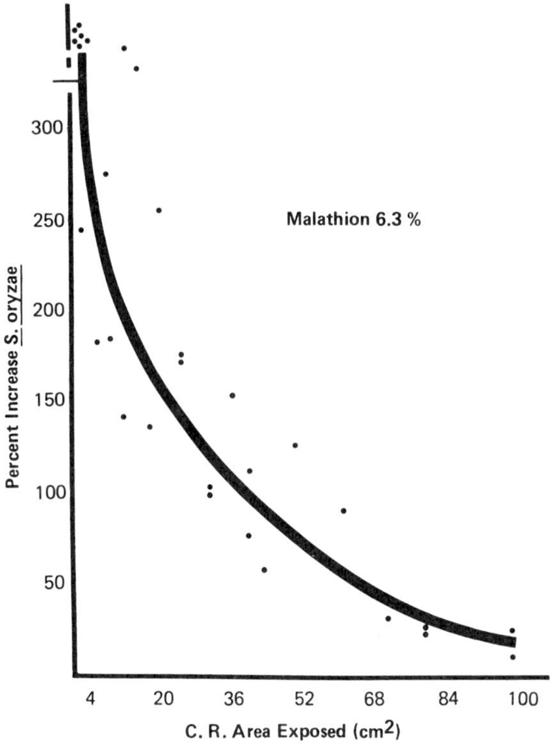

Figure 5 Graphic representation of the relationship of the percentage of population increase of *S. oryzae* and the controlled release area with malathion exposed in rice stored for 7 months.

further insect control. Overall, residues were lower in rice stored with controlled release dispensers containing malathion. The larger the controlled release area used in each storage bag, the higher the resultant residues on the rice. If the area of the controlled release dispenser used is kept constant and the initial concentration of insecticide in the laminate varied, the resultant residues on the rice will be smaller on those samples exposed to the lower level of toxicant. Additional samples are being analyzed.

CONCLUSIONS

Laminated controlled release dispenser materials formulated with chlorpyrifos and malathion show great potential as preventive control measures against weevil infestation in rice packaging. Chlorpyrifos

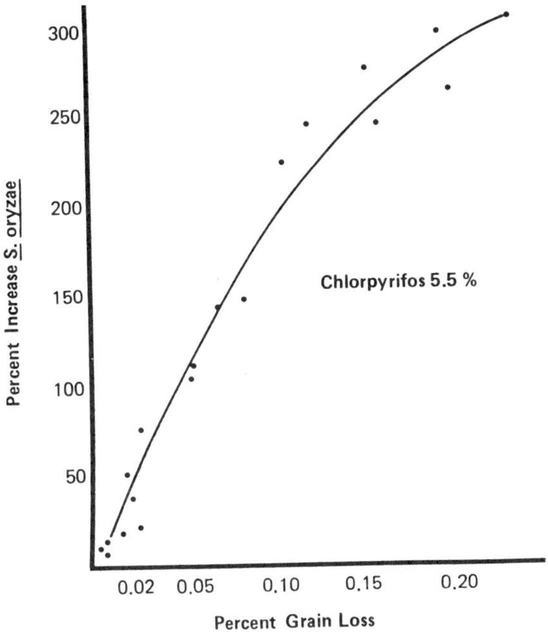

Figure 6 Population increase of *S. oryzae* and the resultant grain loss in rice protected with controlled release dispensers with 5.5% chlorpyrifos in the laminate.

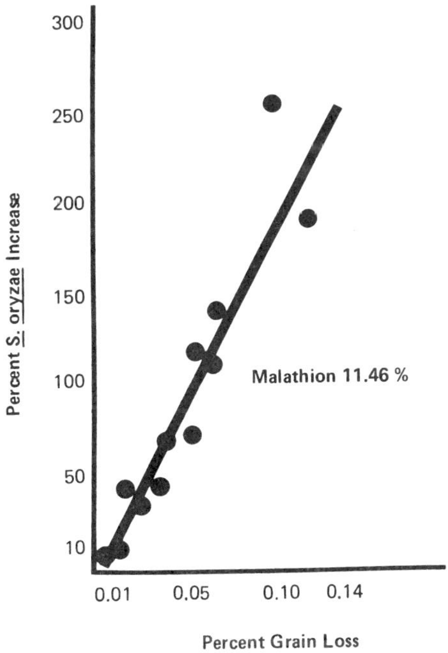

Figure 7 Population increase of *S. oryzae* and resultant grain loss in rice protected with controlled release dispensers with 11.46% malathion in the laminate.

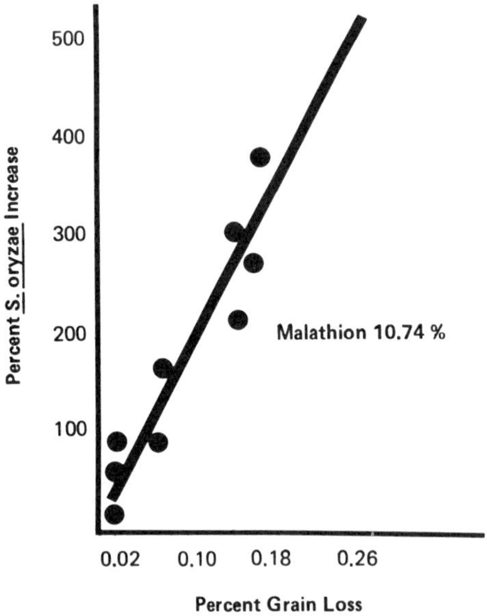

Figure 8 Population increase of *S. oryzae* and resultant grain loss in rice protected with controlled release dispensers with 10.74% malathion in the laminate.

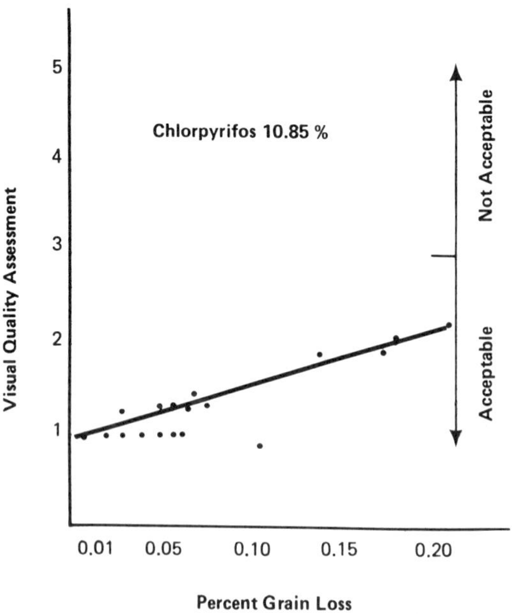

Figure 9 Relationship of visual quality assessment and percentage grain loss by *S. oryzae* feeding in rice in plastic bags with controlled release dispensers containing 10.85% chlorpyrifos.

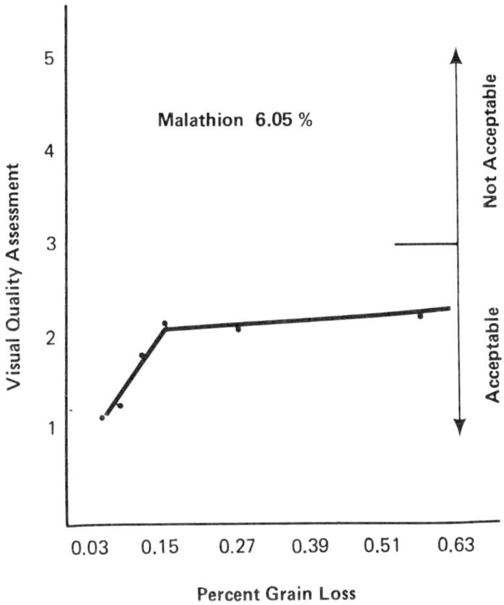

Figure 10 Relationship of visual quality assessment and percentage grain lost by *S. oryzae* feeding in rice in plastic bags with controlled release dispensers containing 6.05% malathion.

Table 3 Rice Visual Quality Assessment Gradient Compared to Controlled Release Dispenser Area

Insecticide in reservoir	Concentration (%)	Controlled release area in cm^2 per bag to obtain a quality rating of: 1.75	1.50
Chlorpyrifos	4.60	20.0	30.0
	5.50	1.8	3.0
	6.30	3.0	3.0
	8.20	7.0	12.0
	10.85	1.7	3.3
	12.00	3.0	3.0
Malathion	6.05	15.0	30.0
	6.4/6.30	46.0	52.0
	10.74	36.0	55.0
	10.87	4.0	10.0
	11.46	28.0	44.0

Table 4 Results of the Laboratory Analysis of Rice Stored with Controlled Release Dispensers for 7 Months

Insecticide concentration in laminate		Area of controlled release dispenser used (cm^2)	Residue in rice (ppm)
Initial	After storage		
		Chlorpyrifos	
8.20	NA[a]	12.6	6.0
10.85	9.61	50.0	15.8
5.50	4.62	80.0	20.9
5.50	4.21	100.0	17.8
5.50	3.46	100.0	15.0
10.85	8.24	100.0	30.6
10.80	6.40	100.0	40.6
5.50	3.40	112.0	20.0
10.80	6.89	112.0	56.7
		Malathion	
6.40	5.16	50.0	0
6.40	5.64	50.0	4.3
10.87	8.49	50.0	11.3
10.87	10.18	80.0	7.9
6.40	4.34	100.0	10.9
6.40	4.40	100.0	10.4
10.87	8.36	100.0	11.3
10.87	10.01	160.0	6.5

[a]Data not available.

at both high and low concentrations appears more efficacious than similar concentrations of malathion in reducing percentage increase of *S. oryzae* populations. However, alterations in controlled release area exposed in treated packaging can be made with both insecticides to obtain a good visual grain quality index rating. At this stage of experimentation, it is difficult to indicate which controlled release formulation, design, or exposed area provides optimum control suitable for practical utilization. Research is continuing in this area.

ACKNOWLEDGMENTS

The authors appreciate the cooperation received from the Malaysian Agricultural Research and Development Institute. Many thanks to Dr. Mohd. Yusof Hashim for his continual support and to Abdul Rahim Muda for his competent technical assistance.

REFERENCES

1. National Academy of Sciences, *Postharvest Food Losses in Developing Countries*, Washington, D.C., 1981.
2. K. L. Harris and C. J. Lindblad, in *Postharvest Grain Loss Assessment Methods*, American Association of Cereal Chemistry, St. Paul, Minn., 1978.
3. T. Sze-Peng, in The Rice Weevil, *Sitophilus oryzae* (L.) on Stored Rice in Malaysia, M.S. thesis, Simon Fraser University, Burnaby, B.C., Canada, 1979.
4. K. I. Singh, *Trop. Stored Prod. Inf.*, *23*:29 (1972).
5. A. Yunus and K. I. Singh, *Dept. Agric., Kuala Lumpur, Malaysia. Entomol. Inf.*, *24*:22 (1968).
6. G. Singh and B. L. Parker, *Malaysia Tumbuh*, *1*:47 (1974), University of Malaya, Kuala Lumpur, Malaysia.
7. G. S. Lim, *Malaysia Agric. Res. Dev. Inst. Rep.* *33*:11 (1975), Serdang, Malaysia.

Chapter 20

Encapsulated Sumithrin: Core Concentration and Biological Activity

HIROSHI FUYAMA, GORO SHINJO, and KOZO TSUJI
Sumitomo Chemical Co., Ltd., Takarazuka, Hyogo, Japan

Microencapsulated pesticides are generally 1- to 100-μm-diameter particles which are composed of pesticides (or pesticide solutions) and wall materials. The wall is a thin polymeric membrane which is generally semipermeable. The pesticides, as core materials, can be released from the microcapsules by diffusing through the wall. The release rate of the pesticides from the microcapsules can be controlled by the chemical structure of the capsule wall, its thickness, and the particle size of the microcapsules.

Encapsulated pesticides have the following characteristics:

1. Improvement in residual activity
2. Stabilization of pesticides against environmental degradation
3. Decrease in mammalian toxicity
4. Decrease in chemical reactivity
5. Occlusion of odor and a decrease of human mucous membrane irritation
6. Decrease in phytotoxicity
7. Decrease in drift phenomena
8. Solidification of liquid pesticides
9. Increase in the number of target organisms

Microencapsulated pesticides are generally formulated as water-based suspensions or microcapsule concentrates, which can be diluted with water prior to the application. They can be applied by spraying with the conventional spraying equipment.

Some encapsulated pesticides are already on the market [1]. Pen. M®, for example, is a microcapsule of methyl parathion. Characteristics of this formulation are a decrease of toxicity and longer residual activity [2-4].

We are now carrying out research work on encapsulation of pesticides [5,6]. In this paper, the results of encapsulation of 3-phenoxybenzyl-d-cis,trans-chrysanthemate (Sumithrin) are discussed. The relationship between active ingredient (A.I.) concentration in the microcapsules and biological efficacy against the German cockroach is considered in detail. The purpose of this research is to develop a formulation which shows consistent efficacy on various kinds of application surfaces.

METHODS AND MATERIALS

Microencapsulation of Sumithrin

According to our previous research work [6], a polyurethane wall was found to be the most suitable for this microcapsule. Therefore, polyurethane microcapsules were used for this research.

Polyurethane microcapsules were prepared by interfacial polyaddition reaction of polyisocyanate (adduct of toluene diisocyanate and trimethyrol propane) and ethylene glycol.

Table 1 shows the ingredients for microencapsulation of Sumithrin. Cyclohexanone was used to dissolve both Sumithrin and polyisocyanate. Cyclohexanone was charged at various rates to prepare microcapsules which had different active-ingredient concentrations as core materials.

Table 1 Components of Sumithrin Microcapsule Concentrate (% w/w)

	Sample number			
	1	2	3	4
Sumithrin A.I.	12.0	10.0	6.25	2.5
Cyclohexanone	0.5	2.5	6.25	10.0
Polyisocyanate	0.8	0.8	0.8	0.8
Ethylene glycol	0.32	0.32	0.32	0.32
Gum arabic	1.0	1.0	1.0	1.0
Water	Balance	Balance	Balance	Balance
	100.00	100.00	100.00	100.00

The procedure for preparing the microcapsules is shown in Fig. 1. The first step of the process is dispersion of an organic mixture (containing Sumithrin, polyisocyanate, and cyclohexanone) into a 2% aqueous solution of gum arabic which was added as a dispersing agent. Then the prescribed amount of ethylene glycol was added into the resulting dispersion under light agitation. The wall-forming reaction was carried out for 2 hr at 60°C. The total weight of the resulting mixture was adjusted by addition of water according to the concentration listed in Table 1. The medium diameter of the microcapsules was 40-50 μm and the range of particle sizes was 3-100 μm.

Analytical Methods

The amounts of Sumithrin and cyclohexanone contained in the microcapsules were separately determined according to the following methods by means of gas chromatography using an internal standard.

Analysis of Sumithrin contained in the microcapsules was determined after extraction. Each microcapsule concentrate was accurately weighed into a centrifuge tube. After centrifugal separation, the supernatant was decanted. The precipitate was extracted with acetone containing triphenylphosphate (as an internal standard) by shaking for 1 hr. The supernatant solution was injected into the gas chromatograph under the following conditions:

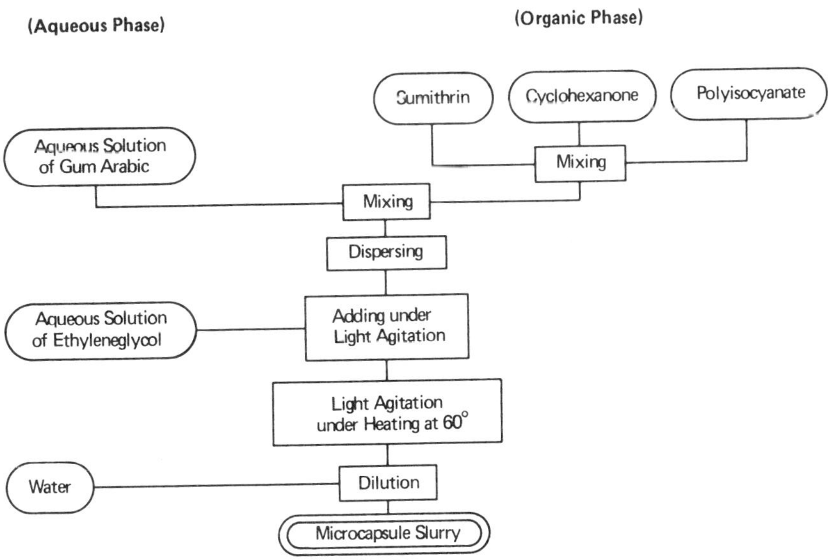

Figure 1 Preparation process of encapsulated Sumithrin (polyaddition reaction).

Apparatus: Shimadzu GC-3BF equipped with a hydrogen flame ionization detector (Shimadzu Seisakusho Ltd., Kyoto, Japan)
Column: glass column 3 mm in inner diameter and 1.2 m in length, packed with 3% silicon XE-60 on Chromosorb W (AW, DMCS, 60-80 mesh)
Temperature: column oven, 193°C; injection port, 265°C
Pressure of carrier gas: nitrogen 1.0 kg/cm^2
Pressure of hydrogen: 0.7 kg/cm^2
Flow rate of air: 40 ml/min

The amount of cyclohexanone contained in the microcapsules was also determined after extraction. Each microcapsule concentrate was weighed accurately into a centrifuge tube. After centrifugal separation, the supernatant liquid was decanted. The precipitate was extracted with acetone containing toluene (as internal standard) by shaking for 1 hr. The extract was then analyzed under the following conditions:

Apparatus: Yanaco GC-550F equipped with a hydrogen flame ionization detector (Yanagimoto Seisakusho Ltd., Kyoto, Japan)
Column: glass column 3 mm in inner diameter and 1.5 m in length, packed with 20% diisodecylphthalate on Celite 545 (60-80 mesh)
Temperature: column, 115°C; injection port, 150°C
Flow rate of carrier gas: nitrogen 25 ml/min
Flow rate of hydrogen: 50 ml/min
Flow rate of air: 40 ml/min

Evaluation of the Biological Efficacy Against German Cockroach (*Blattella germanica*) by the Confined Contact Method

Each microcapsule concentrate was diluted with water to various concentrations and applied uniformly onto the surfaces of plywood panels and overlaid plywood panels (15 × 15 cm) with a microsyringe at the rate of 50 ml/m^2 (1.125 ml per panel).

The panels were applied for biological efficacy measurement at 2 hr and 2 weeks after treatment. During the test period, the panels were kept in the room at 25°C with 50-60% relative humidity.

Experiments were conducted in triplicate using 10 German cockroaches in each trial. The insects were released into a stainless steel ring 5 cm high and 10 cm in diameter, which was put on the treated panel. After 2 hr, they were transferred into the recovery containers for mortality counts (after 72 hr).

The efficacy of emulsifiable concentrate (EC) and wettable powder (WP) was also evaluated in the same way in order to compare with the microcapsule concentrate.

Release Rate of Sumithrin from Two Types of Microcapsule Concentrates

Release rates of Sumithrin from two types of microcapsule concentrates, samples 1 and 2, were determined by chemical analysis according to the following procedure.

The microcapsule concentrates were diluted to 1% w/v A.I. with water. The dilution was applied uniformly into the bottom of five petri dishes (11 cm inner diameter) at the rate of 1 cc per dish (10 mg per dish).

The treated petri dishes were stored in the dark shelf at an ambient temperature (ca. 20°C) and were quickly rinsed with 5 ml of n-hexane per dish into a distilling flask at the end of prescribed periods (2 hr, 1 day, 3 days, 7 days, and 15 days, respectively). The five dishes corresponded to the series of storage periods, respectively.

The collected solutions were evaporated to near dryness by means of a rotary evaporator. The amount of Sumithrin recovered was equivalent to the amount of Sumithrin released during the prescribed period. These values were converted into the release rates (%) by dividing with 10 mg (i.e., total amount of treated Sumithrin per dish).

Figure 2 is the microscopic picture of the microcapsules (sample 1) initially applied into the petri dish. Figure 3 is the one observed

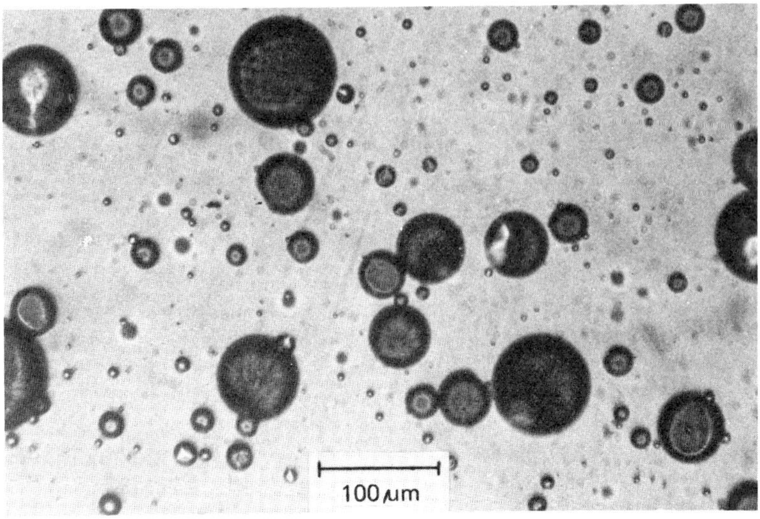

Figure 2 Microscopic picture of the microcapsules (sample 1) initially applied into the petri dish.

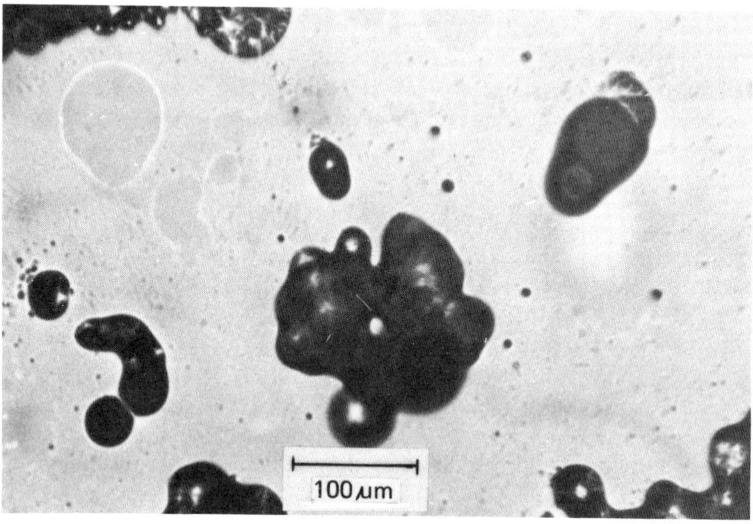

Figure 3 Microscopic picture of the microcapsules (sample 1) after 4 hr.

after 4 hr. As water vaporized with the lapse of time, the particles aggregated and the release Sumithrin was observed just around the particles.

RESULTS AND DISCUSSION

Table 2 shows the charged amounts of Sumithrin and cyclohexanone in 100 g of the reaction mixture and their amounts contained in the microcapsules in 100 g of the microcapsule concentrate which were recovered by chemical analysis.

The amount of cyclohexanone in the microcapsules is smaller than the charged amount. This is due to partial dissolution of cyclohexanone into water in the microencapsulation process, as the solubility of cyclohexanone in water is ca. 50 g/liter at 30°C.

Tables 3 and 4 show the efficacy of four kinds of microcapsule concentrates which contain different amounts of active ingredient against German cockroach on the plywood panel and the overlaid plywood panel, respectively.

It is apparent from Tables 3 and 4 that higher active ingredient concentration in the microcapsules as core material gives better biological efficacy (both initial and residual effects) on both the plywood panel and the overlaid plywood panel.

Table 2 Components of Microencapsulated Sumithrin

	Sample number			
	1	2	3	4
Charged amount (g)				
Sumithrin A.I.	12.0	10.0	6.25	2.50
Cyclohexanone	0.5	2.5	6.25	10.0
Recovered amount (g)				
Sumithrin A.I. in capsule	11.70	9.98	6.28	2.49
Cyclohexanone in capsule	0.225	1.10	2.30	1.95
A.I. concentration in capsule	98.1	90.1	73.2	56.1

Moreover, Fig. 4 shows that the release rate of active ingredient through the microcapsule wall in sample 1 is higher than that of sample 2, especially at the initial stage.

Therefore, it is concluded that biological efficacy depends on the inner active ingredient concentration and that higher inner active ingredient concentration causes the larger amount of release of active ingredient through the capsule wall especially at the initial stage of release, which results in better biological efficacy (both initial and residual effects).

The biological efficacy of EC and WP depends on the kind of the applied surfaces. In the case of WP, efficacy is very good on the plywood panel but not on the overlaid plywood panel, while in the case of EC, efficacy is good on the overlaid plywood panel but not on the plywood panel.

These results may be caused by the fact that the plywood panel easily absorbs liquid materials and that WP can easily be taken away by the cockroaches on the overlaid plywood panel since the surface of the overlaid plywood panel is very smooth.

The encapsulated Sumithrin having higher inner active ingredient concentration (sample 1), on the other hand, shows sufficient efficacy on both the plywood panel and the overlaid plywood panel. Thus it is evident that encapsulation provides consistent biological efficacy on both application panels.

Table 3 Biological Activity of Encapsulated Sumithrin Against German Cockroach by the Confined Contact (2 hr) Method on the Plywood Panel

			Initial effect		Residual effect (2 weeks)	
Sample number	Inner A.I. conc. (%)	Dosage (mg/m^2)	KT_{50}[a] (min)	Mortality (%) (after 3 days)	KT_{50}[a] (min)	Mortality (%) (after 3 days)
1	98.1	500	68	100	>120	93
2	90.1	500	>120	100	>120	43
3	73.2	500	>120	75	>120	35
4	56.1	500	>120	62	>120	35
WP	—	500	29	100	78	88
EC	—	500	>120	77	>120	0

[a]KT_{50}, 50% knockdown time.

Table 4 Biological Activity of Encapsulated Sumithrin Against German Cockroach by the Confined Contact (2 hr) Method on the Overlaid Plywood Panel

			Initial effect		Residual effect (2 weeks)	
Sample number	Inner A.I. conc. (%)	Dosage (mg/m^2)	KT_{50}[a] (min)	Mortality (%) (after 3 days)	KT_{50}[a] (min)	Mortality (%) (after 3 days)
1	98.1	250	72	100	64	100
2	90.1	250	103	100	57	97
3	73.2	250	>120	0	>120	0
4	56.1	250	>120	3	>120	27
WP	–	250	31	100	>120	0
EC	–	250	9.3	100	36	100

[a]KT_{50}, 50% knockdown time.

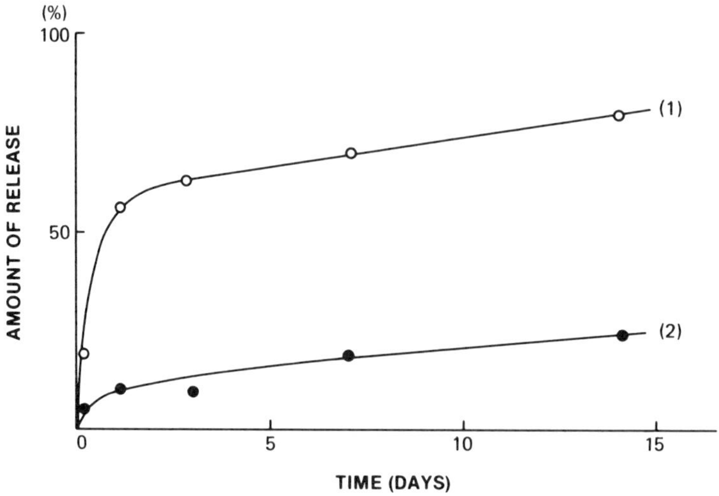

Figure 4 Release behavior of Sumithrin from the microcapsules. The numbers 1 and 2 correspond to the components in Table 1.

ACKNOWLEDGMENTS

The authors wish to express their gratitude to Mr. C. Hirose and Dr. Y. Nishizawa for their kind suggestion and encouragement. The authors are indebted to Sumitomo Chemical Co. Ltd. for permission to publish the results.

REFERENCES

1. K. Tsuji, *Kagaku to Kogyo*, *34*:119 (1981).
2. E. E. Ivy, *J. Econ. Entomol.*, *65*:473 (1972).
3. E. J. Vevai, *Pesticides*, *10*(11):15 (1976).
4. J. R. Lowell, Jr., *9th Int. Congr. Plant Protect.*, Washington, D.C., August 1979.
5. H. Fuyama and K. Tsuji, Japanese Patent, Publication (examined) No. 55-6415 (Sumitomo Chemical Co. Ltd.).
6. H. Fuyama, G. Shinjo, and K. Tsuji, Japanese Patent, Publication (examined) No. 55-38325 (Sumitomo Chemical Co. Ltd.).

Chapter 21

Development of BioLure* Controlled Release Pheromone Products

KELLY L. SMITH and RICHARD W. BAKER Bend Research, Inc., Bend, Oregon

YASUO NINOMIYA Nitto Electric Industrial Co., Ltd., Ibaraki, Osaka, Japan

Insect pheromones have been playing an increasingly important role in insect management in recent years. This is the result of several factors, including their efficacy, specificity, and inherent safety, especially when compared with conventional insecticides. Inefficient or excessive application of insecticides, insect resistance to insecticides, mortality of nontarget organisms, and environmental damage are all either eliminated or substantially reduced by the use of pheromones together with, or in place of, insecticides.

Pheromones have been used in two major applications: detection or monitoring of insect pests, and direct control of insect populations. In monitoring uses, the pheromone is used to attract insects to a trap to aid growers in determining when, or if, insecticide application is necessary. A photograph of an insect trap and pheromone dispensers for monitoring is presented in Fig. 1. An insect control technique known as *mass trapping* consists of using a large number of traps in order to catch a sufficient number of insects to reduce the population. Alternatively, a relatively high concentration of pheromone can be maintained in a field or orchard, which effectively disrupts insect communication and prevents mating; this control technique is called *communication disruption* or *mating disruption*.

Pheromones are expensive, volatile, potent, and in some cases labile compounds. Controlled release is therefore essential for efficient, economical use in insect management. For use in attracting insects to a trap, a dispenser should release the pheromone at an effective rate for a long period of time. In many cases, the release rate must be

*BioLure is a trademark of Bend Research, Inc.

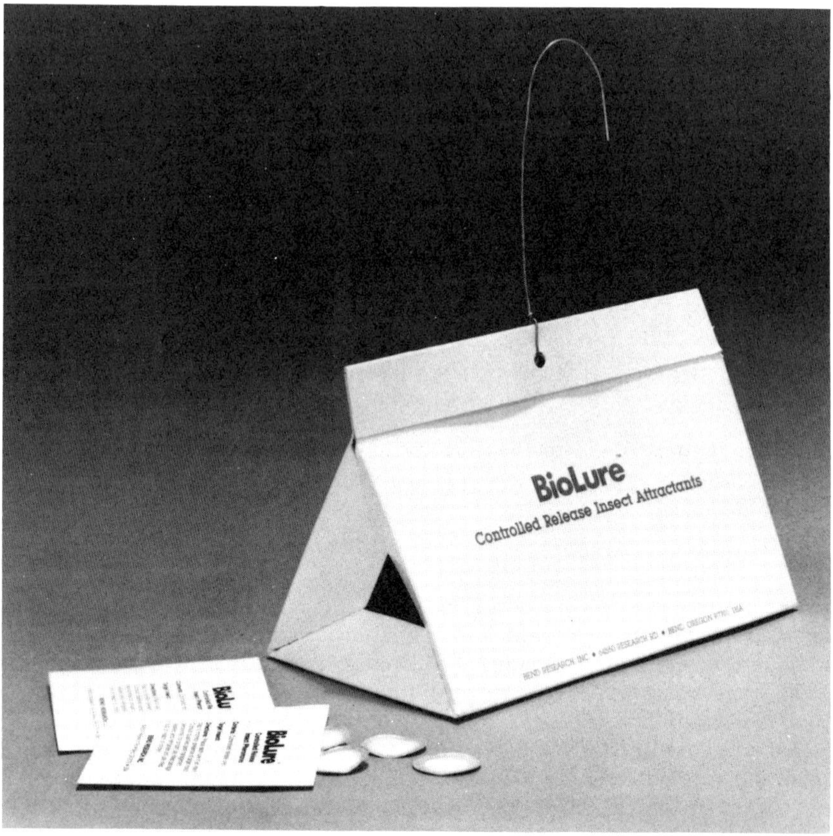

Figure 1 Insect trap and controlled release dispensers for monitoring and detection.

within narrow limits to be effective [1], and it should be relatively constant to obtain consistent results and to avoid wasting the pheromone. Pheromone dispensers commonly used for monitoring have included filter paper, cotton dental wicks, rubber stoppers, glass vials, and plastic vials. These dispensers not only exhibit decreasing release rates with time, but often are inconvenient to use, are effective in the field for relatively short periods, and are not sufficiently reproducible to guarantee consistent trapping results. Such poorly controlled formulations prompted the development of BioLure controlled release insect pheromone dispensers for insect monitoring and detection.

Controlled release is also required in mating disruption in order to provide a prolonged treatment duration and to conserve the pheromone.

The use of pheromones for insect control requires U.S. Environmental Protection Agency (EPA) registration, which has somewhat slowed the introduction of pheromones to this field. However, several products have been introduced in the last three years and are commercially used today. We are currently developing formulations for use in mating disruption that may avoid the problems of currently available products —problems such as short duration of efficacy, difficulty of application, and rapid degradation of labile pheromones.

BIOLURE PHEROMONE DISPENSERS

BioLure pheromone dispensers consist of three primary components: (1) a rate-controlling membrane through which the pheromone diffuses; (2) a reservoir, which contains the pheromone; and (3) an impermeable backing. This structure is shown in Fig. 2. Controlled release from this system occurs by simple Fickian diffusion; as long as pheromone at constant activity remains in the reservoir, the pheromone release rate is constant. This can be expressed mathematically as follows:

$$\frac{dM}{dt} = \frac{ADS}{\ell} \qquad (1)$$

where dM/dt represents the pheromone release rate, A the releasing surface area, D the diffusivity of the pheromone in the membrane, S the pheromone solubility in the membrane, and ℓ the membrane thickness. The grouping DS is usually referred to as the membrane permeability. By using polymeric membranes of different thickness, area, and permeability, pheromones with widely different properties can be released at optimum rates. In addition, the duration of release is dependent only on the initial quantity of pheromone in the reservoir and on the release rate, and can be easily adjusted.

In contrast to the constant release rate obtained with the BioLure sealed-reservoir systems, release rates from other types of pheromone

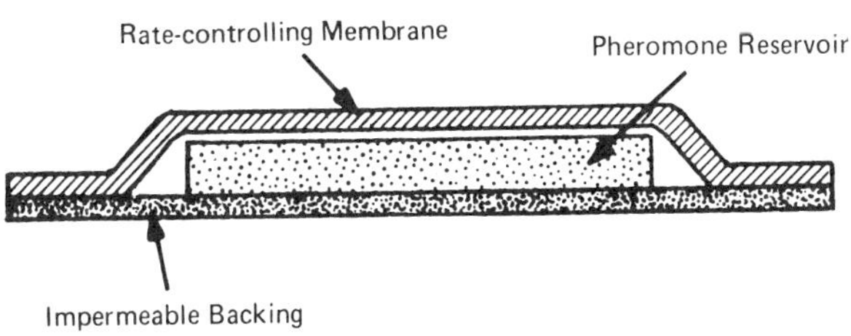

Figure 2 Structure of BioLure pheromone dispensers.

dispensers are not constant, but decrease with time. Rubber stoppers containing dissolved pheromone, which are commonly used as trap lures, release approximately the first half of the pheromone according to the relationship

$$\frac{dM}{dt} = 2M_{\infty}\left(\frac{D}{\pi \ell^2 t}\right)^{1/2} \tag{2}$$

and the last half of the pheromone according to the relationship

$$\frac{dM}{dt} = \frac{8DM_{\infty}}{\ell^2} \exp\left(\frac{-\pi^2 Dt}{\ell^2}\right) \tag{3}$$

where M_{∞} is the mass of pheromone initially present, ℓ the stopper thickness, and t the time [2]. It can be seen from these equations that the release rate decreases continuously with time.

Another common type of pheromone dispenser consists of a membrane-laminated reservoir with unsealed reservoir edges. The pheromone is commonly present in the reservoir at a concentration Co, in excess of its solubility in the reservoir material, C_R. With this dispenser, the pheromone is released both from the membrane surface and from the edges. Because of pheromone release from the edges of the device, the overall release behavior is complex. When Co >> C_R, the release rate can be expressed as follows:

$$\frac{dM}{dt} = \frac{ADS}{\ell} + \frac{A_E}{2}\left(\frac{2D_R C_R Co}{t}\right)^{1/2} \tag{4}$$

where D_R is the diffusivity of the pheromone in the reservoir, and A_E is the total area of the unsealed edge of the reservoir [2]. For dispensers with A >> A_E, the edge effect is minimized, and the release rate can be nearly constant. As A_E approaches A, the release rate becomes increasingly nonlinear.

Another pheromone dispenser in use is a hollow fiber. One end of the fiber is sealed, and the pheromone evaporates from the open end. It has been determined that the rate-controlling step in pheromone release from these fibers is diffusion of pheromone from the pheromone-air interface within the fiber to the end of the fiber. In this case, the release rate decreases with time as pheromone is released and the diffusion path length between the interface and the end of the fiber increases. The release rate falls with time according to a $t^{-1/2}$ dependence [3].

A comparison of the relative release rates from these different dispensers is instructive. By making reasonable assumptions of concentrations, solubilities, diffusivities, and areas, the release rate curves

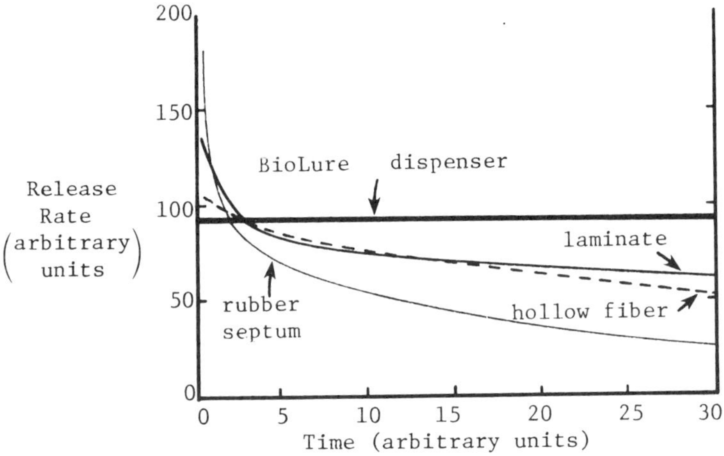

Figure 3 Comparative release rates of pheromone from various dispensers.

shown in Fig. 3 were calculated.* As shown, the rubber stopper exhibits the least constant release rate, and the BioLure dispenser has the only completely constant release rate. Daterman has shown [4] that optimum trap catches of the European pine shoot moth occur over a narrow range of pheromone release rates; either too high or too low a release rate results in a lower trapping efficiency. For insects such as this, the BioLure dispenser can be designed to release at the optimum rate over a full season, and utilization of the expensive pheromone is virtually complete.

Although a substantial amount of work has been published on gas permeation in membranes [5,6], virtually no pheromone permeation data are available in the literature. Our dispenser development efforts therefore entailed extensive release rate studies. A series of polymer membranes with different permeabilities was evaluated for each dispenser. Shown in Fig. 4 are release rates of the cabbage looper pheromone, (Z)-7-dodecenyl acetate (Z7DDA), from several BioLure dispensers. The release rate was varied over two orders of magnitude, and each dispenser released the pheromone at a constant rate, as predicted from Eq. (1). The optimum release rate for attraction of cabbage looper moths is approximately 100 μg/day [7], which was achieved with one of the dispensers. Similar studies were completed for each type of dispenser developed.

---

*Initial "burst" effects, which are dependent on storage conditions, were ignored.

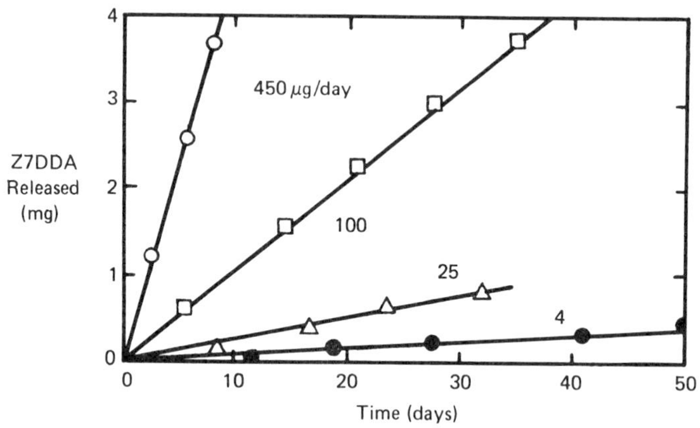

Figure 4 Release of cabbage looper pheromone from experimental BioLure dispensers.

CONTROLLED RELEASE DISPENSERS FOR MATING DISRUPTION

Pheromone dispensers with the same design as those described above can also be used for mating distruption by releasing the pheromone at a higher rate than would be used for attraction. Such a dispenser was designed to release a mimic of the corn earworm pheromone at a rate of 230 μg/day for a disruption study in sweet corn in Florida. The constant release rate of the pheromone mimic, (Z)-9-tetradecenyl formate (Z9TDF), from these dispensers is shown in Fig. 5. These dispensers were placed on the corn plants at two different spacing intervals (1 m and 2 m), and the disruption was monitored with a female-insect-baited trap over a 40-day period prior to harvest. As shown in Fig. 6, 98.6-100% disruption was achieved over the entire period, which indicates excellent potential for protection of the crop [8].

MICROCAPSULE FORMULATIONS

Such hand-applied dispensers may be feasible for use in some cases for disruption, but for most crops aerial broadcast application is more economical. There are several types of sprayable formulations currently available or under development, including hollow fibers, laminated flakes, and microcapsules. Of these, only microcapsules can be sprayed with conventional equipment and have the capability of exhibiting a constant release rate. Because of this, we have under development microcapsule formulations of pheromones for mating disruption.

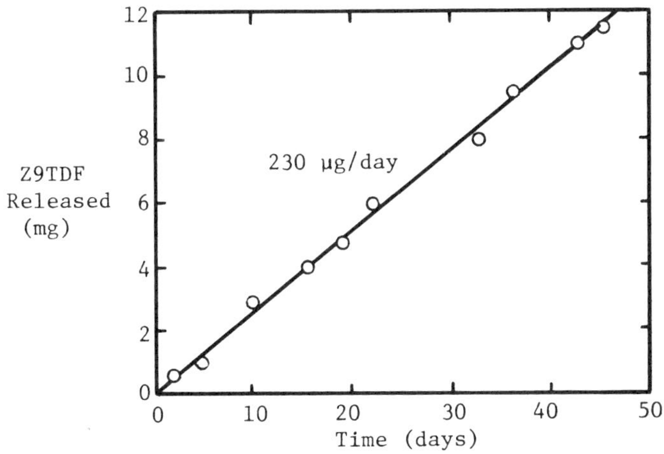

Figure 5 Release of corn earworm pheromone mimic (Z9TDF) from BioLure controlled release dispensers.

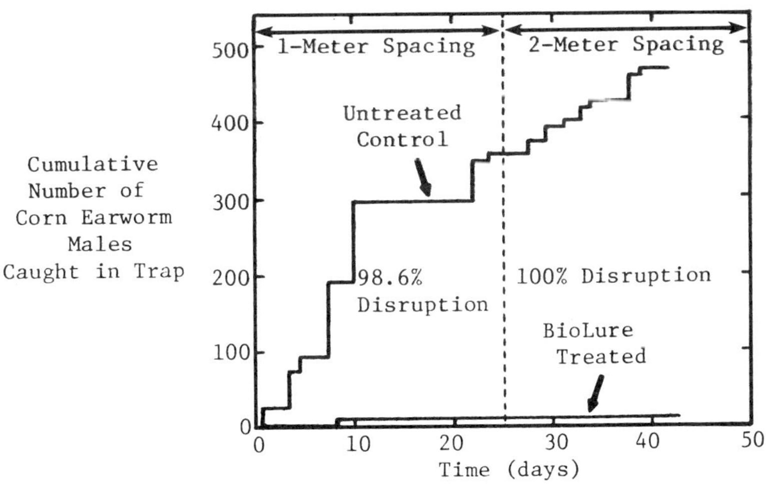

Figure 6 Disruption of pheromone communication in corn earworm with BioLure controlled release dispensers.

The theory of pheromone release from microcapsules is straightforward, and can be summarized by

$$\frac{dM}{dt} = 4\pi DS \frac{r_o r_i}{r_o - r_i} \tag{5}$$

where r_o is the outside radius of the microcapsule wall, and r_i is the inside radius [2]. As in the case of the pheromone dispensers, the pheromone release rate should remain constant as long as pure pheromone remains in the interior. In practice, the release rate from a large quantity of microcapsules is usually not constant, because of variations in microcapsule wall thickness. Shown in Fig. 7 are representative experimental microcapsules containing (E)-9-dodecenyl acetate, the European pine shoot moth pheromone. The range of microcapsule diameters in this sample was from about 80 μm to about 150 μm.

Obtaining a sufficient duration of pheromone release has been a problem with microcapsule formulations reported in the literature [9]. Depending on the insect and host crop, the optimum duration of release can be from about 3 weeks to greater than 10 weeks for mating disruption. Many microcapsule formulations, as well as hollow fibers and flakes, exhibit a much shorter duration, in some cases less than

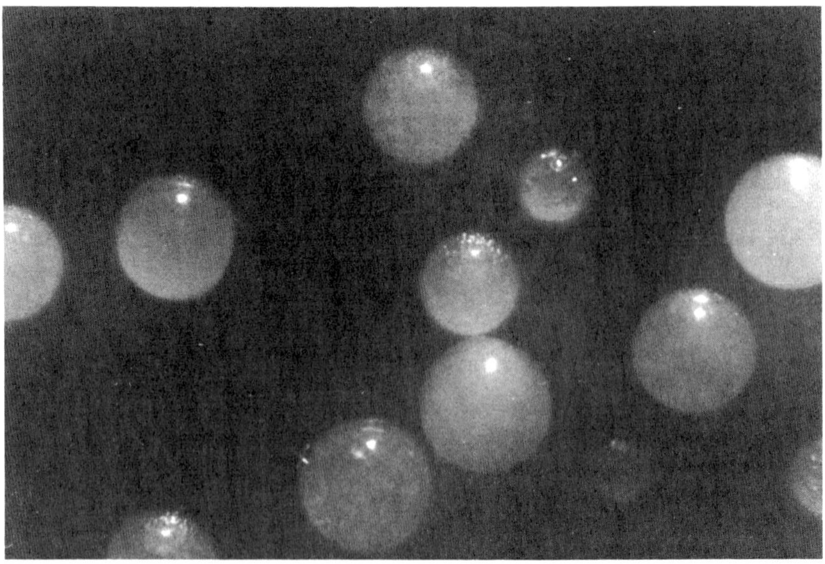

Figure 7 Photomicrograph of microcapsules containing insect pheromones for mating disruption.

2 weeks. By producing microcapsules with walls of low-permeability polymers, we have obtained release durations in excess of 6 weeks. Shown in Fig. 8-10 are release-rate curves of (Z)-9-tetradecenyl acetate (Z9TDA), gossyplure, and disparlure, respectively, from microcapsule formulations. These release rates were not constant over

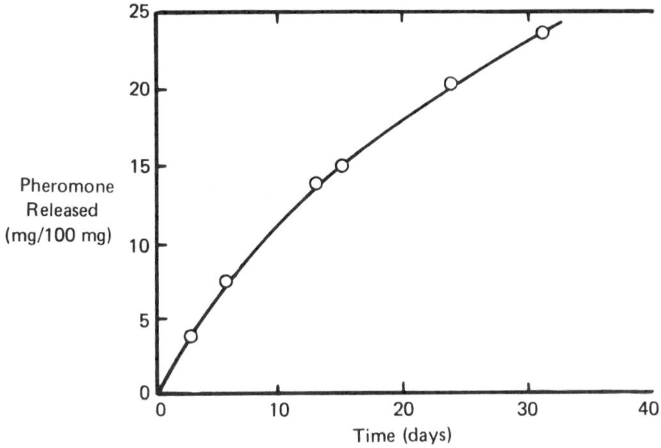

Figure 8 Release of (Z)-9-tetradecenyl acetate from BioLure microcapsules.

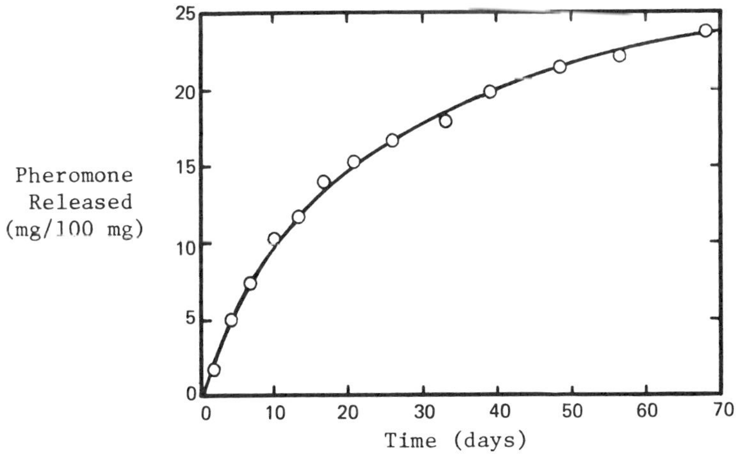

Figure 9 Release of gossyplure from BioLure microcapsules.

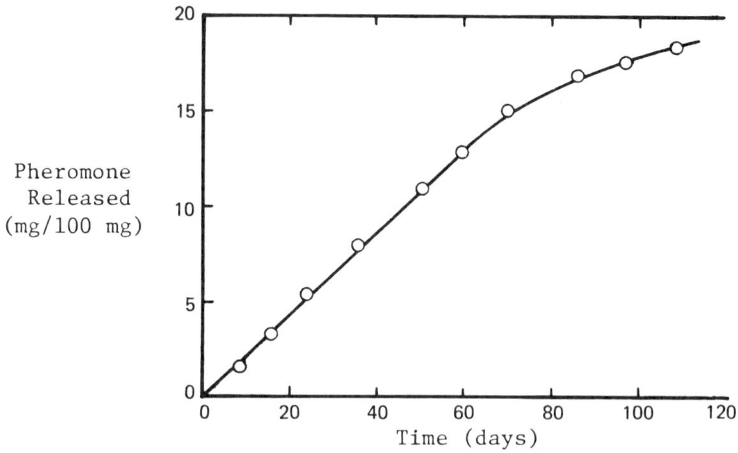

Figure 10 Release of disparlure from BioLure microcapsules.

the entire duration of release, probably due to a range of microcapsule sizes. However, they were reasonably constant, and the microcapsules exhibited prolonged release durations of about 5, 10, and 15 weeks for Z9TDA, gossyplure, and disparlure, respectively. Similar results have been obtained for several other pheromones and attractants. Of course, the release rates and release durations are dependent on temperature and perhaps other environmental conditions, but optimum release behavior for given conditions can be adjusted by varying the microcapsule radii and wall composition.

REFERENCES

1. W. L. Roelofs, *J. Chem. Ecol.*, *4*:685 (1978).
2. R. W. Baker and H. K. Lonsdale, Controlled release: mechanisms and rates, in *Controlled Release of Biologically Active Agents* (A. C. Tanquary and R. E. Lacey, eds.), Plenum Press, New York, 1974, pp. 15-71.
3. T. W. Brooks, Controlled vapor release from hollow fibers: theory and applications with insect pheromones, in *Controlled Release Technologies: Methods, Theory, and Applications*, Vol. 2 (A. F. Kydonieus, ed.), CRC Press, Boca Raton, Fla., 1980.
4. G. E. Daterman, USDA For. Serv. Res. Pap. PNW-180, Portland, Ore., 1974.
5. S. T. Hwang, C. K. Choi, and K. Kammermeyer, *Sep. Sci.*, *9*:461 (1974).

6. H. J. Bixler and O. J. Sweeting, Barrier properties of polymer films, in *The Science and Technology of Polymer Films*, Vol. 2 (O. J. Sweeting, ed.), Wiley-Interscience, New York, 1971, p. 85.
7. R. S. Kaae, H. H. Shorey, and L. K. Gaston, *Science, 179*:487 (1973).
8. E. R. Mitchell and J. H. Cross, USDA, Gainesville, Fla., personal communication.
9. D. G. Campion, R. Lester, and B. F. Nesbitt, *Pestic. Sci.*, *9*:434 (1978).

Chapter 22

Environmental Effects on Long-Term Antifouling Systems

NADIM A. GHANEM College of Engineering, King Saud University, Riyad, Saudi Arabia

MOUNIR M. ABD EL-MALEK and MAGDY H. AYOUB National Research Centre, Dokki, Cairo, Egypt

The subject of antifouling coatings continues to be a matter of great challenge to the polymer chemist, coatings engineer, toxicologist, and marine ecologist. While the need is pressing for protecting the hull from attachment and growth of fouling for extended periods, there are increasing demands for keeping the waters and sediments of commercial harbors and canals clean [1]. These are two contradicting tasks which pose the challenge.

First, protection of the hull while maintaining unpolluted waters and sediments was accomplished by designing antifouling compositions with no toxicity. Trends along this line were summarized together with our own laboratory and environmental investigations; they showed that nontoxic antifouling coatings are attainable [2] and further work has to be done in order to obtain the desired longevity of action. Second, protection of the hull for long periods, irrespective of ecology requirements, was the subject of even greater concern. For example, with the most popular antifouling coatings, those based on cuprous oxide as the toxin, protection for longer times was achieved through scrubbing the film with wire brushes. This was done after use to expose the remaining stored toxin. Another recent attempt was to include a biochemical ingredient which was claimed [3] to extend copper activity for a longer period. Poisoning the sulfate-reducing bacteria prevents the action of oxide in store, and thereby prevents the formation of insoluble copper sulfide. Our earlier studies in connection with increasing the effective life of the coating dealt with the effect of (1) rosin as a seawater-soluble pore-promoting ingredient [4], (2) the chemical nature of the pasticizer [5], and (3) the content of cuprous oxide [6]. These studies were performed in the laboratory, and throughout the year in regions of high fouling intensity [7,8]. It was shown that 13 months was the maximum protection period in raft testing of antifouling coatings prepared with cuprous oxide as the sole toxin.

In the present work, an attempt to increase the effective protection period was performed with two binder mixtures which interact differently with the seawater environment. All other ingredients were maintained constant and were reduced to the minimum required for a true antifouling paint. The condition of the film was examined at regular intervals to determine the implication of the different interactions of the binder mixture with seawater and the antifouling effectiveness of the whole film after long periods of exposure to the marine environment.

It is noteworthy that cuprous oxide was the only pigment used in this series of compositions. It acted as its own extender and filler in addition to being the toxic ingredient, and was used at the highest tolerable ratio, about 81.5% by weight (equal to about 46% by volume). This ratio was kept constant in all the compositions tested and thus the comparison is entirely between the two binder mixtures.

Rosin, a natural resin composed mainly of abietic acid, is invariably used in antifouling formulations. It dissolves slowly in seawater, which is usually slightly basic. To determine its role as a supporting resin to the two binder mixtures under investigation, it was used in three different proportions with each binder mixture (thus expanding the number of compositions to six). These compositions are given in Table 1.

MATERIALS AND METHODS

Materials

Resin 1 is a copolymer of vinyl chloride and vinyl isobutyl ether,* and plasticizer 1 is poly(vinyl methyl ether).* Resin 1 and plasticizer 1 constitute the insoluble portion of the binder constituents in compositions I, II, and III. Plasticizer 1, although soluble in water, was found insoluble when used in conjunction with resin 1 [9]. Compositions I, II, and III thus become swellable in water by the aid of the highly flexible ether bonds in both resin 1 and plasticizer 1. The only soluble ingredient is rosin.

*BASF Company AG, Ludwigshafen, West Germany.

Table 1 Antifouling Compositions with Fixed Cuprous Oxide Contents and Varying Binder Mixtures

Ingredient (wt %)	Composition number					
	I	II	III	IV	V	VI
Resin 1	10.40	8.10	3.10	–	–	–
Plasticizer 1	4.50	2.90	2.80	–	–	–
Resin 2	–	–	–	10.40	8.10	3.10
Plasticizer 2	–	–	–	4.50	2.90	2.80
Rosin ww	4.20	8.10	12.20	4.20	8.10	12.20
Cuprous oxide	80.90	80.90	81.90	80.90	80.90	81.90
Additives	0.10	0.10	0.10	0.10	0.10	0.10
Pigment/binder (wt)	4.2:1	4.2:1	4.3:1	4.2:1	4.2:1	4.3:1
Cu_2O (vol %)	45.80	45.33	46.21	46.69	45.99	46.25
Rosin in binder (wt %)	22.00	42.00	67.00	22.00	42.00	67.00

Resin 2 is a copolymer of vinyl chloride and vinyl acetate*, and plasticizer 2 is tricresyl phosphate, recommended for use in conjunction with resin 2. Cuprous oxide was of pigment-grade micronized quality.† Rosin was of the water-white (ww) grade.

Resin 2 and plasticizer 2 constitute the insoluble portion of the binder constituent in compositions IV, V, and VI. Both resin 2 and plasticizer 2 are slowly hydrolyzable in seawater (pH 8.1-8.5) through cleavage of the ester linkages. Hydrolysis of resin 2 leaves behind polyol segments

$$\left(CH_2-\underset{\displaystyle Cl}{\underset{|}{CH}}-CH_2-\underset{\displaystyle OH}{\underset{|}{CH}} \right)_n$$

which may contribute to the dissolution of the whole macromolecule. Hydrolysis of plasticizer 2 in seawater gives the soluble phosphoric acid and cresols.

*The Union Carbide Company, New York, New York.
†The Nordox Company, Norway.

Methods

Methods of paint and panel preparation for testing in the laboratory and in the raft have been described in detail [5-7]. The glycine test was utilized as an accelerated screening test method for preliminary determination of the effectiveness of new antifouling compositions. The test depends on immersing a small painted panel in an alkaline sodium chloride solution (pH 10.5) of sodium glycinate under specified conditions for a predetermined period of time [10]. When greater than 1 mg of copper/cm^2 leaches from the surface in 3 days without visual erosion of the film, the film is considered suitable for further testing.

The acid/alkali test provides another rapid test for selection of new antifouling compositions suitable for further testing [11]. The test depends upon two successive extractions of the paint film. The first is in seawater acidified to pH 4 with hydrochloric acid and the second is in distilled water adjusted to pH 10.5 with sodium hydroxide. The copper leaching rate is determined after each extraction. Acid extraction removes surface copper and alkali extraction removes surface rosin.

The normal laboratory leaching rate test simulates the paint film in a testing raft with no temperature fluctuations, living organisms, silt, currents, tides, and so on. It is performed for the period of time required for effective performance of the coating in actual practice, which is at least 1 year. The test depends on measuring periodically the amount of copper leached out of the film in $\mu g/cm^2$ per day. A release rate of at least 10 μg Cu/cm^2 per day is considered to be effective in repelling fouling organisms and hence their settling and growth [12].

All copper determinations were performed spectrophotometrically using a modified preparation of sodium diethyldithiocarbamate as a complexing agent under standardized conditions [13]. Next to the ultimate actual performance of a ship on duty, raft testing is considered the best test for effectivity of a new antifouling composition. The testing raft [7] floating in the eastern harbor of Alexandria was employed for the present series of experiments. This site is one of the most fouling intensive locations in the whole world [14].

RESULTS AND DISCUSSION

The six compositions prepared are given in Table 1. Compositions I, II, and III were prepared with resin 1 and plasticizer 1, while compositions IV, V, and VI were prepared with resin 2 and plasticizer 2 (see the materials section). Compositions I and IV have the same low rosin content, while compositions II and V, and compositions III and VI, have medium and high rosin contents, respectively.

Typical results of the glycine test are summarized in Table 2. The amount of copper released from each composition and the physical

Table 2 Glycine Test Results

Composition number	Resin, plasticizer	Glycine acc. test ($mg\ Cu/cm^2/3$ days)
I	1,1	2.331
IV	2,2	3.593
III	1,1	4.226
VI	2,2	4.592

integrity of the films after the test indicate that all films are good candidates for further testing. However, it may be predicted that compositions IV and VI, prepared with resin 2 and plasticizer 2, may be consumed earlier because they release copper faster than corresponding compositions I and III prepared with resin 1 and plasticizer 1. Also, as expected, compositions III and VI prepared with high rosin release more copper than I and IV prepared with low rosin and hence may be depleted more rapidly in actual practice.

The results of the acid-alkali test are given in Table 3. In view of the reasonable leaching rates both after the acid and alkali extractions and the physical integrity of the films, all compositions can be recommended for further testing. The results show that the leaching rates of composition I is somewhat greater than its counterpart IV, and release from composition III is greater than composition VI both after acid and after alkali extractions. Therefore, compositions I and III should last longer than compositions IV and VI, respectively, before

Table 3 Normal Leaching Rates (L.R.) After Acid and Alkali Extractions

Composition number	Resin, plasticizer	L.R. ($\mu g/cm^2/day$) after extraction with:	
		Acid	Alkali
I	1,1	19.23	25.85
IV	2,2	17.23	19.61
III	1,1	47.20	57.82
VI	2,2	43.46	47.20

they (compositions I and III) reach the minimum effective leaching rate of 10 μg/cm^2 per day. It cannot be concluded from the instantaneous test, however, that compositions III and VI, prepared with a high rosin content, would last longer than compositions I and IV, prepared with a low rosin concentration. A normal laboratory leaching rate test over an extended period of time was used to verify this result.

The normal laboratory leaching rate test was performed for a period of 1 year and the results are summarized in Figs. 1 and 2. All compositions gave leaching rates well above the optimal of 10 μg/cm^2 per day of copper. However, it is obvious that composition I is more slowly depleted than its counterpart composition IV, which means that it should last longer. This, however, does not apply as readily when comparing compositions III with VI, probably in view of their elevated rosin content, which is manifested in the very high leaching rates during the initial period of immersion (see Fig. 2). Such high rates would deplete the copper and hence the lifetime of the film would be reduced.

The appearance of the coatings after immersion in the testing raft for increasing periods of time was recorded photographically. Figures 3 and 4 represent the appearance of two stands carrying panels coated with compositions I to VI after 405 days (13-1/2 months) and 436 days (14-1/2 months) of immersion in the testing raft located in Alexandria

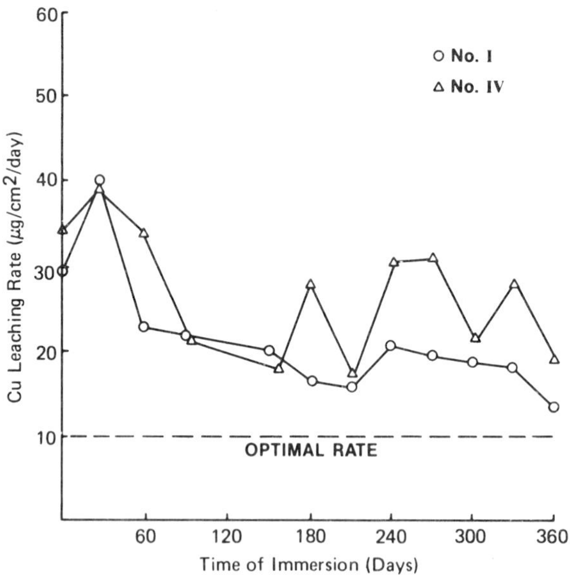

Figure 1 Normal leaching rates of compositions I and IV.

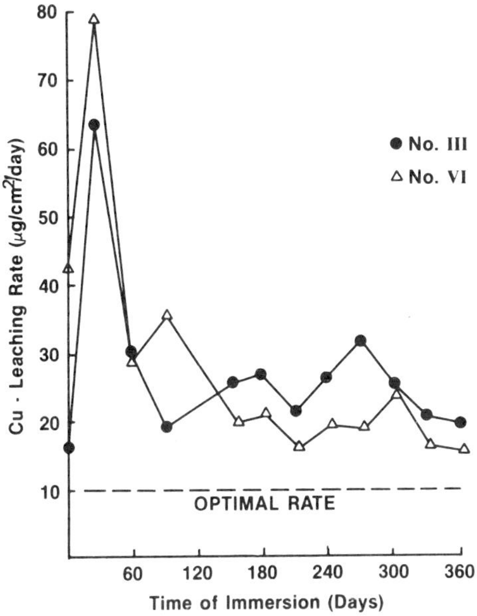

Figure 2 Normal leaching rates of compositions III and VI.

harbor [7] All panels were painted face and back in duplicate, resulting in four film surfaces for examination with each composition. Additionally, panels bearing compositions I and VI were placed in each stand for double checking.

It is evident from the pictures that composition VI had exhausted both its copper and its protecting power much earlier than the others; its high rosin content and the hydrolyzable nature of the resin and plasticizer must have been the reason for the limited protection. Compositions V and IV follow in the scale of short-time effectivity. Both are prepared with a hydrolyzable binder but have lower rosin contents (see Table 1).

In contrast, compositions I, II, and III, prepared with the nonhydrolyzable binder mixture, resist fouling more effectively, and it is hard to distinguish their effectiveness. It is concluded that resin 1 with plasticizer 1 makes a better combination for long-term protection even when a high rosin content is included. The latter point is important from the commercial point of view since rosin is a much cheaper constituent than the insoluble part of the binder mixture.

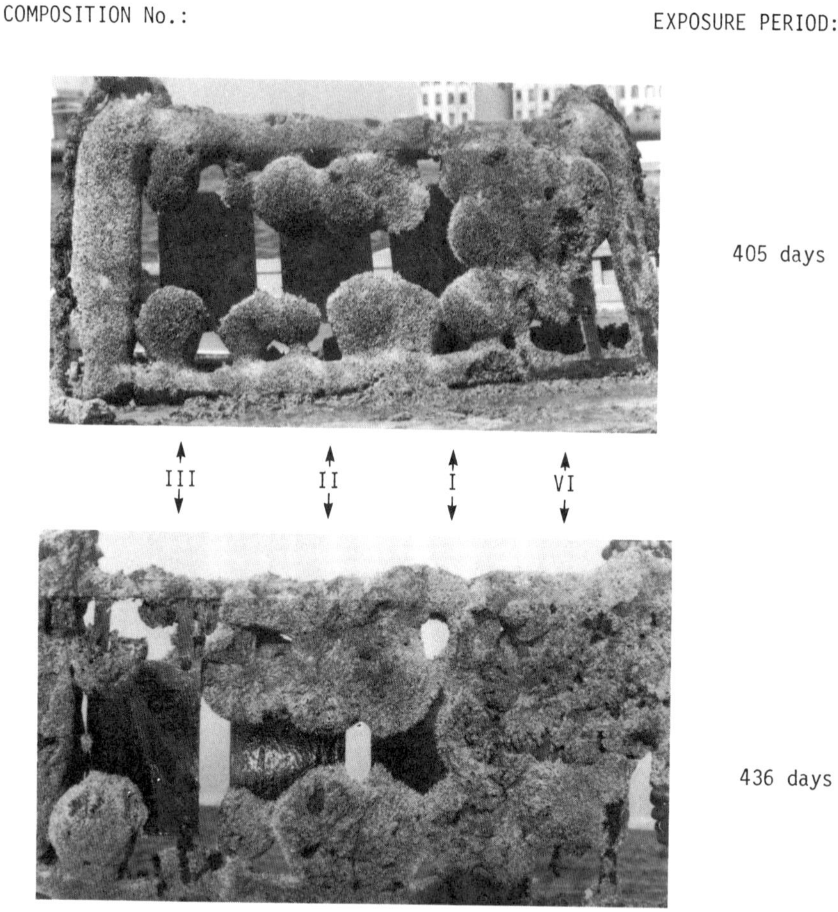

Figure 3 Antifouling compositions I, II, III, and VI after 405 days and 436 days of raft testing in Alexandria harbor.

SUMMARY AND CONCLUSIONS

In regions of temperate waters, relatively higher salinity, and high fouling intensity, such as those encountered in the Mediterranean Sea and Red Sea harbors, antifouling coatings based on cuprous oxide must fulfill certain requirements in order to give protection periods exceeding 1 year. It has been shown that besides a high content of a fine grade of cuprous oxide and a moderate amount of rosin, only special binders and plasticizers can achieve this goal. These polymeric

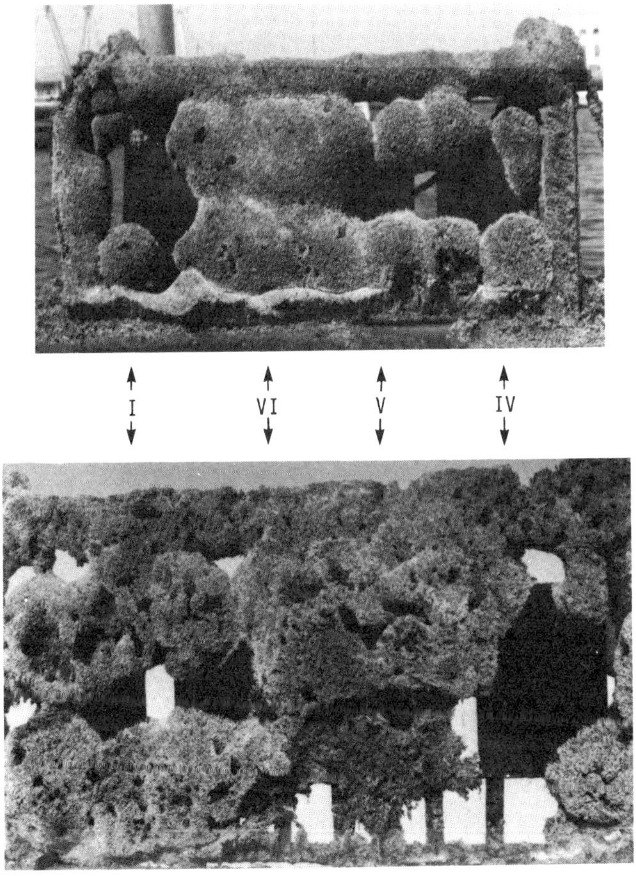

Figure 4 Antifouling compositions IV, V, VI, and I after 405 days and 436 days of raft testing in Alexandria harbor.

materials are insoluble but swellable and wettable enough to keep the copper active in the film and provide more uniform release rates in the sea. Resin 1 and plasticizer 1, both containing flexible ether linkages, are examples of materials that complement each other and provide a good binder for antifouling coatings for long-term effectiveness.

REFERENCES

1. N. A. Ghanem, *Proc. 15th FATIPEC Congr.*, Vol. 1, Amsterdam, June 8-13, 1980, pp. 212-243.
2. N. A. Ghanem, N. H. El-Awady, M. M. El-Awady, and W. S. El-Hamouly, *J. Coatings Technol.*, in press (1982).
3. D. Tinsley, *Fairplay Int. Shipping Wkly*, *31*:20 (July 1980).
4. M. M. Abd El-Malek and N. A. Ghanem, *Proc. 4th Int. Congr. Mar. Corrosion-Fouling*, Juan-les-Pins, France, June 1976, Vol. 33 (1977). (Published by CREO, Boulogne, France.)
5. N. A. Ghanem, M. M. Abd El-Malek, M. A. Abou-Khalil, and M. M. El-Awady, *Ind. Eng. Chem. Product Res. Dev.*, *17*:44 (1978).
6. N. A. Ghanem and M. M. Abd El-Malek, *J. Coatings Technol.*, *50*(645):60 (1978).
7. M. M. Abd El-Malek and N. A. Ghanem, *J. Paint Technol.*, *47*(608):75 (1975).
8. A. F. A. Ghobashy, M. M. El-Komy, and Sh. M. Ramadan, *Proc. 5th Int. Congr. Mar. Corrosion-Fouling*, Barcelona, Spain, May 1980.
9. N. A. Ghanem, M. M. Abd El-Malek, and N. A. Rizk, to be Published.
10. Z. Hippe, A. Jedlenski, J. Korat, and K. Uhorez, *J. Oil Colour Chem. Assoc.*, *45*:653 (1962).
11. F. M. Marson, *J. Oil Colour Chem. Assoc.*, *47*:323 (1964).
12. Woods Hole Oceanographic Institution, *Marine Fouling and Its Prevention*, U.S. Naval Institute, Annapolis, Md., 1952.
13. N. A. Ghanem and M. M. Abd El-Malek, *J. Chem., EGYPT Arab Rep.*, *9*(3):377 (1966).
14. A. H. Megally, M.Sc. thesis, University of Alexandria, 1970.

Chapter 23

Bioactive Polymer-Wood Composites

ROGER M. ROWELL United States Department of Agriculture, Forest Products Laboratory, Madison, Wisconsin

Wood is a three-dimensional polymeric composite comprised primarily of cellulose, hemicellulose, and lignin. These polymers make up the cell wall and are responsible for most of the physical and chemical properties exhibited by wood. Wood can also be considered as a substrate for further chemical composite formations. Basically, two types of composites can be formed with wood: monomer or polymer grafting to reactive groups on the cell wall polymers and nongrafted bulk polymer formation in the void structure of wood.

Compounds bonded or grafted to cell wall polymers can be biologically active. For this discussion, a bioactive chemical will be broadly defined as any chemical that inhibits wood degradation by organisms. By this definition these chemicals would not necessarily be toxic to the organisms, but in this study chemicals used were known to be toxic to wood-attacking organisms in the free state and the mechanism of effectiveness was probably due to toxicity. It is possible that the chemicals are toxic while still bound to the cell wall but the toxicity is more likely due to release of the chemical into the surrounding wood structure.

Filling the voids in wood with bulk polymers containing bioactive compounds grafted onto or copolymerized with carrier polymers would inhibit attack in the same way as would bioactive materials grafted onto wood. The Forest Products Laboratory has had an active research program in both wood cell wall grafting and wood lumen polymer-filling technologies for several years. This chapter concerns part of the research done in the area of lumen polymer-filling technology.

BACKGROUND

The voids in wood, mainly lumens, can hold a considerable amount of chemicals. In southern pine earlywood, for example, with a density of 0.33 g/cm^3, the void volume is 0.77 cm^3/cm^3 (2.3 cm^3/g). Latewood, with a density of 0.70 g/cm^3, has a void volume of 0.52 cm^3/cm^3 (0.74 cm^3/g). Filling the void structure of wood with a monomer, followed by polymerization, results in a wood-polymer composite in which there is no attachment between the bulk polymer and the cell wall.

Most of the work done at this Laboratory has been with methyl methacrylate (MMA) as the bulk polymer.

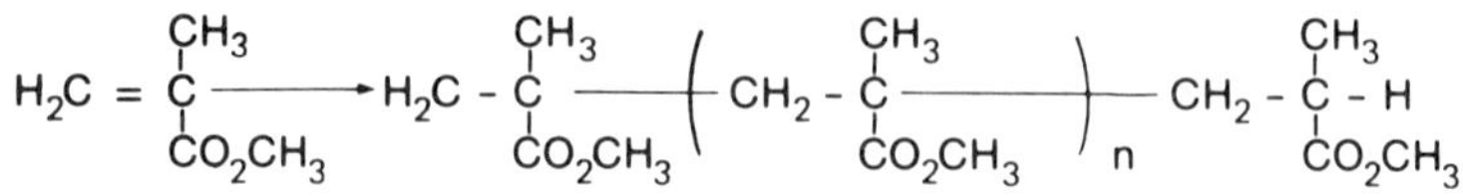

Methacrylate and acrylate esters other than the methyl can be synthesized. Bioactive materials can be esterified onto acryloyl or methacryloyl chlorides or acrylic or methacrylic acids, and these substituted monomers can be incorporated in a treating solution with methyl methacrylate as the main carrier monomer.

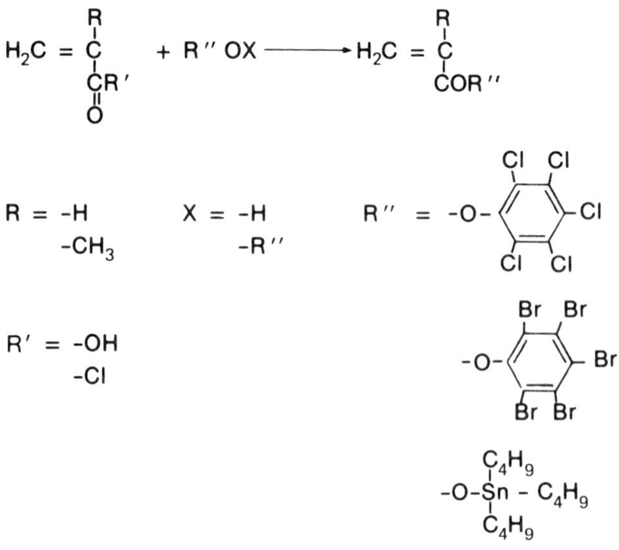

Wood can be impregnated with MMA monomer containing an acrylate or methacrylate bioactive ester using a vacuum method [1,2]. The monomers are then copolymerized in an oven at 60°C, where a free-radical catalyst initiates the reaction. Weight gains of over 100%

polymer add-on are possible. Autoradiography of tritium-labeled MMA (tritium on the methyl ester carbon) shows the bulk of the polymerized MMA to be located in the lumen and not in the cell wall [3].

Organotin acrylate and methacrylate esters have been polymerized in wood [4] and have been found to be effective preservatives [5]. Biocidal methacrylates have also been applied in the form of surface films and found to be effective antifouling materials [6-8].

Treatment of wood that results in methacrylate bulk polymers in the void structure has several advantages. At high polymer loading the diffusion coefficient is greatly reduced, which means that even though little or no dimensional stability is achieved by the treatment, there is a greatly restricted rate of moisture pickup [9]. There is an increase in modulus of elasticity and rupture, higher fiber stress of proportional limit, higher work to maximum load, higher maximum crushing strength, and a greatly increased hardness index over untreated wood [9,10].

Even though the mechanical properties are greatly increased with methacrylate treatments, the disadvantages are the high weight increase in the treated wood and the high cost of the treatment. Even so, treatment of wood with MMA in combination with slow-release bioactive chemicals attached may find application in marine structures because of the improved mechanical properties and resistance to marine organism attack.

This chapter reports on the results of the synthesis of acrylate and methacrylate esters of pentachlorophenol, pentabromophenol, and tributyltin oxide, subsequent treatment of southern pine with these bioactive monomers incorporated into a methyl methacrylate-treating system, and biological testing of the resulting treated wood.

MATERIALS AND METHODS

Synthesis of Acrylate and Methacrylate Monomers

Pentachlorophenol Acrylate (PCPA) Into a two-neck round-bottom flask (250 ml) was placed 100 ml of dry chloroform, 13.3 g (0.05 mol) of pentachlorophenol (PCP), and 8.5 ml (0.06 mol) of triethylamine (TEA). To this was added, dropwise, 5.0 ml (0.06 mol) of acryloyl chloride with stirring. The rate of addition was such that the temperature did not exceed 35°C. After all the acryloyl chloride had been added, the solution was stirred for an additional hour at room temperature. The chloroform solution was then added to 750 ml of ice water, stirred, and the chloroform layer separated. The chloroform solution was washed twice with water, separated, and dried over sodium sulfate. The chloroform was removed under water aspiration at 50°C and the resulting solid dissolved in hot ethyl ether. Upon cooling, white crystals (9.2 g) were obtained (mp 81°C; 58%). Thin layer chromatography

(TLC) on silica-gel-coated TLC sheets in a solvent system of hexane/chloroform (1:1 v/v) showed an R_f of 0.74 for PCPA and R_{PCP} of 3.1. The R_f of PCP is 0.25. Location of compounds on TLC plates was determined under short-wave ultraviolet (UV) light. A second crop of crystals was obtained by concentrating the mother liquor from the first crystallization and redissolving in a small amount of hot ether. Upon cooling, 3.1 g of additional PCPA was isolated. Total yield was 12.3 g (theoretical 16.0 g) or 77%.

It should be noted that in the literature [11] benzene is used as a solvent in this reaction. With benzene, upon addition of the acryloyl chloride, a white precipitate occurs which forms a gel and is very hard to stir. The precipitate is triethylamine hydrochloride, which can be filtered after the reaction is complete. This does not occur in chloroform, making this the preferred solvent. The literature reports [11] that after recrystallization of a brownish solid from ethyl ether a waxy white solid (mp 58°C) was obtained. This melting point is considerably lower than that obtained in these experiments.

Pentachlorophenol Methacrylate (PCPM) The same procedure was used as for PCPA except that 6 ml of methacryloyl chloride was added to the PCP and TEA in chloroform at such a rate that the temperature did not exceed 40°C. After isolation as before, drying over sodium sulfate, removal of chloroform under water aspiration, dissolving in hot ethyl ether, and cooling, 12.9 g (theoretical 16.7 g) or 77% of white crystalline PCPM was obtained with a melting point of 90-91°C. TLC showed an R_f of 0.74 and an R_{PCP} of 3.1. There was minor unknown by-product with an R_f of 0.63. Recrystallization removed this contaminate.

Pentabromophenol Acrylate (PBPA) The same procedure was used as for PCPA except 24.4 g of pentabromophenol (PBP) and 5 ml of acryloyl chloride was used. The PBP is not as soluble as PCP in the chloroform/TEA solution. Stirring until solution was achieved was done before the acryloyl chloride was added. Concentration of the isolated chloroform solution gave a white solid which was dissolved in hot ethyl ether. Cooling yielded white crystalline PBPA 19.8 g (theoretical 27.1 g) or 81.4% (mp 150-151°C). TLC showed an R_f of 0.64, an R_{PBP} of 1.9 with an R_f for the PBP of 0.34.

Pentabromophenol Methacrylate (PBPM) The same procedure was used for PCPA except that 24.4 g of PBP and 6 ml of methacryloyl chloride were used. Stirring until solution was achieved was done before the methacryloyl chloride was added. The isolated chloroform solution was dark orange in color and was dried over sodium sulfate and decolorized with charcoal. Concentration to dryness, dissolving in a large amount of hot ethyl ether, and cooling gave 19.8 g (theoretical 27.8) or 71% of PBPM as a white crystalline material (mp 140-141°C). Thin-layer chromatography (TLC) of PBPM gave an R_f of 0.67 and an R_{PBP} of 2.1. There was a minor by-product with an R_f of 0.54. Recrystallization removed this contaminant.

Tri-n-Butyltin Acrylate (TBTOA) This procedure is a modification of the methods of Montermosa [12] and Mendoza [13]. Acrylic acid, 4.8 g (4.6 ml, 0.034 mol) was added to a solution of 20 g (17.1 ml, 0.034 mol) of tri-n-butyltin oxide (TBTO) dissolved in 50 ml of carbon tetrachloride. The mixture was refluxed for 3 hr. The by-product water was removed from the solution with sodium sulfate. The carbon tetrachloride was removed under water aspiration, yielding 25 g of a semicrystalline solid. Dissolution of the solid in hot hexane followed by cooling and filtration yielded 7.8 g of a white crystalline material (TBTOA) with a melting point of 69-71°C. Reconcentration of the hexane mother liquor yielded a second crop of crystals (6.9 g) to give a total yield of 14.7 g (theoretical 24.2) or 60.7%. Recrystallization from hot hexane gave needlelike crystals of the pure monomer (mp 74°C; lit. mp 74° [14]).

Tri-n-Butyltin Methacrylate (TBTOM) This procedure is a modification of the methods reported earlier [12,13]. Acryloyl chloride, 5.8 g (5.7 ml, 0.034 mol), was added to a solution of 20 g (17.1 ml, 0.034 mol) of TBTO dissolved in 60 ml of carbon tetrachloride cooled at 5°C at such a rate that the temperature did not go over 30°C. The temperature was then maintained at 30°C for 3 hr. By-product water was removed using sodium sulfate. Carbon tetrachloride was removed under water aspiration. The semicrystalline syrup was dissolved in hot carbon tetrachloride and cooled to -15°C and crystallization occurred. The mother liquor was separated by decantation and the crystals washed with cold carbon tetrachloride. The needlelike crystals were recrystallized from hot carbon tetrachloride at -15°C to give 16.9 g (theoretical 25.2 g) or 67% of TBTOM (mp 18°C; lit. mp 18°C [14]).

Preparation of Treating Solutions

Pentachlorophenol Methacrylate (PCPM) Solution 1 (theoretical 6.62% Cl): PCPM (100 g) was dissolved in 400 ml of methyl methacrylate (MMA). To this solution was added 25 ml (5%) of trimethylol propane trimethacrylate (TMPT) as a crosslinking agent and 1.25 g (0.25%) of azobisisobutyronitrile (Vazo) catalyst. When this solution was cooled for storage, part of the PCPM precipitated from solution. Redissolution was achieved by stirring and warming to 25°C.

Solution 2 (theoretical 3.31% Cl): solution 1 (400 ml) was added to 400 ml MMA plus 20 ml TMPT and 1 g Vazo.

Solution 3 (theoretical 1.65% Cl): solution 2 (400 ml) was added to 400 ml MMA plus 20 ml TMPT and 1 g Vazo.

Pentabromophenol Methacrylate (PBPM) Solution 1 (theoretical 4.49% Br): PBPM (92 g) was dissolved in 800 ml MMA. To this was added 50 ml TMPT and 2.25 g Vazo. When this solution was cooled for storage, part of the PBPM precipitated from solution. Redissolution was achieved by stirring and warming to 25°C.

Solution 2 (theoretical 2.24% Br): solution 1 (400 ml) was mixed with 400 ml MMA plus 20 ml TMPT and 1 g Vazo.

Solution 3 (theoretical 1.12% Br): solution 2 (400 ml) was mixed with 400 ml MMA plus 20 ml TMPT and 1 g Vazo.

Solution 4 (theoretical 0.56% Br): solution 3 (400 ml) was mixed with 400 ml MMA plus 20 ml TMPT and 1 g Vazo.

Tributyltin Methacrylate (TBTOM) Solution 1 (theoretical 7.9% Sn): TBTOM (300 g) was dissolved in 600 ml MMA. To this was added 45 ml TMPT and 2.25 g Vazo catalyst.

Solution 2 (theoretical 3.95% Sn): solution 1 (400 ml) was mixed with 400 ml of MMA plus 20 ml TMPT and 1 g Vazo.

Solution 3 (theoretical 1.975% Sn): solution 2 (400 ml) was mixed with 400 ml of MMA plus 20 ml TMPT and 1 g Vazo.

Wood Treatments

Southern pine specimens to be treated (soil block samples 3/4 in. × 3/4 in. × 3/4 in.; marine specimens 1½ in. × 1/4 in. × 6 in., six to eight growth rings per inch) with MMA alone or with a bioactive methacrylate were placed in a treating chamber and the system evacuated for 1 hr. The selected methacrylate solution was poured into a separatory funnel and then admitted to the treating chamber until the solution covered the samples. A weight on top of the samples prevented them from floating in the solution. The vacuum was released and the chamber exposed to atmospheric pressure. The specimens continued to soak for 1 hr. They were then removed, wiped of excess monomer, immediately wrapped in aluminum foil, and placed in a chamber at 60°C for 18 hr to allow the monomer to polymerize. The foil was removed, the specimens scraped of excess surface polymer, oven dried, and weighed. Seven samples were treated with each of the solution levels. The highest and lowest weight gain specimens were ground to 40 mesh, combined, and submitted for either chlorine, bromine, or tin analysis.

Exposure Tests

Soil Block Standard soil block tests were run according to specifications as outlined in ASTM D 1413, "Standard Method of Testing Wood Preservatives by Laboratory Soil-Block Cultures" [15]. Southern pine blocks untreated (control) and treated with the MMA solutions to various weight percent gains (WPG) were placed in test with the brown-rot fungus *Gloeophyllum trabeum* (Pers. ex Fr.) Murr. (Madison 617). Specimens were removed after 12 weeks and the extent of decay determined on an oven-dry weight loss.

Marine Standard marine exposure tests were run according to specification as outlined in ASTM D 2481, "Standard Method of Accelerated Evaluation of Wood Preservatives for Marine Service by Means of Small-Size Specimens" [16]. Specimens untreated (control) and treated with the MMA solutions to various WPGs were placed in test in warm coastal Atlantic waters (Key West, Florida). Inspections were made semi-annually starting in January 1980. Marine borer attack on each panel was rated: 10, no more than trace attack; 9, light attack; 7, moderate attack; 4, heavy attack; and 0, destroyed by attack.

RESULTS AND DISCUSSION

The synthesis of acrylic and methacrylic acid esters of pentachlorophenol, pentabromophenol, and tri-n-butyltin oxide were straightforward, and all compounds were crystalline and easily purified (Table 1). Purity of the PCP and PBP esters was determined by using light to locate the compounds on the TLC plates. TBTO esters do not respond to UV light.

Because very little difference in biological activity would be expected between acrylate and methacrylate derivatives, the methaacrylate series was used to treat wood in a methyl methacrylate solvent system. Three different concentrations of PCPM, four different concentrations of PBPM, and three different concentrations of TBTOM were prepared in methyl methacrylate (Table 2).

No increase in wood volume occurred during treatment with the methacrylate solutions, which indicated that little or no cell wall penetration occurs. The monomer is contained in the voids, and in situ polymerization leaves the bulk polymer in the void structure of wood. Large variations in weight gain result from each treatment, as indicated by high standard deviations (Table 2). The highest and lowest weight gain samples were ground to 40 mesh, combined, and submitted for analysis for either chlorine, bromine, or tin (Table 2). X-ray analysis of these samples showed that the level of the element analyzed for was close to the theoretical amount of each element present in each solution.

Table 1 Yield and Melting Points of Acrylate and Methacrylate Monomers

	Acrylate		Methacrylate	
Bioactive compound	Yield (% of theoretical)	mp (C°)	Yield (% of theoretical)	mp (C°)
Pentachlorophenol (PCP)	77	81 (PCPA)	77	90-91 (PCPM)
Pentabromophenol (PBP)	81	150-151 (PBPA)	71	140-141 (PBPM)
Tributyltin oxide (TBTO)	61	74 (TBTOA)	67	18 (TBTOM)

Table 2 Characteristics of Southern Pine Specimens Treated with Bioactive Methacrylates

Treating solution[a]	Average weight gain[b] (%)	SD[c]	X-ray analysis[d] Cl (%)	Br (%)	Sn (%)
MMA	62.6	11.6	–	–	–
PCPM/MMA					
1:4	75.3	16.9	7.09	–	–
1:8	54.8	13.9	4.30	–	–
1:16	69.6	8.6	2.11	–	–
PBPM/MMA					
1:8	68.6	11.3	–	8.56	–
1:16	71.4	16.4	–	3.33	–
1:32	72.3	15.0	–	1.42	–
1:64	68.4	16.5	–	0.83	–
TBTOM/MMA					
1:2	84.8	27.5	–	–	5.82
1:4	73.9	18.6	–	–	2.61
1:8	68.1	11.4	–	–	1.30

[a]MMA, methyl methacrylate; PCPM, pentachlorophenol methacrylate; PBPM, pentabromophenol methacrylate; TBTOM, tributyltin oxide methacrylate.
[b]Average of all seven samples treated.
[c]Standard deviation.
[d]Analysis run on highest and lowest weight gain samples obtained from each treating solution. Value given is average of these two samples.

Twelve-week soil block tests of untreated specimens, MMA-treated specimens, and PCPM, PBPM, or TBTOM in combination with MMA show that, whereas the control lost 42% by weight during this test, the MMA-treated specimens lost less than half this amount (Table 3). All levels of MMA-PCPM and MMA-PBPM treatments are not significantly different from MMA alone, indicating that the resistance to biodegradation of the treated wood is probably due to restriction in moisture caused by the bulk polymer and not due to any release of the toxic chemical. The PCP and PBP esters seem to be stable under these conditions and do not release the active biocide. This is not the case with TBTOM. All levels of MMA-TBTOM were effective in preventing attack by the brown-rot fungus.

Table 3 Weight Loss of Bioactive Methacrylate-Treated Southern Pine in Soil Block Test with *Gloeophyllum trabeum*

Treatment[a]	Average weight gain (%)	Average weight loss[b] in 12 weeks (%)
Control	0	41.9
MMA	61.6	17.3
PCPM/MMA		
1:4	76.0	17.0
1:8	56.1	9.0
1:16	69.5	14.5
PBPM/MMA		
1:8	65.5	9.6
1:16	69.8	15.0
1:32	69.4	12.0
1:64	66.5	10.8
TBTOM/MMA		
1:2	86.0	0.1
1:4	72.9	0
1:8	69.1	0

[a]MMA, methyl methacrylate; PCPM, pentachlorophenol methacrylate; PBPM, pentabromophenol methacrylate; TBTOM, tributyltin oxide methacrylate.
[b]Ovendried basis.

Marine tests show that, after only 1 year, the control specimens were largely destroyed by limnoria and teredine borers (Table 4). Specimens containing the largest amount of PCPM and highest two amounts of PBPM show no attack, while light attack occurred on a few specimens at the lower two amounts of PCPM and PBPM. All levels of TBTOM are effective in preventing attack by marine organisms. MMA alone is somewhat effective in preventing attack but, under these conditions, is apparently not as effective as those MMA solutions that contain an active biocide ester. All of these specimens are still in test.

Future research in this area will be directed toward preparing wood treated to high levels of bioactive acrylates and methacrylates but at lower overall weight gains of bulk polymer.

Table 4 Rating of Samples of Bioactive Methacrylate-Treated Southern Pine in Marine Exposure

Treatment[a]	Average weight gain (%)	Number of samples rating[b]				
		10	9	7	4	0
Controls	0	–	–	2	–	11
MMA	80.3	3	2	–	–	–
PCPM/MMA						
1:4	80.5	5	–	–	–	–
1:8	83.5	4	1	–	–	–
1:16	81.3	4	1	–	–	–
PBPM/MMA						
1:8	82.7	5	–	–	–	–
1:16	87.1	5	–	–	–	–
1:32	82.8	4	1	–	–	–
1:64	77.3	3	2	–	–	–
TBTOM/MMA						
1:2	82.6	5	–	–	–	–
1:4	79.6	5	–	–	–	–
1:8	72.6	5	–	–	–	–

[a]MMP, methyl methacrylate; PCPM, pentachlorophenol methacrylate; PBPM, pentabromophenol methacrylate; TBTOM, tributyltin oxide methacrylate.

[b]Grading system for limnoria and teredine attack rating: 10, no more than trace attack; 9, light attack; 7, moderate attack; 4, heavy attack; 0, destroyed by attack.

REFERENCES

1. J. A. Meyer, *For. Prod. J.*, *15*(9):362 (1965).
2. J. A. Meyer, *Am. Chem. Soc. Symp. Ser.*, *43*:301 (1977).
3. T. K. Timmons, J. A. Meyer, and W. A. Côté, Jr., *Wood Sci.*, *4*(1):13 (1971).
4. B. K. Garg, J. Corredor, and R. V. Subramanian, *J. Macromol. Sci.-Chem.*, *A11*(9):1567 (1977).
5. R. V. Subramanian, J. A. Mendoza, and B. K. Garg, *Proc. 5th Int. Symp. Controlled Release Bioact. Mater.*, Gaithersburg, Md., August 1978, pp. 6.8-6.24.
6. F. W. Harris, *Proc. Symp. Controlled Release Pestic. Symp.*, University of Akron, Akron, Ohio, September 1976, pp. 1.33-1.43.

7. G. A. Stahl and C. U. Pittman, Jr., *Proc. Symp. Paint Res. Inst.*, *135*:62 (1977).
8. J. A. Montemarano and E. J. Dyckman, *Proc. Controlled Release Pestic. Symp.*, University of Akron, Akron, Ohio, September 1974, pp. 21.2-21.9.
9. R. M. Rowell, R. Moisuk, and J. A. Meyer, *Wood Sci.*, *15*(2): (1982).
10. J. E. Langwig, A. Meyer, and R. W. Davidson, *For. Prod. J.*, *18*(7):33 (1968).
11. C. U. Pittman, Jr., G. A. Stahl, and H. Winters, *J. Coatings Technol.*, *50*(636):49 (1978).
12. J. C. Montermosa, J. M. Andrews, and L. P. Marinelli, *J. Polym. Sci.*, *32*(125):523 (1958).
13. J. A. Mendoza, M.S. thesis, Washington State University, 1977.
14. V. N. Kotrelev, S. P. Kalinina, G. I. Kuznetsov, I. V. Laine, and A. I. Borisova, *Vysokomol. Soedin.*, *3*:1128 (1961).
15. American Society for Testing and Materials, ASTM Stand. Des. D 1413, Philadelphia, 1976.
16. American Society for Testing and Materials, ASTM Stand. Des. D 2481, Philadelphia, 1976.

Chapter 24

Bayluscide and Controlled Release Tin Formulations as Molluscicides and Larvicides

PONGPEN SA-NGUANKUL, E. S. UPATHAM, and NOUWARATH SUKHAPANTH Mahidol University, Bangkok, Thailand

MEDICAL IMPORTANCE

In Thailand, some common species of medically important snails are *Bithynia (Digoniostoma) siamensis siamensis*, *B.s. goniomphalos*, *B. funiculata*, *Indoplanorbis exustus*, and *Lymnaea (Radix) auricularia rubiginosa*.

B.s. siamensis, *B.s. goniomphalos*, and *B. funiculata* act as the first intermediate host of *Opisthorchis viverrini* in the central, northeastern, and northern parts of Thailand. Humans can acquire this liver fluke infection by eating improperly cooked cyprinoid fish contaminated with the fluke's metacercariae [1,2]. *I. exustus* is the intermediate host of *Schistosoma spindale*, the blood fluke of water buffaloes and cattle [3]. It can also act as the first and second intermediate hosts of *Hypodereum conoideum* and *Echinostoma* spp., the intestinal flukes of ducks [4] and rats and ducks [5,6], respectively, which can be transmitted to humans.

L.a. rubiginosa serves as intermediate hosts of a few flukes such as *S. incognitum*, the blood fluke of bandicoots and field rats [7], *Orientobilharzia harinasutai*, the blood fluke of water buffaloes [8], and *Trichobilharzia maegraithi*, the blood fluke of ducks [9]. In addition, it can act as the first intermediate host of *Fasciola* spp., the liver flukes of cattle and humans, and as the second intermediate hosts of *H. conoideum* [4] and *Echinostoma* spp. [5,6].

Some common species of medically important mosquitoes in Thailand are *Anopheles (Cellia) dirus*, *Aedes aegypti*, and *Culex quinquefasciatus*.

An. dirus is a carrier of *Plasmodium falciparum* which produces human malaria, especially in forest hill regions [10,11]. *Ae. aegypti* acts as the principal vector of dengue virus and chikungunya virus which causes hemorrhagic fever infections in urban and rural populations [12]. *C. quinquefasciatus* is the major vector of Bancroftian filariasis in the Oriental Region [13].

This chapter reports the results of laboratory testing of Bayluscide versus controlled release formulations of bis(tri-n-butyltin) oxide and tributyltin fluoride on the snails *B.s. siamensis*, *I. exustus*, and *L.a. rubiginosa*, and on the mosquito larvae of *An. dirus*, *Ae. aegypti*, and *C. quinquefasciatus*.

MATERIALS AND METHODS

Molluscicides

Bayluscide Bayluscide (Bayer 6076) is the ethanolamine salt of 5,2-dichloro-4-nitrosalicylanilide in the form of an emulsifiable concentrate (25% active ingredient) which is produced by Bayer Company, Leverkusen, West Germany.

Organotin Compounds The commercial organotin molluscicide formulations evaluated against snails and mosquito larvae were BioMet SRM and CBL-9B. BioMet SRM is 6% bis(tri-n-butyltin) oxide (TBTO). It was formulated in natural, sinking rubber pellets manufactured by M & T Chemicals, Rahway, New Jersey. CBL-9B is 20% tributyltin fluoride (TBTF). It was formulated in natural, floating rubber pellets manufactured by the Creative Biology Laboratory, Barberton, Ohio.

Experimental Animals

Snails The snails used in this study were adult *Bithynia (Digoniostoma) siamensis siamensis* (size: 7-9 mm), *Indoplanorbis exustus* (10-12 mm), and *Lymnaea (Radix) auricularia rubiginosa* (10-12 mm). They were collected in the field, were maintained in glass aquaria under laboratory conditions for a few days prior to exposure, and were fed lettuce leaves.

Mosquito Larvae The molluscicides were evaluated against laboratory-bred second instar larvae of *An. (Cellia) dirus*, *Ae. aegypti*, and *C. quinquefasciatus*. Prior to exposure, the larvae were maintained in aluminum pans each measuring 24 cm × 37 cm × 8 cm in size; the larvae were fed crushed hamster or dog food.

Snail Bioassays

Bayluscide Each species of snails were exposed to various concentrations of Bayluscide for 24 hr using 1-liter glass jars. A 10-fold dilution series of 0.01, 0.1, 1.0, 10.0, and 100 mg/liter was performed.

After the critical range was determined, a twofold series of 0.01, 0.02, 0.04, 0.08, 0.16, 0.32, 0.64, and 1.28 mg/liter was used. For each species of snails, a total number of 480 snails were tested: 400 for the experimental and 80 for the control groups. Eight replicates with 10 snails each were performed at each concentration. Then the snails were washed thoroughly in dechlorinated tap water and transferred into other sets of jars for a 48-hr recovery. During the recovery period, the snails were fed lettuce leaves.

After the 48-hr recovery period, the mortality of snails was recorded and the LC_{50} values were determined using probit analysis described by Finney [14].

Organotin Compounds Dosages of the two controlled release molluscicides, from 1 to 25 mg/liter with 5-mg/liter intervals, were calculated according to the percentage active ingredient of each molluscicide (pellet dosages) and placed in 1-liter jars containing dechlorinated tap water. The jars were covered with cotton gauze to prevent the snails from crawling out. For each dose, eight replicates with 10 snails each were performed. Eighty control snails, with 10 snails per replicate, were maintained in dechlorinated tap water. For each species of snails, a total number of 560 snails was used. During the treatments, snails were continuously exposed to various concentrations, and were fed lettuce leaves. Every 24 hr, mortality of the snails was observed and recorded, dead snails removed, and lettuce leaves were changed to prevent fouling of the water until all of them died.

Mosquito Bioassays

Bayluscide The second instar larvae of three mosquito species were exposed to concentrations of Bayluscide, ranging from 0.01 to 100 mg/liter with 10-fold increase intervals, for a period of 24 hr. After 24 hr of exposure, the larvae were washed in dechlorinated tap water and transferred to another set of containers containing 250 ml of water for recovery. Food was given as required. After a 48-hr recovery period, mortality of the larvae in each concentration was observed and recorded to determine the relationship between the percentage mortality of the larvae and concentrations of the toxicant. Subsequently, dosage-mortality curves and an LC_{50} were achieved by probit analysis [14]. Afterward, the larvae were not discarded, but were continuously observed until all of them died or emerged as adults. For each concentration, four replicates with 20 larvae each were performed. Eighty control larvae, with 20 larvae per replicate, were kept in dechlorinated tap water. For each species of mosquitoes, a total number of 480 larvae was used.

Organotin Compounds Concentrations ranging from 1 to 25 mg/liter, with 5-mg/liter intervals, were tested against the mosquito larvae in 1-liter jars containing dechlorinated tap water. The rubber pellets of

TBTO and TBTF were accurately weighed and added to each jar. Control jars with no toxic-containing rubber were maintained under identical conditions. For each concentration, four replicates with 20 larvae each were performed. For each species of mosquitoes, a total number of 560 larvae was used. During the exposure periods, the mosquito larvae were fed with crushed, dry powdered dog food or hamster food. The newly emerged pupae were washed in water, and were then transferred into small vials covered with cotton gauze for adult emergence. Accumulative mortality of each developmental stage was recorded daily until all of them died or developed into adults. The abnormalities of molting and physical structures of life stages of the mosquitoes were also observed.

Laboratory Conditions

During the course of this study, each experiment was carried out under the same laboratory conditions as follows: room temperature 28.0-30.0°C; water temperature 27.0-30.5°C; and pH 7.5-7.8.

RESULTS

Experiment 1: Effects of Bayluscide on Snails

The results on effects of Bayluscide on snails were analyzed statistically using probit analysis, as shown in Table 1 and Fig. 1. The LC_{50} values of *B.s. siamensis*, *I. exustus*, and *L.a. rubiginosa* were 0.149, 0.171, and 0.145 mg/liter, respectively. The LC_{50} values of *I. exustus* was highest, while the LC_{50} values of *B.s. siamensis* and *L.a. rubiginosa* differed slightly. Therefore, *I. exustus* seemed to be less sensitive to Bayluscide than other snails.

It was observed that the snails that nearly died excreted a lot of mucus around their apertures. The succumbed snails of all three species contracted their head-foot portions deeply into the shells.

Table 1 Effects of Bayluscide on Snails Expressed as LC_{50} Values[a]

Snail species	LC_{50} (mg/liter) and 95% confidence limits	Slope functions
B.s. siamensis	0.149 (0.146-0.152)	21.45
I. exustus	0.171 (0.165-0.177)	11.81
L.a. rubiginosa	0.145 (0.131-0.160)	4.33

[a]The exposure time and recovery period were 24 and 48 hr, respectively.

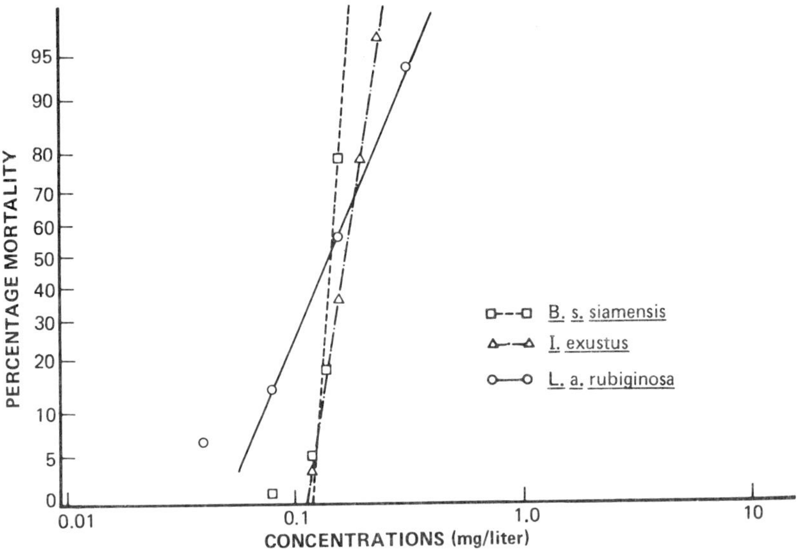

Figure 1 Dosage-mortality lines of snails exposed to Bayluscide.

In case of *I. exustus*, bleeding also occurred. During the recovery period, there was a difference in the rate of food consumption among the snails exposed to various concentrations of Bayluscide. The rate of food consumption appeared indirectly proportional to the concentration of Bayluscide: snails exposed to low concentrations consumed more food than snails exposed to high concentrations.

Experiment 2: Effects of Controlled Release TBTO and TBTF Molluscicide Pellets on Snails

The results on effects of controlled release molluscicides TBTO and TBTF pellets on *B.s. siamensis*, *I. exustus*, and *L.a. rubiginosa* are given in Figs. 2-7. The LC_{50} values of TBTO and TBTF were 1 mg/liter at 4 days and 25 mg/liter at 2 days for *B.s. siamensis*; 1 mg/liter at 2 days and 25 mg/liter at 1 day for *I exustus*; and 1 mg/liter and 25 mg/liter, both at 1 day, for *L.a. rubiginosa*. *L.a. rubiginosa* were the most sensitive and *B.s. siamensis* the least sensitive to TBTO and TBTF. The order of sensitivity of the experimental snails to both chemicals was as follows: *L.a. rubiginosa* > *I. exustus* > *B.s. siamensis*. *B.s. siamensis* and *I. exustus* were more sensitive to TBTF than to TBTO, but *L.a. rubiginosa* was equally sensitive to both chemicals. There was no mortality observed within 24 hr of the exposure time. The snails were still vigorous and consumed a lot of food. In all cases,

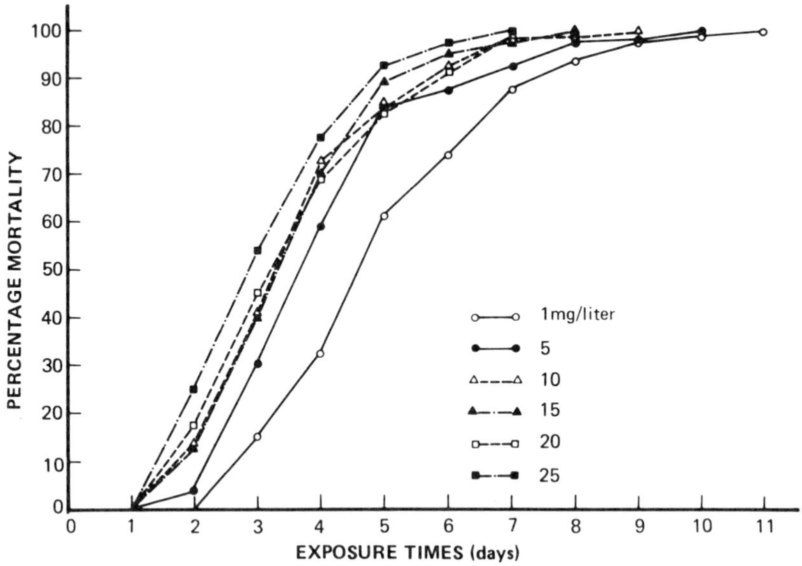

Figure 2 Mortality curves of *B.s. siamensis* exposed to six dosages of controlled release TBTO.

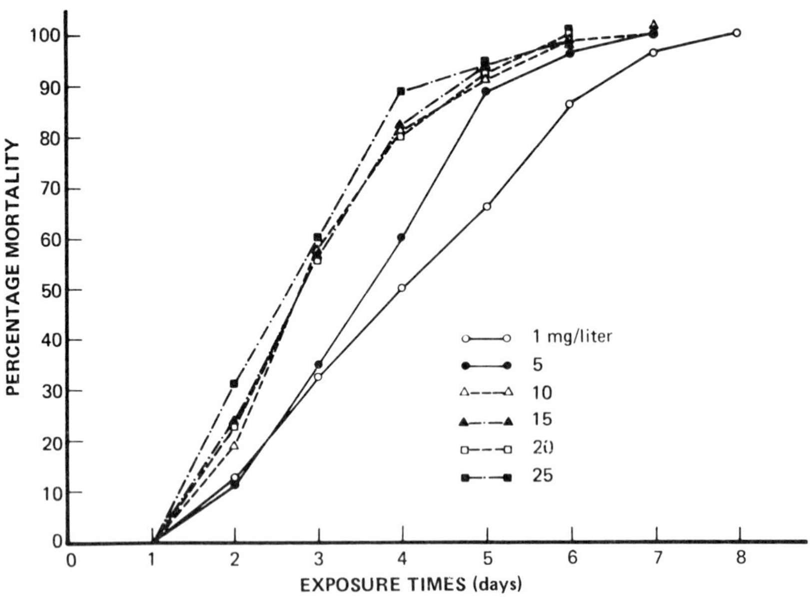

Figure 3 Mortality curves of *B.s. siamensis* exposed to six dosages of controlled release TBTF.

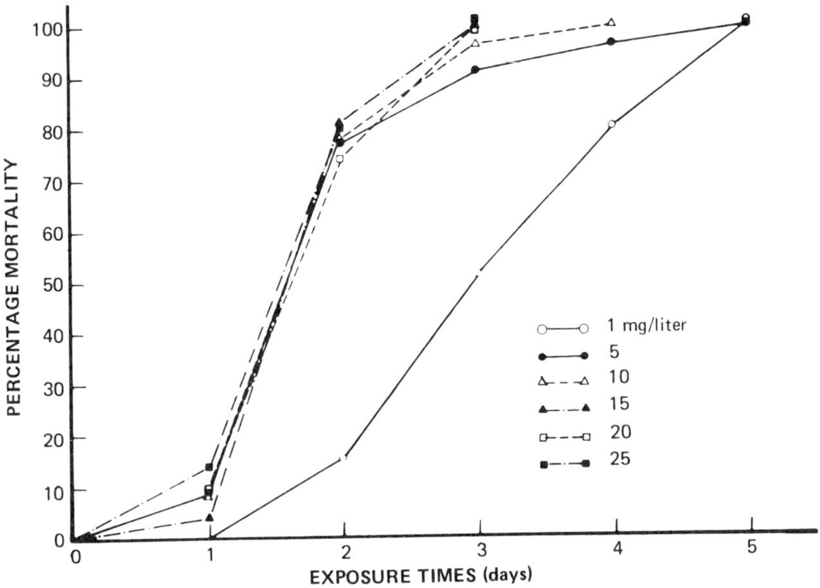

Figure 4 Mortality curves of *I. exustus* exposed to six dosages of controlled release TBTO.

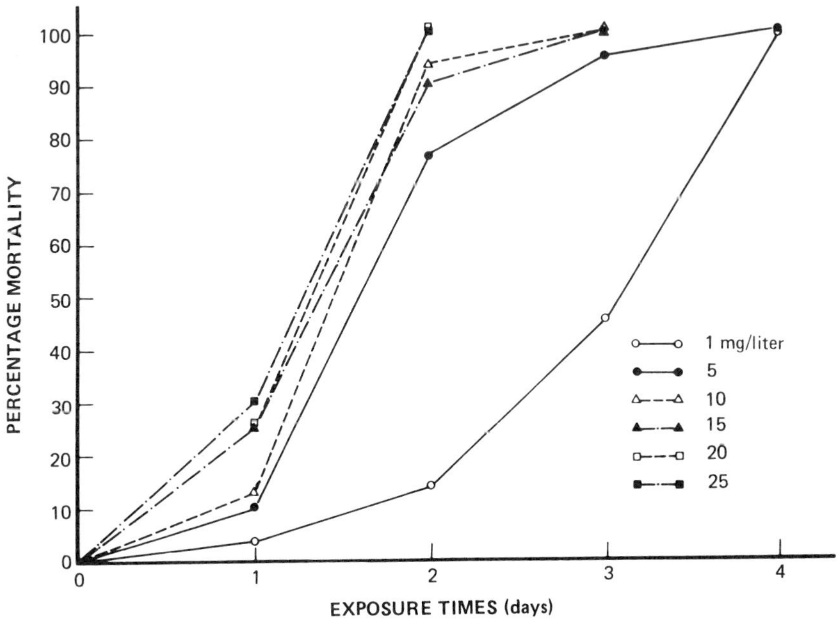

Figure 5 Mortality curves of *I. exustus* exposed to six dosages of controlled release TBTF.

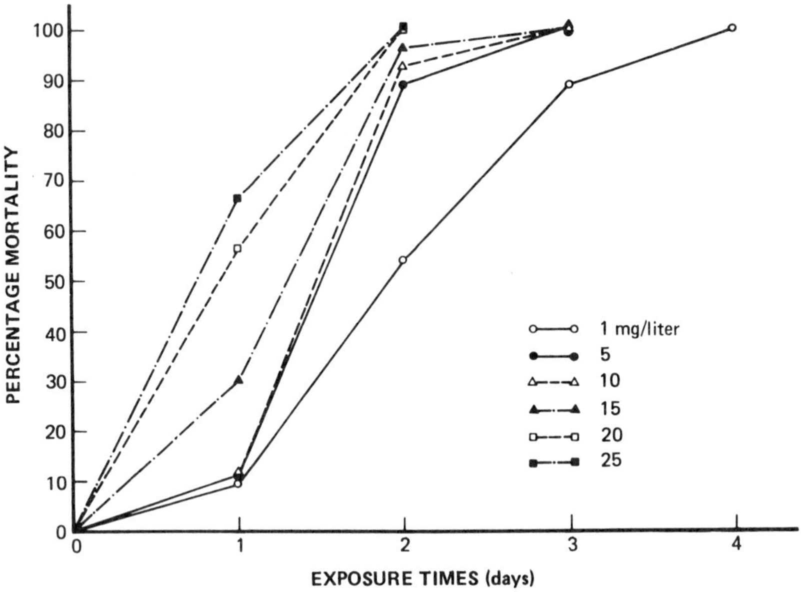

Figure 6 Mortality curves of *L. a. rubiginosa* exposed to six dosages of controlled release TBTO.

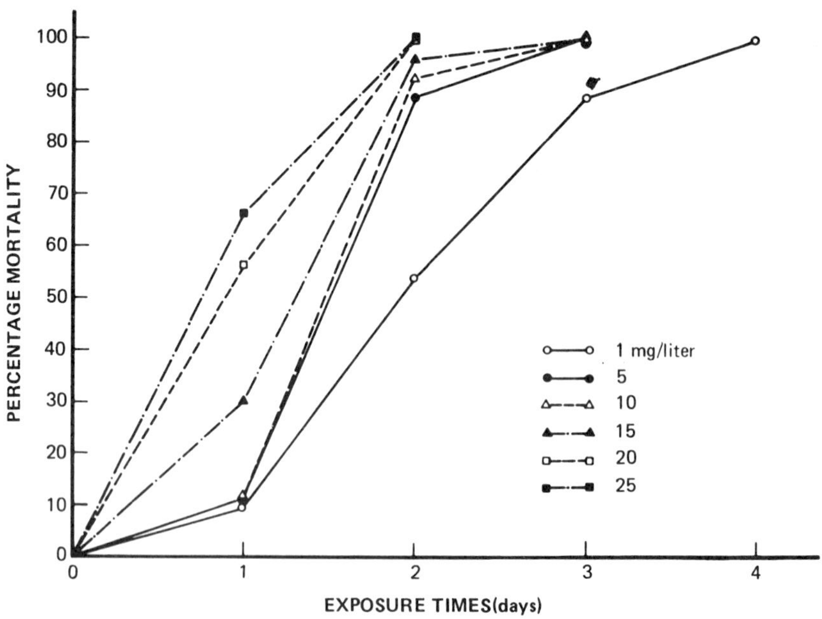

Figure 7 Mortality curves of *L. a. rubiginosa* exposed to six dosages of controlled release TBTF.

after the prolonged exposure to both controlled release formulations, the snails became inactive and extended their head-foot portions out of the shells, and excreted a copious quantity of mucus, especially *I. exustus* and *L. a. rubiginosa*. All of the succumbed snails died with their head-foot portions extended and much enlarged.

Experiment 3: Effects of Bayluscide on Mosquito Larvae

The results on effects of Bayluscide on mosquito larvae were analyzed statistically using probit analysis, and are shown in Table 2 and Fig. 8. The LC_{50} values of *An. dirus*, *Ae. aegypti*, and *C. quinquefasciatus* exposed to Bayluscide were 0.219, 0.509, and 0.285 mg/liter, respectively. *An. dirus* was the most sensitive to Bayluscide.

The effects of Bayluscide on the development of the second instar larvae of mosquitoes are shown in Table 3. At the high concentrations, 10 and 100 mg/liter, all larvae of *An. dirus* and *C. quinquefasciatus* died, whereas 10% (8/80) of the larvae of *Ae. aegypti* survived but died during the pupal stage. At the lowest concentration tested, 0.01 mg/liter, 20-50% of the larvae survived, 20-40% pupated, and 3-17% emerged as adults. Among the three species of mosquito larvae tested, *An. dirus* was the most sensitive to Bayluscide. It was observed that low concentrations of Bayluscide retarded the development and caused molting abnormalities in metamorphosis. Moreover, the adults failed to escape from the pupal molts completely during the course of emergence. Sometimes, the anterior parts, such as the head and thorax, and some parts of the abdomen came out of the pupal molt, but the posterior part remained inside.

Experiment 4: Effects of Controlled Release TBTO and TBTF Molluscicide Pellets on Mosquito Larvae

The results on effects of controlled release TBTO and TBTF molluscicide pellets on mosquito larvae of *An. dirus*, *Ae. aegypti*, and *C. quinquefasciatus* are given in Figs. 9-14. The LC_{50} values of TBTO

Table 2 Effects of Bayluscide on Mosquito Larvae Expressed as LC_{50} Values[a]

Mosquito species	LC_{50} (mg/liter) at 24 hr and 95% confidence limits	Slope functions
An. dirus	0.219 (0.128-0.373)	0.648
Ae. aegypti	0.509 (0.349-0.744)	0.989
C. quinquefasciatus	0.285 (0.185-0.441)	0.859

[a]The exposure time and recovery periods were 24 and 48 hr, respectively.

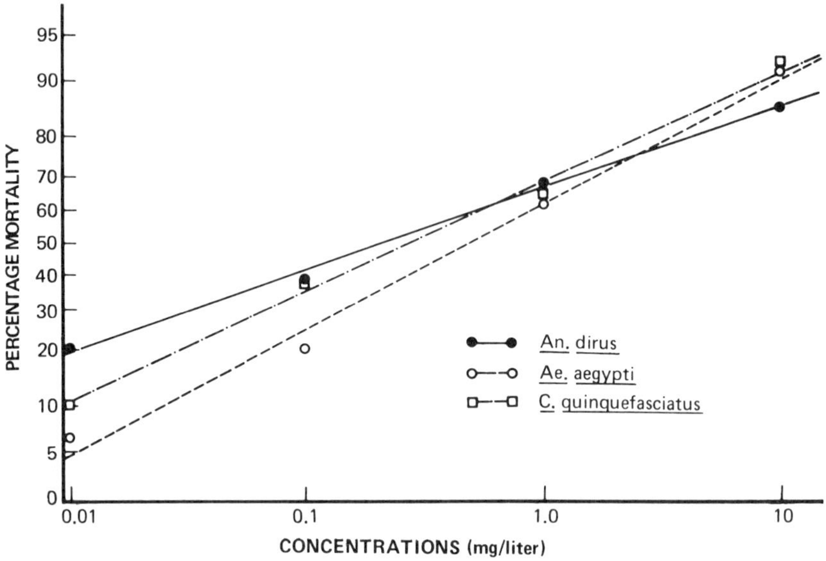

Figure 8 Dosage-mortality lines of mosquito larvae exposed to Bayluscide.

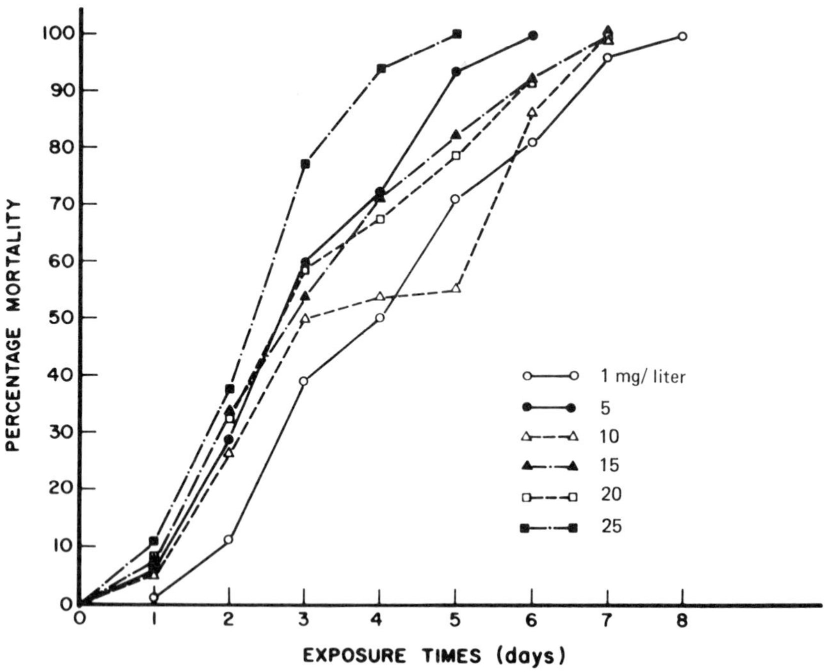

Figure 9 Mortality curves of *An. dirus* expcsed to six dosages of controlled release TBTO.

Table 3 Effects of Bayluscide on the Development of the Second Instar Larvae of Mosquitoes

Mosquito species	Bayluscide conc. (mg/liter)	Number dead larvae	Number larvae pupated	Number dead pupae	Number adults emerged	Number dead adults	Total number dead
An. dirus	0	11	69	10	59	0	21
	0.01	68	12	8	3	1	77
	0.10	7[illegible]	7	5	1	1	79
	1.0	7[illegible]	2	2	0	0	80
	10.	8[illegible]	0	0	0	0	80
	100.	8[illegible]	0	0	0	0	80
Ae. aegypti	0	12	68	3	65	0	14
	0.01	40	32	12	14	6	66
	0.10	60	20	12	4	4	76
	1.0	67	13	10	2	1	78
	10.	72	8	8	0	0	80
	100.	80	0	0	0	0	80
C. quinquefasciatus	0	17	63	3	60	0	20
	0.01	55	25	11	11	3	69
	0.10	68	12	6	4	2	76
	1.0	78	2	1	0	1	80
	10.	80	0	0	0	0	80
	100.	80	0	0	0	0	80

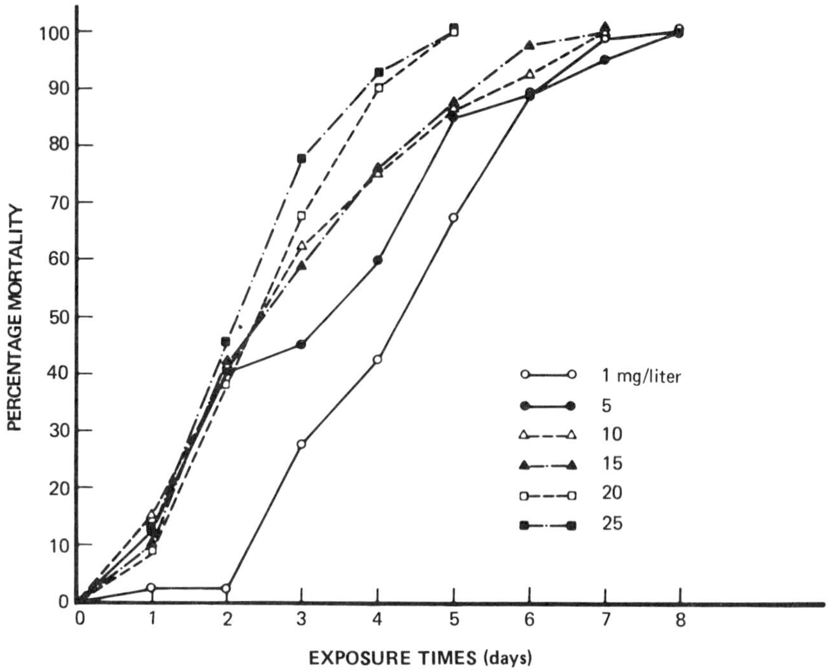

Figure 10 Mortality curves of *An. dirus* exposed to six dosages of controlled release TBTF.

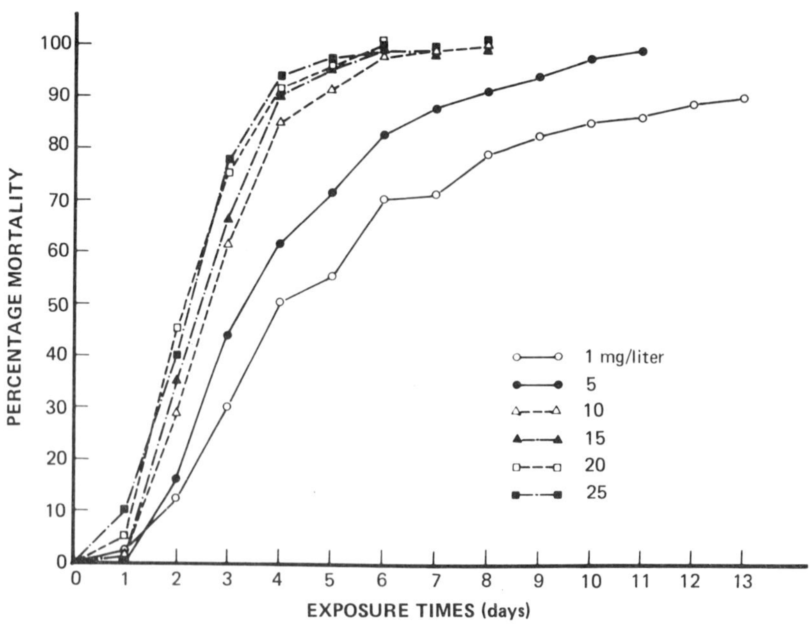

Figure 11 Mortality curves of *Ae. aegypti* exposed to six dosages of controlled release TBTO.

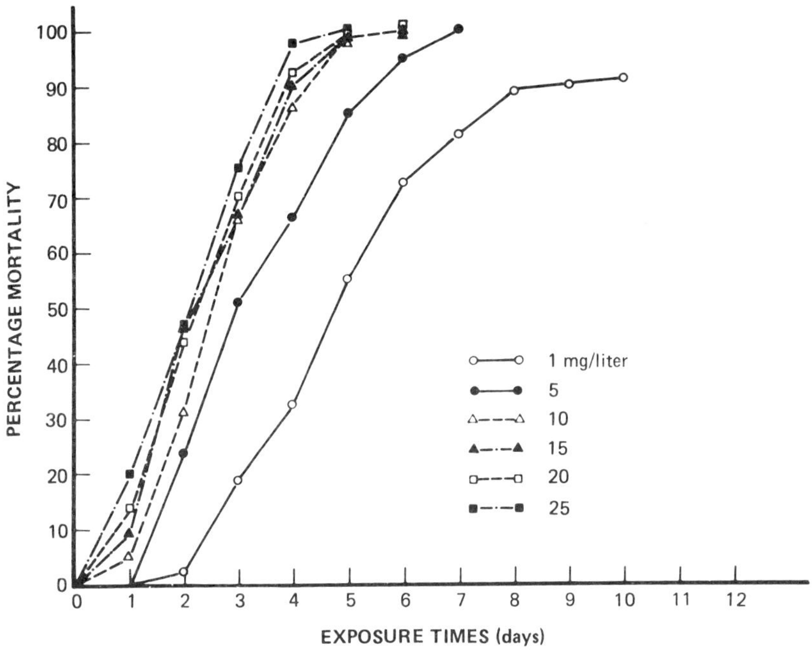

Figure 12 Mortality curves of *Ae. aegypti* exposed to six dosages of controlled release TBTF.

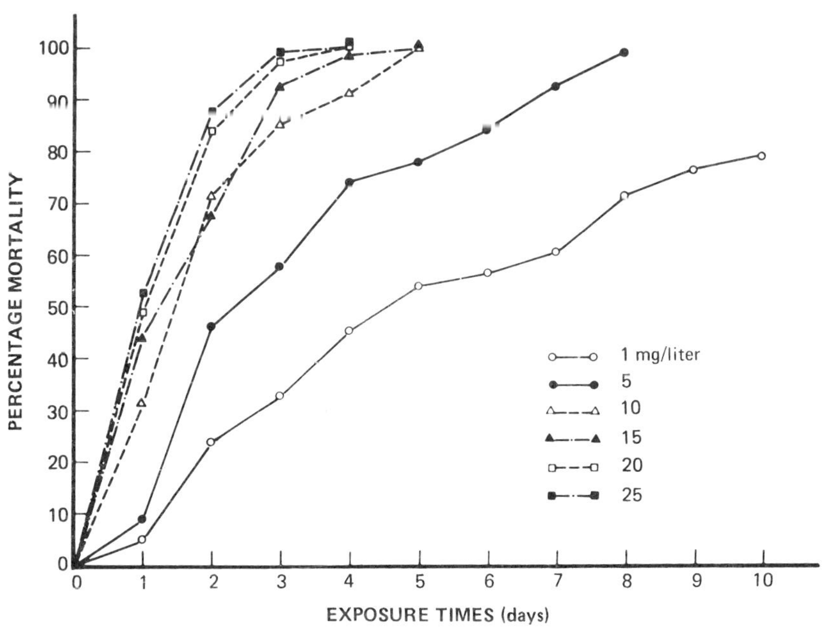

Figure 13 Mortality curves of *C. quinquefasciatus* exposed to six dosages of controlled release TBTO.

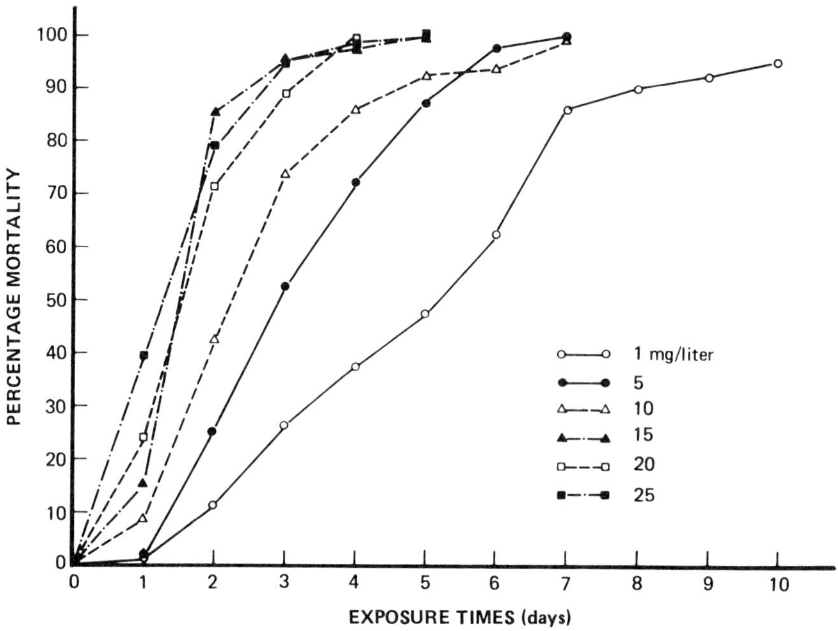

Figure 14 Mortality curves of *C. quinquefasciatus* exposed to six dosages of controlled release TBTF.

and TBTF were 1 mg/liter at 4 days and 25 mg/liter at 2 days for larvae of *An. dirus* and *Ae. aegypti*; and 1 mg/liter at 4 days and 25 mg/liter at 1 day for larvae of *C. quinquefasciatus*. They were about equally sensitive to TBTO and TBTF.

The effects of TBTO and TBTF on the developmental stages of mosquito larvae are shown in Tables 4 and 5. At high concentrations (pellet dosages), from 5 to 25 mg/liter, most of the larvae died. Although a few of them developed to fourth instars, they did not pupate. At the lowest concentration tested, 1 mg/liter, 7-35% of the mosquito larvae survived and pupated, and 2-21% emerged as adults. In the case of *An. dirus* and *C. quinquefasciatus*, it was observed that low dosages of both chemicals retarded their development and caused molting abnormalities in metamorphosis which resulted in a large number of deaths between the larval and pupal stages, either completely unmelanized as white pupae or completely melanized as brown pupae. Some of the surviving pupae tolerated and continued their development to complete metamorphosis to become normal adults, while some of them became abnormal adults during the course of the adult emergence. For example, the abnormal adult partly emerged from the pupal molt, only head and thorax freed except the abdomen. In

Table 4 Effects (in %) of Controlled Release TBTO on the Development of the Second Instar Larvae of Mosquitoes

Mosquito species	TBTO conc. (mg/liter)	Number dead larvae (%)	Number larvae pupated (%)	Number dead pupae (%)	Number adult emerged (%)	Number dead adults (%)	Total number dead (%)
An. dirus	0	13 (16.25)	67 (93.75)	9 (11.25)	58 (72.5)	0	22 (27.5)
	1	65 (81.25)	15 (18.75)	13 (16.25)	2 (2.5)	2 (2.5)	80 (100)
	5	80 (100)	0	0	0	0	80 (100)
	10	80 (100)	0	0	0	0	80 (100)
	15	80 (100)	0	0	0	0	80 (100)
	20	80 (100)	0	0	0	0	80 (100)
	25	80 (100)	0	0	0	0	80 (100)
Ae. aegypti	0	13 (16.25)	67 (93.75)	1 (1.25)	66 (82.5)	0	14 (17.5)
	1	63 (78.75)	17 (21.25)	7 (8.75)	8 (10)	0	72 (90)
	5	75 (93.75)	5 (6.25)	4 (5)	1 (1.25)	0	79 (98.75)
	10	80 (100)	0	0	0	0	80 (100)
	15	80 (100)	0	0	0	0	80 (100)
	20	80 (100)	0	0	0	0	80 (100)
	25	80 (100)	0	0	0	0	80 (100)
C. quinquefasciatus	0	10 (12.5)	70 (87.5)	9 (11.25)	61 (76.25)	0	19 (23.75)
	1	52 (35)	28 (35)	8 (10)	17 (21.25)	3 (3.75)	63 (78.75)
	5	72 (90)	8 (10)	7 (8.75)	1 (1.25)	0	79 (98.75)
	10	80 (100)	1 (1.25)	1 (1.25)	0	0	80 (100)
	15	80 (100)	0	0	0	0	80 (100)
	20	80 (100)	0	0	0	0	80 (100)
	25	80 (100)	0	0	0	0	80 (100)

Table 5 Effects (in %) of Controlled Release TBTF on the Development of the Second Instar Larvae of Mosquitoes

Mosquito species	TBTF conc. (mg/liter)	Number dead larvae (%)	Number larvae pupated (%)	Number dead pupae (%)	Number adult emerged (%)	Number dead adults (%)	Total number dead (%)
An. dirus	0	18 (22.5)	60 (75)	7 (8.75)	55 (68.75)	0	25 (31.25)
	1	74 (92.5)	6 (7.5)	6 (7.5)	0	0	80 (100)
	5	80 (100)	0	0	0	0	80 (100)
	10	80 (100)	0	0	0	0	80 (100)
	15	80 (100)	0	0	0	0	80 (100)
	20	80 (100)	0	0	0	0	80 (100)
	25	80 (100)	0	0	0	0	80 (100)
Ae. aegypti	0	9 (11.25)	71 (88.75)	7 (8.75)	64 (80)	0	16 (20)
	1	72 (90)	8 (10)	1 (1.25)	7 (8.75)	0	73 (91.25)
	5	80 (100)	0	0	0	0	80 (100)
	10	80 (100)	0	0	0	0	80 (100)
	15	80 (100)	0	0	0	0	80 (100)
	20	80 (100)	0	0	0	0	80 (100)
	25	80 (100)	0	0	0	0	80 (100)
C. quinquefasciatus	0	17 (21.25)	63 (78.75)	9 (11.25)	54 (67.5)	0	26 (32.5)
	1	59 (73.75)	21 (26.25)	14 (17.5)	4 (5)	3 (3.75)	76 (95)
	5	79 (98.75)	1 (1.25)	1 (1.25)	0	0	80 (100)
	10	77 (96.25)	3 (3.75)	2 (2.5)	1 (1.25)	0	79 (98.75)
	15	79 (98.75)	1 (1.25)	1 (1.25)	0	0	80 (100)
	20	80 (100)	0	0	0	0	80 (100)
	25	80 (100)	0	0	0	0	80 (100)

general, an adult started to emerge at the anterior end of pupae, but sometimes the abnormal adult emerged at the middle region of its body; the abdomen came out of the pupal molt except that the anterior and posterior parts were still inside. In addition, it was occasionally observed that a normal adult almost completely emerged from a pupal molt, but the tarsi of the hind pair of legs remained attached to the pupal exuvium. Such adults could not fly and thus died. From the results obtained, it was noted that the controlled release TBTO and TBTF showed similar effects, such as molting abnormalities and death, but the chemicals did not cause structural abnormalities of the mosquitoes.

DISCUSSION

The LC_{50} values of three species of vector snails exposed to Bayluscide in the present study indicated that the LC_{50} value of *I. exustus* differed slightly from the LC_{50} values of *B.s. siamensis* and *L.a. rubiginosa*, but there was no significant difference in the LC_{50} values of the two latter species. The dosage-mortality relationship showed that all probit regression lines of the three species of snails had relatively steep slopes (b = 21.4534, 11.8135, and 4.3328), which indicated that Bayluscide was highly effective against the snails. The mortality rates of snails increased rapidly as the chemical concentrations increased. *L.a. rubiginosa*, with a low LC_{50} value, tended to have a shallower slope than *I. exustus*, with high LC_{50} value. However, *B.s. siamensis*, with a low LC_{50} value, had a very steep slope.

Concerning Bayluscide, other investigators reported that the LC_{50} values of adult snails such as *Bi. glabrata* [15], *Bi. sudanica tanganyicensis*, *Bu. (Physopsis) nasutus productus* [16], and *L. ollula* [17] were 0.045, 0.074, 0.084, and 0.05 mg/liter, respectively. The LC_{50} values of the snails tested to Bayluscide in the studies mentioned above were relatively lower than the LC_{50} values of the snails tested in the present study. The variation in the sensitivity of snails to Bayluscide has never been elucidated. However, Walker [18] suggested that the variation may be due to the ionic contents of the body fluids of different species of snails, and to the chemical constituents of the water used in the experiment. The lethal mechanism of Bayluscide in the snails that has been studied previously suggested that the inhibition of succinate oxidation may be the cause of death [19]. Moreover, the rapid retraction of snails into their shells when exposed to the chemical may inhibit oxygen consumption in the snails [20]. The nearly dead snails excreted a lot of mucus around their apertures, which may cause a suffocating effect by preventing the exchange of ions and gases across the epithelium [21,22].

Controlled release TBTO and TBTF with the same butyl radical showed relatively equal efficacy as molluscicide. However, TBTF seemed to be more effective than TBTO because it took less time to kill 100% of the snails; for instance, all *B.s. siamensis*, *I. exustus*, and *L.a. rubiginosa* were killed within 11, 5, and 4 days, respectively, when exposed to TBTO and within 8, 4, and 4 days when exposed to TBTF. These results agreed with the observation by Walker [23] that the mortality rate of *Bi. glabrata* was more rapid when exposed to TBTF than TBTO. It is interesting to note that the mortality rates of the snails exposed to both TBTO and TBTF were consistent: *B.s. siamensis* was the least sensitive and *L.a. rubiginosa* was the most sensitive. Although the mode of action of organotin compounds is not yet clearly understood, it was presumed that the toxicant caused chronic intoxication in snails through slow and accumulative actions [24,25]. Juijten [26] suggested that the cause of snail death may be the inhibition of oxidative phosphorylation.

Laboratory study on the effect of Bayluscide on the larvae of *An. dirus*, *Ae. aegypti*, and *C. quinquefasciatus* showed that *Ae. aegypti* was less sensitive than others. The dosage mortality relationship showed that the probit regression lines for each species tested had shallow slopes (b = 0.64, 0.989, and 0.859). *An. dirus* and *C. quinquefasciatus*, with similarly low LC_{50} values, had shallower slopes than *Ae. aegypti* with a slightly higher LC_{50} value. At high concentrations, all the larvae died between larval and pupal development when exposed to Bayluscide. At low concentrations, from 0.01 to 1 mg/liter, most of them died in the early stages of development; however, a few survived and died at later stages, owing to abnormal molting. It was apparent that the abnormalities occurring in the test species were similar and did not differ from those exposed to controlled release molluscicides.

The LC_{50} values of mosquito larvae exposed to Bayluscide were considerably higher than those of the snails. This indicated that Bayluscide was not only an effective molluscicide but also could be a mosquito larvicide. However, a concentration of Bayluscide which is needed to kill mosquito larvae will be higher than that needed to kill snails.

At high dosages of TBTO and TBTF, all the *An. dirus* larvae were killed after 8 days, the *Ae. aegypti* larvae after 13 and 12 days, and *C. quinquefasciatus* larvae after 10 days. At low dosages, mortality rates of the mosquito larvae did not reach 100% because some of them developed to normal adults. The effects of TBTO and TBTF on the mosquito larvae differed slightly, from 8 to 12 days. The larvae of *An. dirus* were more sensitive to both TBTO and TBTF than those of *Ae. aegypti* and *C. quinquefasciatus*. At a concentration of 1 mg/liter, 18.8% and 7.6% of the *An. dirus* larvae pupated when exposed to TBTO and TBTF, respectively. At the same concentration, 21.3% and 10% of the *Ae. aegypti* larvae pupated when exposed to TBTO and TBTF, respectively. In addition, at 5 mg/liter, 6.3% of the *Ae. aegypti* larvae pupated when exposed to TBTO. Regarding *C. quinquefasciatus*, 35%

and 26.3% of the larvae pupated when exposed to 10 mg/liter TBTO and 15 mg/liter TBTF, respectively. In the case of *Ae. aegypti*, no molting abnormalities were observed because the survived pupae developed into normal adults. Thus it may be concluded that low dosages of TBTO and TBTF caused larval death and retarded normal development in the mosquitoes studied. Furthermore, the mosquitoes died in their early developmental stages when they were exposed to high concentrations of TBTO and TBTF. The lethal mechanism of organotin compounds for mosquitoes has never been explained fully; however, Cardarelli [27] suggested that a proteolytic activity in connective and other tissues may be the cause of death.

The mosquito mortalities were not consistent when they were exposed to either TBTO or TBTF. At concentrations of 1 and 5 mg/liter TBTO, *Ae. aegypti* larvae were the least sensitive and *An. dirus* larvae were the most sensitive. At 10, 15, and 25 mg/liter TBTO, *Ae. aegypti* larvae were still the least sensitive, but *C. quinquefasciatus* larvae were the most sensitive. At 20 mg/liter TBTO, *An. dirus* larvae were the least sensitive and *C. quinquefasciatus* larvae were still the most sensitive. TBTF exhibited different patterns from TBTO. At 1 mg/liter TBTF, *Ae. aegypti* and *C. quinquefasciatus* larvae were the least sensitive and *An. dirus* larvae were the most sensitive. At 5 mg/liter TBTF, *An. dirus* larvae were the least sensitive and *Ae. aegypti* and *C. quinquefasciatus* larvae were the most sensitive. At 10 mg/liter TBTF, *An. dirus* and *C. quinquefasciatus* larvae were the least sensitive and *Ae. aegypti* larvae were the most sensitive. At 15 and 20 mg/liter TBTF, *C. quinquefasciatus* larvae were the most sensitive, whereas *An. dirus* and *Ae. aegypti* larvae were the least sensitive. At 25 mg/liter TBTF, they were equally sensitive. Laboratory studies on the controlled release molluscicides TBTO and TBTF also suggested that they were effective as molluscicide and mosquito larvicide, and that the mosquito larvae were less sensitive to them than the snails.

SUMMARY

1. Conventional (Bayluscide) and controlled release (tri-n-butyltin oxide and tributyltin fluoride) molluscicides were laboratory tested against three species of medically important snails and mosquito larvae. The effects of the molluscicides were expressed as lethal concentration (LC_{50}) values in mg/liter for the conventional type and in days for the controlled release type.
2. The LC_{50} values of *B.s. siamensis*, *I. exustus*, and *L.a. rubiginosa* exposed to Bayluscide were 0.1489, 0.1709, and 0.1447 mg/liter, respectively.
3. The LC_{50} values of snails when exposed to controlled release TBTO and TBTF were 4 days at 1 mg/liter and 2 days at 25 mg/liter for *B.s. siamensis*; 2 days at 1 mg/liter and 1 day at 25

mg/liter for *I. exustus*; and 1 day at both 1 and 25 mg/liter for *L.a. rubiginosa*.

4. The LC_{50} values of the larvae of *An. dirus*, *Ae. aegypti*, and *C. quinquefasciatus* exposed to Bayluscide were 0.2186, 0.5092, and 0.2852 mg/liter, respectively.
5. The LC_{50} values of the mosquito larvae when exposed to controlled release TBTO and TBTF were 4 days at 1 mg/liter and 2 days at 25 mg/liter for the larvae of *An. dirus* and *Ae. aegypti*, and 4 days at 1 mg/liter and 1 day at 25 mg/liter for the larvae of *C. quinquefasciatus*. They were about equally sensitive to both chemicals.
6. These two types of molluscicides showed high molluscicidal and larvicidal activities. The dosages required to kill snails were lower than those required to kill mosquito larvae. They interrupted molting in the mosquito larvae and produced abnormal adults. The effects of interrupting molting were similar in all cases.

ACKNOWLEDGMENTS

The authors thank Nate Cardarelli at the Environmental Management Laboratory of the University of Akron, Ohio, and the Bayer Company, Liverkusen, West Germany, for providing controlled release molluscicides TBTO and TBTF and Bayluscide, respectively. Much appreciation is expressed to Departments of Medical Entomology of Armed Forces Research Institute of Medical Science and Faculty of Tropical Medicine, Mahidol University, for providing mosquito larvae.

This investigation was supported by the UNDP/World Bank/WHO Special Programme for Research and Training in Tropical Diseases.

REFERENCES

1. C. Harinasuta and S. Vajrasthira, *Ann. Trop. Med. Parasitol.*, *54*:100 (1960).
2. D. E. Wykoff, C. Harinasuta, P. Juttijudata, and M. M. Winn, *J. Parasitol.*, *51*:207 (1965).
3. C. Harinasuta, M. Kruatrachue, and S. Sornmani, *J. Trop. Med. Hyg.*, *68*:125 (1965).
4. M. A. Yokogawa, C. Harinasuta, and P. Charoenlarp, *Jap. J. Parasitol.*, *14*:148 (1965).
5. K. J. Lie, *Trop. Geogr. Med.*, *11*:17 (1963).
6. M. Bhaibulaya, P. Charoenlarp, and C. Harinasuta, *J. Med. Assoc. Thailand*, *47*:720 (1964).
7. H. F. Lee and D. E. Wykoff, *J. Parasitol.*, *52*:323 (1966).
8. M. Kruatrachue, M. Bhaibulaya, and C. Harinasuta, *Ann. Trop. Med. Parasitol.*, *59*:181 (1965).

9. M. Kruatrachue, M. Bhaibulaya, C. Chesdapan, and C. Harinasuta, *Ann. Trop. Med. Parasitol.*, *62*:67 (1968).
10. J. E. Scanlon and U. Sandhinand, *J. Med. Entomol.*, *2*:61 (1965).
11. R. N. Wilkinson, D. J. Gould, P. Boonyakanist, and H. E. Segal, *J. Med. Entomol.*, *14*:666 (1978).
12. S. B. Halstead, S. Udomsakdi, J. E. Scanlon, and S. Rohitayodhin, *Am. J. Trop. Med. Hyg.*, *18*:1022 (1969).
13. M. O. T. Lyenger, *Bull. WHO*, *9*:731 (1953).
14. D. J. Finney, *Probit Analysis*, 2nd ed., Cambridge University Press, Cambridge, 1964.
15. R. F. Sturrock, G. Barnish, and E. S. Upatham, *Int. J. Parasitol.*, *4*:231 (1974).
16. G. Webbe and R. F. Sturrock, *Ann. Trop. Med. Parasitol.*, *58*: 234 (1964).
17. Y. Harada, *Jap. J. Parasitol.*, *23*:285 (1974).
18. K. E. Walker, in *Proc. Controlled Release Pestic. Symp.*, University of Akron, Akron, Ohio, September 1976.
19. M. M. Ishak, A. A. Sharaf, A. M. Mohamed, and A. H. Mousa, *Com. Gen. Pharmacol.*, *1*:201 (1972).
20. T. von Brand, B. Mehlman, and M. O. Nolan, *J. Parasitol.*, *35*: 475 (1949).
21. T. C. Cheng and J. Sullivan, in *Molluscicides in Schistosomiasis Control* (T. C. Cheng, ed.), Academic Press, New York, 1974.
22. T. C. Cheng and J. Sullivan, in *Proc. Controlled Release Pestic. Symp.*, University of Akron, Akron, Ohio, September 1974.
23. K. E. Walker, in *Proc. Controlled Release Pestic. Symp.*, Oregon State University, Corvallis, Oregon, August 1977.
24. C. J. Shiff, C. Yiannakis, and R. C. Evans, in *Proc. Controlled Release Pestic. Symp.*, Wright State University, Dayton, Ohio, 1975.
25. T. Quick and N. F. Cardarelli, in *Proc. Controlled Release Pestic. Symp.*, Oregon State University, Corvallis, Oregon, August, 1977.
26. J. G. A. Juijten, *Organotin Compounds*, *2*:940 (1972).
27. N. F. Cardarelli, *Mosquito News*, *38*:328 (1978).

Chapter 25

Analyses of Volatile Model Compounds in Accurel® Porous Materials

TIMOTHY D. DAVIS and WILLIAM R. BRADE Armak Company, McCook, Illinois

Evaporation rate studies were performed to investigate the potential of Accurel®* porous thermoplastic polymers as controlled release devices for agents that are active in the vapor state. The polymer used in these tests was polypropylene with a void volume of 75%.

A porous disk which was 25 mm in diameter and 3 mm thick was prepared. The same material was also ground to produce a powder that was less than 106 μm in diameter. These samples were then loaded with up to three times their own weight of active material.

A number of common solvents were used as the model compounds in these initial studies. Most of these materials are highly volatile and thus made it possible to run a large number of rather short experiments while improving our experimental procedures. Furthermore, the physical properties of the model compounds are well known and available for interpreting the results.

MATERIALS

Porous Polymer Description

Accurel is Armak Company's family of porous polymers based on the work of Castro [1]. These polymers have microporous structures of essentially spherical, interconnected void spaces. The porous nature of 75% void material is shown in the scanning electron micrograph illustrated in Fig. 1.

*Accurel is the trademark of Armak Company, a part of Akzona, Inc.

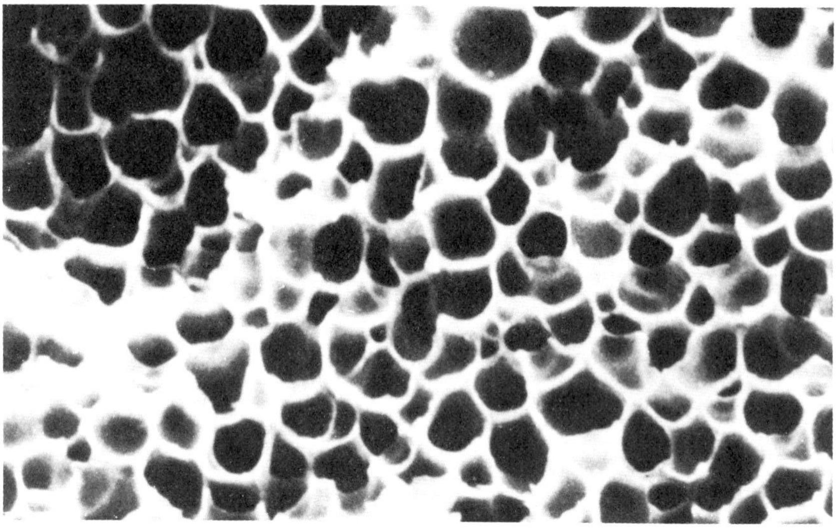

Figure 1 Scanning electron micrograph of 75% void Accurel. (Courtesy of Armak Company, McCook, Illinois.)

Void volume can be controlled over a range 30-90%. The median size of cells and interconnecting pores can be made to vary widely from system to system. Within any given system, however, the cell and pore size distribution are quite narrow. The variations possible are shown in Table 1.

Polymer selection will determine the Accurel systems intrinsic mechanical, thermal, electrical, and chemical properties. The versatility of these materials is demonstrated by the number of polymers that lend themselves to this new type of matrix formation. All the polymers listed in Table 2 can be manufactured in Accurel configurations, but the greatest developmental work has focused on the polyolefin group.

The porous polymeric structure is obtained by heating a polymer and a compatible liquid, as discussed by Castro [1], to a temperature sufficiently high to form a homogeneous solution. The solution is then poured into a mold and is cooled until a solid mass is formed. The details of this procedure are more fully described in Refs. 1 and 2. Finally, the compatible liquid is removed from the resulting solid by solvent extraction to form the microporous polymer. The solid product may be in the form of films, rods, tubes, cast shapes, pellets, or powder, as illustrated in Fig. 2.

If the active agent that is to be loaded into the porous matrix also happens to be a compatible liquid, the active agent can be directly incorporated at the time of manufacture. In this case, the solvent

Table 1 Accurel Matrix Properties

Controlled parameter	Range
Void space	30-90%
Median pore size	0.10-11.0 μm
Median cell size	1.0-30 μm
Pore size distribution	85% within one decade

Source: Courtesy of Armak Company, McCook, Illinois.

Table 2 Accurel Polymer Types

Polyolefins
Polyethylene (low and high density)
Polypropylene
Polystyrene
Copolymers
Styrene butadiene rubber
Ethylene/acrylic acid salts
Condensation polymers
Nylon 11
Polycarbonate
Polyphenylene oxide
Polymer blends
Polystyrene/polyphenylene oxide

Source: Courtesy of Armak Company, McCook, Illinois.

extraction step is eliminated. The animal repellent methyl nonyl ketone, for example, is a compatible liquid useful for making a porous polymer.

EXPERIMENTAL

The porous polymer used in this work was a 75% void formulation based on polypropylene. This material was examined in two formats. A disk with the characteristics listed in Table 3 was prepared. The same material was also ground to produce a powder less than 106 μm in diameter with the characteristics shown in Table 4.

These samples were loaded with up to three times their own weight with solvent. The evaporation rates of solvents from the disk and

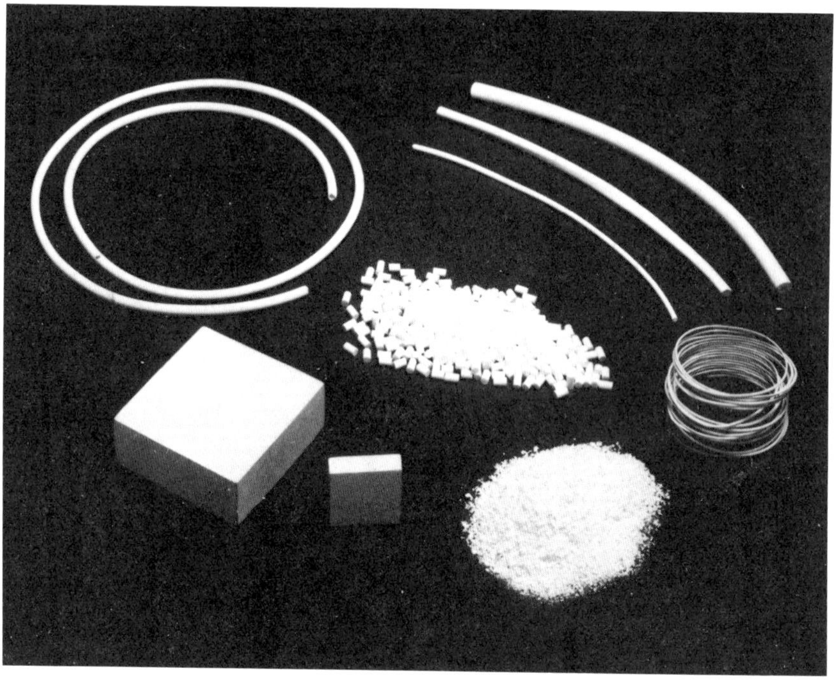

Figure 2 Typical shapes that can be fabricated. (Courtesy of Armak Company, McCook, Illinois.)

from some powder samples were measured at room temperature by means of a recording balance. The evaporation rates of other solvents from the powder were measured at 30°C by capturing the evaporated solvent on activated carbon tubes.

Apparatus

Evaporation rates of solvents from the disk were measured by placing the disk on edge on the pan of a Mettler PT 320 top-loading balance. The balance was equipped with a Mettler GC 20 digital-analog converter to provide a signal to a Gould 105 strip chart recorder. With this equipment it was possible to obtain a continuous recording of the amount of solvent evaporated. The Mettler balance was also used to measure the evaporation rates of the more volatile solvents from Accurel powder.

Evaporation rates of the less volatile solvents loaded on Accurel powder were measured by a different method. Approximately 0.100 g of powder was spread over the bottom of an aluminum pan, which was then inserted into a glass chamber. The chamber was comprised of two

Table 3 Characteristics of Accurel Disk

Diameter (cm)	2.54
Thickness (cm)	0.30
Void volume (%)	75
Void volume (cm^3)	1.14
Mass (g)	0.34
Average cell size (μm)	4.9
Average pore size (μm)	0.64

Table 4 Characteristics of Accurel Powder

Particle size range (μm)	-106 + 10
Average particle size (μm)	50
Void volume (%)	75
Average cell size (μm)	4.9
Average pore size (μm)	0.64

Kontes glass joint adapters with a volume of approximately 120 cc. The chamber was housed in a constant-temperature cabinet maintained at 30°C. Metered air was drawn through a charcoal tube at the entrance of the chamber to remove contaminants, passed over the sample, and then passed through a charcoal tube that adsorbed the evaporated solvent. During a run, the charcoal adsorption tubes were changed at predetermined intervals and the contents were analyzed by gas chromatography.

The charcoal tubes were broken and the contents (approximately 100 mg) placed in 14-ml vials containing 10 ml of carbon disulfide. The vials were then sealed with butyl rubber septums. Samples were removed from the vial with a hypodermic syringe and injected into a Hewlett-Packard 5750 chromatograph with an 1/8 in. diameter × 6 ft stainless steel column packed with 10% Carbowax 20M on Chromosorb WHP 80/100 mesh. The injector temperature and detector temperature were 280 and 300°C, respectively. The column temperature was varied between 110 and 160°C for the various solvents.

An airflow rate of 1 liter/min (STP) was maintained. Preliminary tests indicated that a twofold increase in airflow rate did not alter the evaporation rate.

Solvent Loading

The Accurel disk was loaded with solvent by immersing it in the solvent for eight hours. In each test, the volume of solvent imbibed by the disk was equal to the void volume of the disk. Since the polymer is hydrophobic, a different procedure was necessary to load the disk with water. The disk was first loaded with 95% ethanol and was then immersed in a beaker of water. The water in the beaker was exchanged several times to allow all the ethanol to diffuse out of the disk.

The powder was loaded with solvent by placing 0.5 g of powder in a small bottle. A volume of solvent slightly in excess of the void volume of the powder was added drop by drop. The bottle was sealed and placed in a 4-oz jar. The jar was secured to a stirring motor and was slowly rotated end over end for 8 hr. Four small strips of filter paper were then placed in the sample bottle to adsorb excess solvent, and the sample was allowed to equilibrate for at least 24 hr.

RESULTS

Disk Experiments

The rate-controlling mechanism describing the evaporation of solvent from the disk is assumed to be the diffusion of solvent vapor through an air solvent film surrounding the disk. The equation describing the steady-state evaporation of solvent through a gas film is

$$N = \frac{DP}{RTS} \tag{1}$$

where N = molar evaporation rate
P = vapor pressure
D = diffusion coefficient of solvent through air
R = gas constant
T = absolute temperature
S = film thickness

In this equation it is assumed that the solvent concentration is zero at the air-film boundary. Although Eq. (1) applies to the steady state, it can be used to describe the initial evaporation of solvent from the disk. However, the film thickness and the wetted area of the disk would change with time.

The initial evaporation rates of solvents from the disk are listed in Table 5 together with the diffusion coefficients of the solvents through air reported by Perry et al. [3]. The diffusion coefficients were corrected to the indicated temperatures by using the $T^{3/2}$ relationship between temperature and diffusivity [4].

Table 5 Initial Evaporation Rates from Accurel Disk

Solvent	Amount loaded (mg moles)	Initial rate mg moles (cm^2/min)	Diffusion coefficient (cm^2/sec)	Vapor pressure (mm Hg)	Temperature (°C)
N-Hexane	8.74	0.0715	0.080	150	25
Acetone	15.5	0.0826	0.124	200	22
Methanol	28.0	0.0666	0.150	120	25
Ethanol	19.5	0.0315	0.116	57	23
Toluene	10.7	0.0172	0.085	25	24
Water	50.0	0.0197	0.251	22	25
N-Butanol	11.6	0.0053	0.080	6.5	24
N-Nonane	6.3	0.0036	0.060	5	26
N-Octane	7.0	0.0097	0.057	13.5	25

A plot of the initial evaporation rate N expressed in molar units versus the product of vapor pressure and diffusion coefficient is shown in Fig. 3. The linear relationship between these quantities would seem to support the film diffusion assumption.

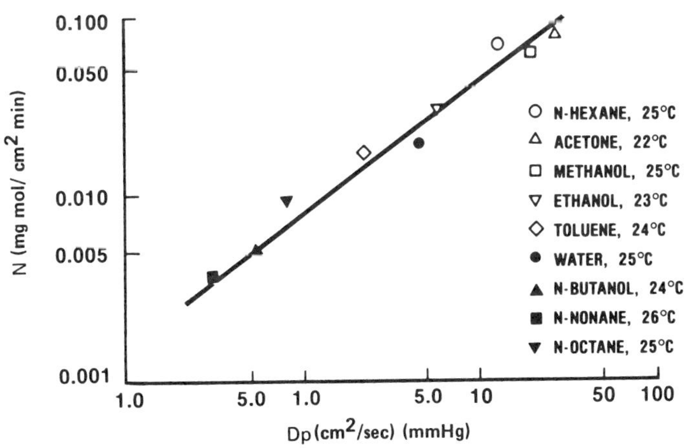

Figure 3 Initial evaporation rates from disk.

The evaporation curves for all the solvents tested are plotted in Figs. 4-6. To convert these plots from fraction evaporated to a specific weight, one can multiply the fraction evaporated by the total amount of solvent loaded (Table 5).

In order to predict evaporation rates of untested solvents, the times at which 0.25, 0.50, 0.75, and 0.90 of each solvent had evaporated were plotted in Fig. 7 against the vapor pressure (P) divided by the total solvent loaded on the disk (W). From this family of curves, one can plot an evaporation curve for any solvent. In Fig. 8, the curves represent evaporation rates predicted in this manner.

Powder Experiments

The evaporation rates of solvents from Accurel powder are summarized in Fig. 9, where the half-time, or the time at which half of the solvent has evaporated, is plotted against the solvent vapor pressure. The

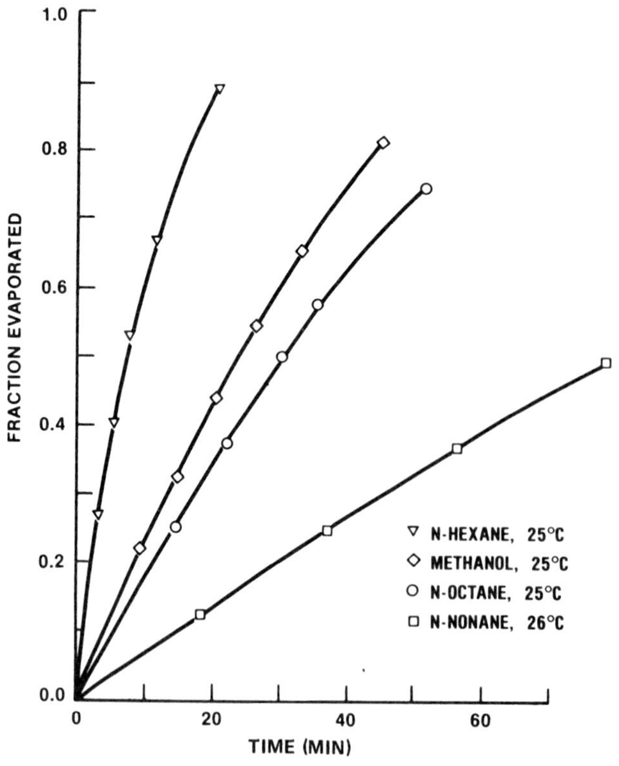

Figure 4 Evaporation of solvents from disk.

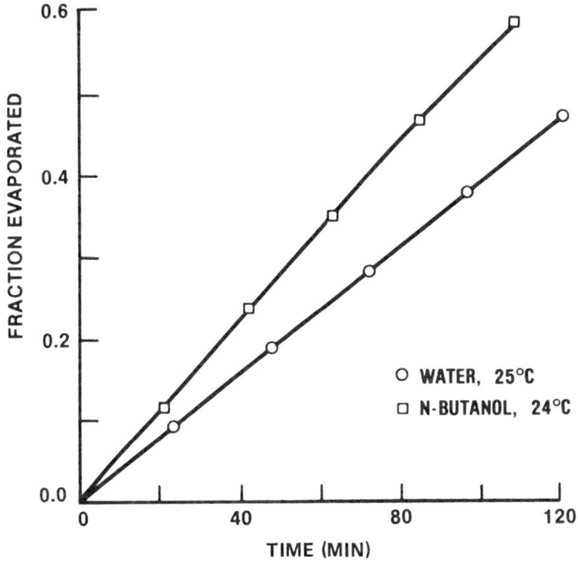

Figure 5 Evaporation of solvents from disk.

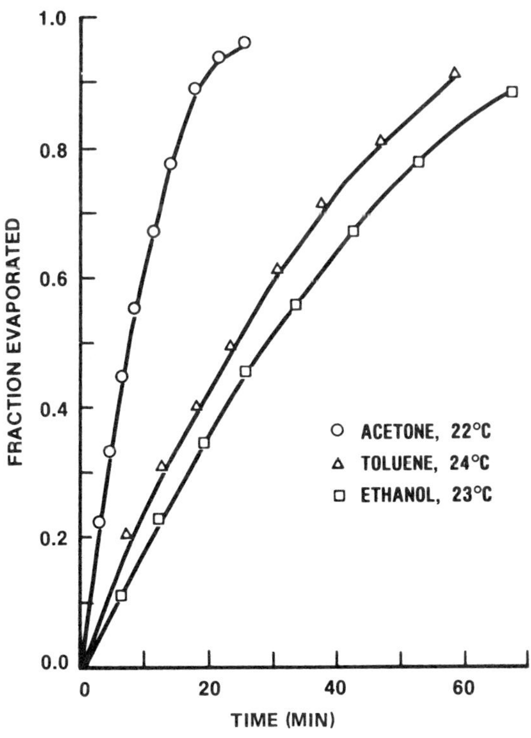

Figure 6 Evaporation of solvents from disk.

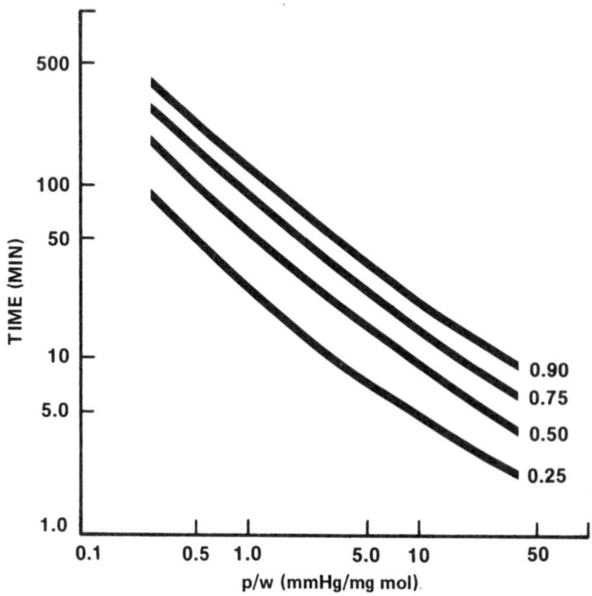

Figure 7 Fraction evaporated-time cross plot.

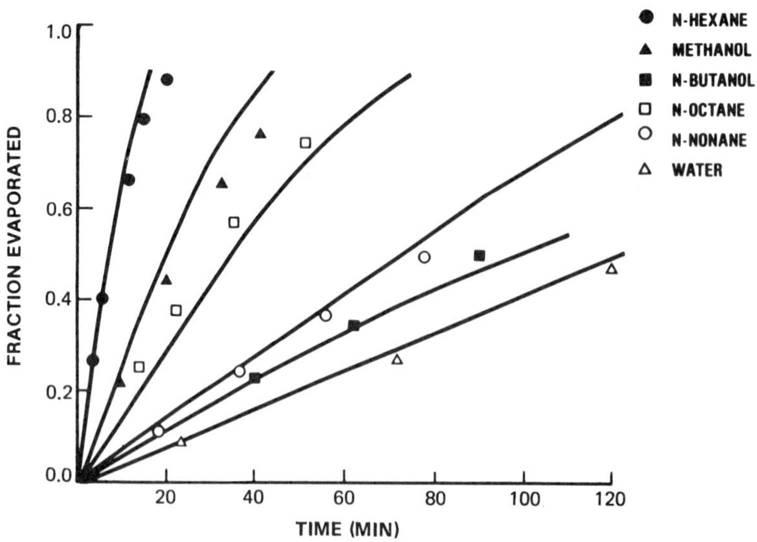

Figure 8 Predicted evaporation rates from disk.

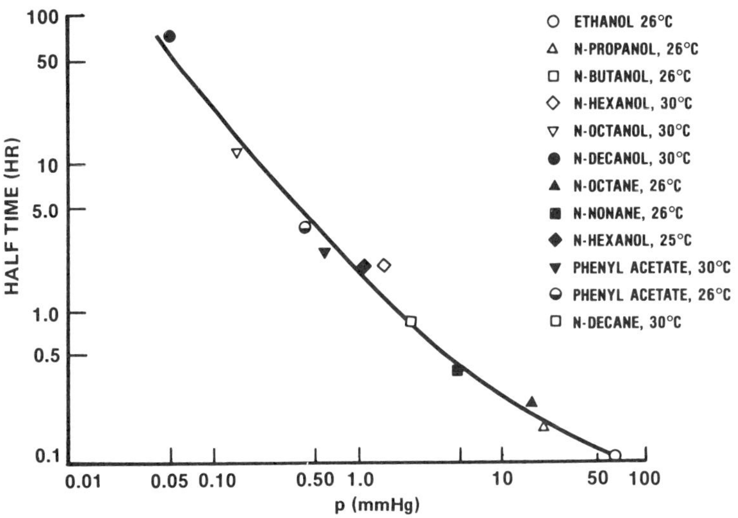

Figure 9 Evaporation half-times.

half-times can be read from plots of the original data (Figs. 11-14). For each test, the total amount of solvent contained by the powder was approximately 0.75 g/g of loaded powder.

If one constructs a plot such as Fig. 9 for $t_{0.25}$, $t_{0.5}$, $t_{0.75}$, and $t_{0.9}$, it is possible to draw an evaporation rate curve for an unknown solvent if its vapor pressure is known. In Fig. 10, the solid lines represent the predicted evaporation rate curves. A major difficulty with this procedure is obtaining accurate vapor pressure data. Vapor pressures of less volatile solvents were obtained by plotting literature values against the reciprocal of absolute temperature on semilog paper to obtain a linear relationship. In some cases it was necessary to extrapolate quite far to arrive at the desired values; thus the extrapolated vapor pressures can be subject to error. Nevertheless, this procedure can be quite useful in predicting approximate evaporation curves of untested solvents.

SUMMARY

Porous thermoplastic polymers with void volumes up to 90% can be produced. These materials can be fabricated into films, slabs, tubes, rods, and micrometer-sized powders.

Evaporation rates of volatile solvents from porous polypropylene in powder and disk forms were measured. It was determined that the

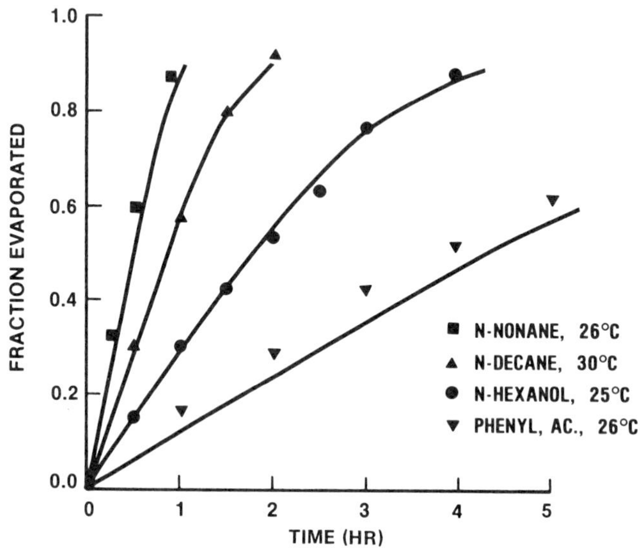

Figure 10 Predicted evaporation rates from powder.

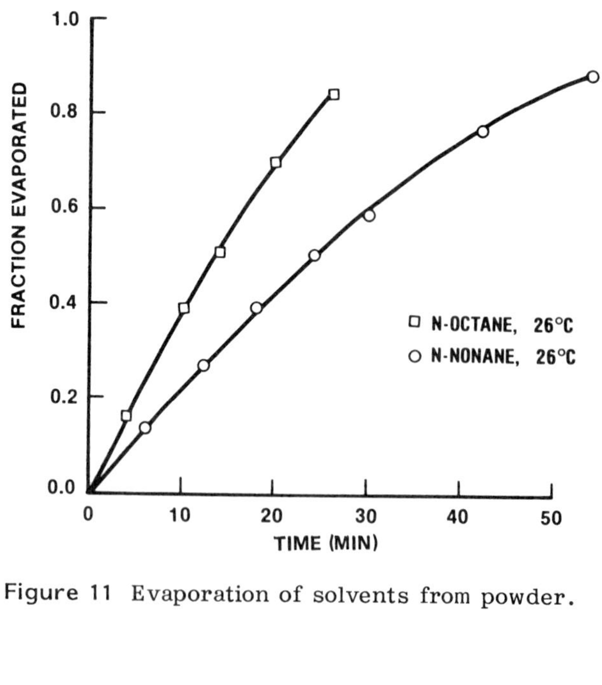

Figure 11 Evaporation of solvents from powder.

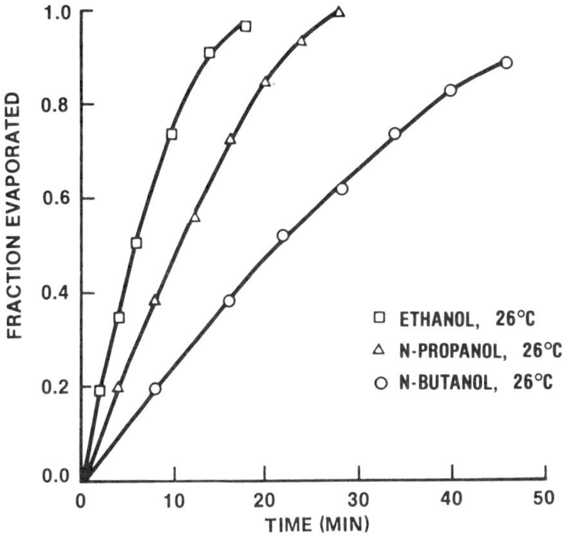

Figure 12 Evaporation of solvents from powder.

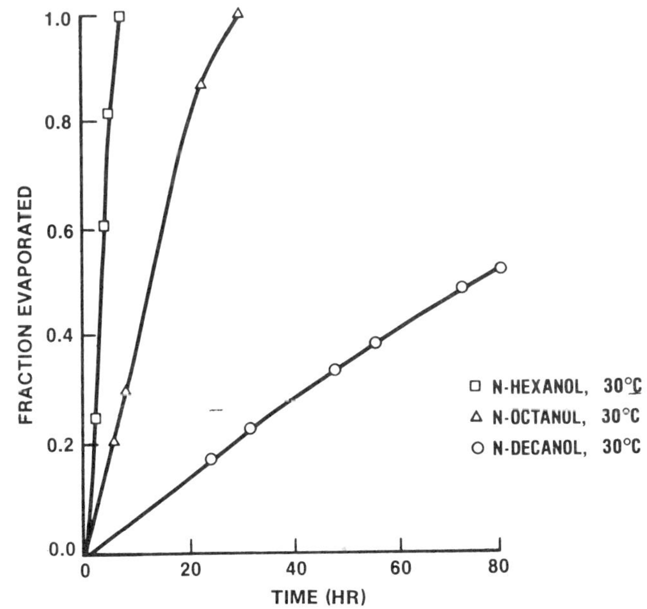

Figure 13 Evaporation of solvents from powder.

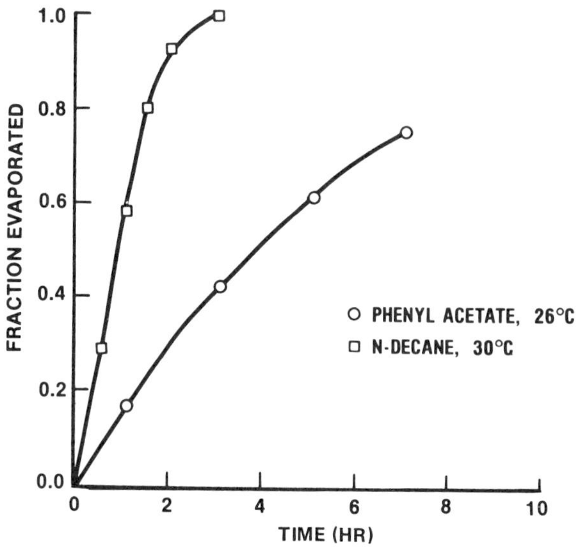

Figure 14 Evaporation of solvents from powder.

evaporation rate can be correlated with solvent vapor pressure. A method for the estimation of evaporation rates of solvents with vapor pressures within the range of this study is proposed.

REFERENCES

1. A. J. Castro, U.S. Patent No. 4,247,498 (1981).
2. W. Worthy, *Chem. Eng. News*, *56*:23 (December 11, 1978).
3. R. Perry, C. Chilton, and S. Kirkpatrick, *Chemical Engineers Handbook*4th ed., McGraw-Hill, New York, 1963, pp. 14-23.
4. R. Treybal, *Mass Transfer Operations*, McGraw-Hill, New York, 1955, p. 23.

Index